Communication *and* Education Skills *for* Dietetics Professionals

FIFTH EDITION

Communication *and* Education Skills *for* Dietetics Professionals

FIFTH EDITION

Betsy B. Holli, EdD, RD, LDN
Professor Emeritus
Department of Nutrition Sciences
Dominican University
River Forest, Illinois

Julie O'Sullivan Maillet, PhD, RD, FADA
Professor and Associate Dean Academic Affairs and Research
University of Medicine & Dentistry of New Jersey
School of Health Related Professions
Newark, New Jersey

Judith A. Beto, PhD, RD, LDN, FADA
Professor and Chairperson
Department of Nutrition Sciences
Director, Didactic Program in Dietetics
Dominican University
River Forest, Illinois

Richard J. Calabrese, PhD
Professor
Department of Communication
Dominican University
River Forest, Illinois

Wolters Kluwer | Lippincott Williams & Wilkins
Health
Philadelphia • Baltimore • New York • London
Buenos Aires • Hong Kong • Sydney • Tokyo

Acquisitions Editor: David B. Troy
Managing Editors: Matthew J. Hauber, Elizabeth Connolly
Marketing Manager: Katie Schauer
Designer: Stephen Druding
Compositor: International Typesetting and Composition

Fifth Edition

Library of Congress Cataloging-in-Publication Data
Communication and education skills for dietetics professionals / Betsy B. Holli . . . [et al.]. — 5th ed.
     p. ; cm.
   Rev. ed. of: Communication and education skills for dietetics professionals/Betsy B. Holli, Richard J. Calabrese, Julie O'Sullivan Maillet. 4th ed. c2003.
   Includes bibliographical references and index.
   ISBN-13: 978-0-7817-7434-5
   ISBN-10: 0-7817-7434-9
  1. Communication in diet therapy. 2. Patient education. 3. Interpersonal communication. I. Holli, Betsy B. II. Holli, Betsy B. Communication and education skills for dietetics professionals.
   [DNLM: 1. Diet Therapy. 2. Communication. 3. Counseling—methods. 4. Patient Care Planning. 5. Patient Education as Topic—methods. WB 18 C734 2008]
   RM214.3.H65 2008
   615.8'54—dc22

                                    2007052678

DISCLAIMER

Care has been taken to confirm the accuracy of the information present and to describe generally accepted practices. However, the authors, editors, and publisher are not responsible for errors or omissions or for any consequences from application of the information in this book and make no warranty, expressed or implied, with respect to the currency, completeness, or accuracy of the contents of the publication. Application of this information in a particular situation remains the professional responsibility of the practitioner; the clinical treatments described and recommended may not be considered absolute and universal recommendations.

The authors, editors, and publisher have exerted every effort to ensure that drug selection and dosage set forth in this text are in accordance with the current recommendations and practice at the time of publication. However, in view of ongoing research, changes in government regulations, and the constant flow of information relating to drug therapy and drug reactions, the reader is urged to check the package insert for each drug for any change in indications and dosage and for added warnings and precautions. This is particularly important when the recommended agent is a new or infrequently employed drug.

Some drugs and medical devices presented in this publication have Food and Drug Administration (FDA) clearance for limited use in restricted research settings. It is the responsibility of the health care provider to ascertain the FDA status of each drug or device planned for use in their clinical practice.

To purchase additional copies of this book, call our customer service department at **(800) 638-3030** or fax orders to **(301) 223-2320.** International customers should call **(301) 223-2300.**

Visit Lippincott Williams & Wilkins on the Internet: http://www.lww.com. Lippincott Williams & Wilkins customer service representatives are available from 8:30 am to 6:00 pm, EST.

The publication of the fifth edition of *Communication and Education Skills for Dietetics Professionals* marks the 22nd anniversary of the publication of the book. We are humbled by the fact that so many have found the book useful and pleased that many students have profited by it. This edition builds on the strengths of the previous editions.

Our primary goal has been to update the content so it remains current with the core communication skills essential for competent professional practice. The book defines these skills, gives examples, and demonstrates how to use them effectively.

Communication is basic to the relationship the professional has with clients. The American Dietetic Association (ADA) recognizes a number of communication skills as important for practitioners, enabling them to remain in the forefront of health promotion, disease prevention, and treatment; these skills are referred to in the chapters throughout the book.

The impact of nutrition counseling and education on promoting healthy lifestyles depends on how well nutrition information is communicated. Providing people with information on what to eat is insufficient as many already know what to eat. Communication is more effective when the foods and nutrition professional uses individual-appropriate models, theories, and strategies that promote and facilitate behavioral changes to more healthful food choices.

Interventions may focus on decisional balance (pros/cons) in motivational interviewing, behavior modification, cognitive evaluation and restructuring, improving self-efficacy, relapse prevention, goal setting, self-monitoring and self-management, nutrition education, and the like. We use these communication and education strategies based on theories and models that promote behavioral change, such as the Transtheoretical Model (Stages of Change) and Health Belief Model.

The ultimate goal or outcome criterion is sustained behavioral change with an early goal of changing to a more healthful diet and lifestyle. Nutrition education and counseling intervention strategies, for example, are useful for the epidemic of obesity as well as for the effects on type 2 diabetes mellitus, hypertension, and heart disease. We evaluate the effectiveness of our interventions and document the outcomes.

In providing our science-based information, our interventions can focus on the many factors influencing food choices. Besides knowledge, these include skills; available resources; lifestyle, family, socioeconomic, cultural, and motivational factors; educational level; and other psychological and environmental influences. As the U.S. population continues to diversify, certain ethnic and racial minorities are growing at a more rapid pace than the majority population, thus requiring culturally sensitive strategies used by culturally competent practitioners.

Professionals in management positions use many of the same communication and education principles in developing working relationships with employees. Skills in communication, conducting personnel interviews, counseling, and training and education are needed. Cultural diversity is also an issue to be addressed.

The chapter content and references have been updated with web addresses providing additional resources. The profession is moving in new directions, and the fifth edition reflects this progression. The Nutrition Care Process (NCP) and model, including the four steps of nutrition assessment, nutrition diagnosis using the PES statement (Problem, Etiology, and Signs/Symptoms), nutrition intervention, and nutrition monitoring and evaluation are incorporated.

Although three of the steps are well known to practitioners, nutrition diagnosis represents a new component that is evolving. We have incorporated it when applicable. The nutrition diagnosis statement, also referred to as the PES statement, identifies and labels the problems found through analysis of the nutrition assessment data and identifies the aim or the nutrition intervention. A standardized nutrition diagnosis language attempts to clearly describe nutrition problems the food and nutrition professional is responsible for treating independently. As a new language it will continue to evolve. The ADA welcomes suggestions.

ADDITIONAL RESOURCES

Communication and Education Skills for Dietetics Professionals, fifth edition, include additional resources available on the book's companion website at http://thepoint.lww.com/Holli5e.

Instructors

Approved adopting instructors will be given access to the following additional resources:

- Instructor's Manual, including additional case studies
- PowerPoint presentations
- Image Bank
- WebCT and Blackboard Ready Cartridge

Students

Students who have purchased *Communication and Education Skills for Dietetics Professionals,* fifth edition, have access to the following additional resources:

- Case Studies
- Review and Discussion Questions

See the inside front cover of this text for more details, including the passcode you will need to gain access to the website.

ACKNOWLEDGMENTS

In the fifth edition we welcome a new coauthor, Judith A. Beto, PhD, RD, FADA, Professor and Chairperson, Department of Nutrition Sciences and Director, Didactic Program in Dietetics at Dominican University.

In updating the content for this fifth edition, staff from the School of Health Related Professions at the University of Medicine and Dentistry of New Jersey (UMDNJ) participated. Diane Rigassio Radler, MS, RD, CDE, continues as a contributor of Chapter 6 (Counseling for Behavior Modification). M. Geraldine McKay, M Ed, RD assisted with the update of Chapter 10 (Principles and Theories of Learning) and Joyce A. O'Connor, Dr PH, RD updated Chapter 8 (Cross-Cultural and Life-Span Counseling). Finally, Angelina Nagel, a graduate student recommended changes in some of the case studies to add the Nutrition Care Process.

We thank Elizabeth Connolly of Lippincott Williams & Wilkins for her assistance throughout the preparation of the manuscript and ancillaries. Anonymous reviewers made helpful suggestions for this edition. We appreciate the assistance of The School of Health Related Professions at the University of Medicine and Dentistry of New Jersey for photographs and the U.S. Department of Agriculture photography service.

CONTENTS

CHAPTER **15**   Planning, Selecting, and Using Instructional Media   337

CHAPTER 1

Challenges for Dietetics Professionals

OBJECTIVES

- Discuss the origins of people's food habits or behaviors.
- Identify problems of dietary adherence.
- Describe the use of the Scope of Dietetics Practice Framework and the Nutrition Care Process.
- Describe why communication is so important to the profession of dietetics.

"There is more than a verbal tie between the words common, community, and communication. . . . Try the experiment of communicating, with fullness and accuracy, some experience to another, especially if it be somewhat complicated, and you will find your own attitude toward your experience changing."

—JOHN DEWEY

Food selection is a part of a complex behavioral system that is shaped by a vast array of variables. Food is essential for life. It is a powerful symbol of cultural identity, a ritual object, and a product to be purchased. There are pleasures in eating and sometimes guilt from eating. Dietary patterns affect our health and are important factors in the risk for several major chronic diseases. Successful nutrition counseling requires understanding of why clients eat the way they do and then use of this knowledge to develop appropriate interventions.

This chapter discusses the origins of people's food habits, often described as food behaviors. Dietetics practitioners work with people to successfully make changes in their food habits as measured by diet adherence, using strategies to motivate and improve people's success at change. The American Dietetic Association (ADA) and its Commission on Accreditation of Dietetics Education have since the beginning of the profession in 1917 stressed communication knowledge and skills as essential for successful professional practice.

ORIGINS OF FOOD HABITS OR BEHAVIORS

Why do people eat the way they do? In physiological response to hunger, of course, but food choices and eating are far more complex. Cultural, social, economic, environmental, and other factors are involved in food selection in addition to individual choice, patterns, and personal taste. Understanding people's food choices is essential before planning an appropriate nutrition intervention.

The goal of nutrition counseling and education is to help clients modify and manage food choices and eating behaviors so that individuals improve their health. However, psychologists tell us that food and language are the "cultural traits humans learn first, and the ones that they change with the greatest reluctance."[1] A major influence is the food eaten during childhood that forever defines what is familiar and brings comfort. Food preferences from childhood continue to be exhibited by adults, showing the profound role that early family experiences have in shaping food habits. Changing one's dietary choices is possible but not easily accomplished, and some intervention strategies are more effective than others.

Food has been influencing cultures for centuries.[2] Culture is the sum total of a group's learned and shared behavior. It is acquired by people living their everyday lives and provides a sense of identity, order, and security. As a group phenomenon, culture is learned from others and transmitted formally and informally to the next generation. These learned traditions are not static; they are dynamic with some changes accepted over time. All cultural and ethnic groups sustain their identities, in part, through their food practices, values, and beliefs. Family and culture determine what foods are appropriate and inappropriate. This makes it especially important to develop good food habits in the home.

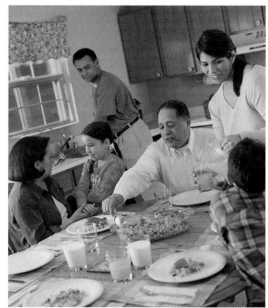

Food habits come from family habits and cultural groups.
Source: United States Department of Agriculture.

Does the person eat tortillas, croissants, cornbread, bagels or bread; hamburgers, sushi, moussaka, curry, bratwurst, pierogies, tacos, lasagna, or pizza; potato, rice, or pasta? Asian diets use rice as a staple, whereas Italians use pasta, for example. American children enjoy a peanut butter–and–jelly sandwich, whereas children from other cultures may have never heard of it. Americans, however, experiment with foods and mix the foods from a variety of cultural traditions, thus making eating practices a diverse cultural smorgasbord. Regional areas of the United States, such as Tex-Mex, New England, the Midwest, and the Southwest also may affect one's food choices. Examples of regional

SELF-ASSESSMENT

List three things that influence your choices of foods.

foods are New England clam chowder, Boston baked beans, Southern grits, New Orleans jambalaya, Texas chili, California sourdough bread, and a Wisconsin fish boil.

FOOD KNOWLEDGE AND BELIEFS

Social changes are determining what, where, when, and why people eat. Lifestyles are less formal. Our social occasions, parties, birthdays, holidays, and anniversaries center around food. Eating in restaurants, eating while grocery shopping, eating during weekend activities, and eating while traveling add challenges to our selection of healthful food choices. Preplanning for these circumstances helps. Food expresses friendship and hospitality, shows concern, and is a status symbol. Prestige is indicated by using expensive meats, fine wines, caviar, and exotic foods along with taking an exotic vacation, eating in a trendy restaurant, and having an expensive car.

How much do people already know about food and nutrition? How do nutrition knowledge, attitudes, and thoughts about food affect one's food choices? What behaviors are people willing to change? What are their beliefs about the relationship of food and health? These are some of the questions that must be answered before dietetics professionals can understand individuals well enough to begin talking with them about the challenges of changing their food choices. The goal of nutrition counseling and education is to help individuals change their food and eating behaviors so that they select healthful choices. The more knowledge one has about people and their personal needs and practices, the more effective the counseling intervention will be.[3] The goal of this book is to enhance success in communicating when counseling and educating individuals or groups.

In 2007, the International Food Information Council Foundation conducted the second Food & Health Survey about Americans' views of health, weight, and nutrition. Key findings included:[4]

- Seventy-five percent are concerned about their weight, and 56% are trying to lose weight.
- Sixty percent of those trying to lose weight are trying to reduce calories, and 23% are increasing activity.
- Only 11% knew the recommended calories for their height and age.
- Seventy-two percent are concerned about types and amount of fat they consume, with 87% aware of trans fat.
- Seventy percent are concerned about the amount of sugar they consume.
- Food decisions are strongly based on taste and price, but "healthfulness" has increased to 65%.
- Ninety percent thought breakfast was the most important meal, but only 49% consistently had breakfast.

- Snacking is an important component of the American diet, with 93% snacking at least once a day, the mean being 2.5 snacks per day, and 19% snacking more than four times per day.

Other surveys have found:

- Over 38% of our food dollar was spent out of the home in 1998, the last statistic from the Economic Research Service.[5]
- The take in–take out trend is increasing, with restaurants targeting foods that can easily be brought home or back to work.[6]

The interest in healthy eating is there but obesity continues to rise.[7] As dietetics professionals, our job is to capitalize on the interest in food and nutrition and provide the counseling and educational methods to promote behavior change. This huge task needs to be accomplished through professionals within and outside dietetics for the health of the public.

HEALTH BELIEFS

A person's beliefs about health may influence his or her food choices. The Health Belief Model is a framework to predict whether a person would or would not change an activity or behavior to benefit his or her health. "Perceived susceptibility" to illness was the "strongest predictor for preventive health behaviors" and the "strongest predictor for sick-role behavior was the perceived benefits."[8]

Having positive rather than negative cognitions or thoughts helps a person to make changes. There is a big difference between "Nutrition is important and this is worth the effort for my health" and "It's too much trouble and I feel ok anyway." One study found that some women linked the word "diet" to losing weight, whereas men disliked the word. "Food choices" or "choose a meal" were suggested as alternatives.[9] Cognitions may be influenced by attitudes and feelings. Therefore, attitudes are thought to influence peoples' decisions and actions. People may eat not only for physiological reasons such as hunger, but for psychological reasons, such as anxiety, depression, loneliness, stress, and boredom as well as from positive emotional states, such as happiness and celebrations. Food may assuage guilt as well as lead to guilt feelings.[10]

Knowledge of what to eat is certainly a first step in influencing healthful food choices, but it is probably overrated. There are individuals who know what to eat and do not do it. When people do not eat properly, some counselors redouble their efforts in educating as if the problem is lack of knowledge. The relationship between what people know about food and nutrition and what they eat is a very weak one. Other factors may be taking precedence and need to be explored. Knowledge helps only when people are willing and motivated to change.

Thus, there are many influences on food choices, including cognitive, sociocultural, physical, and geographical factors. The nutrition counselor needs to explore all of them to understand the client, the client's motivation for change, and the appropriate intervention to use. **Figure 1-1** summarizes some of the variables motivating changes in people's food choices and health behaviors. Discussion of variables continues in the chapters that follow.

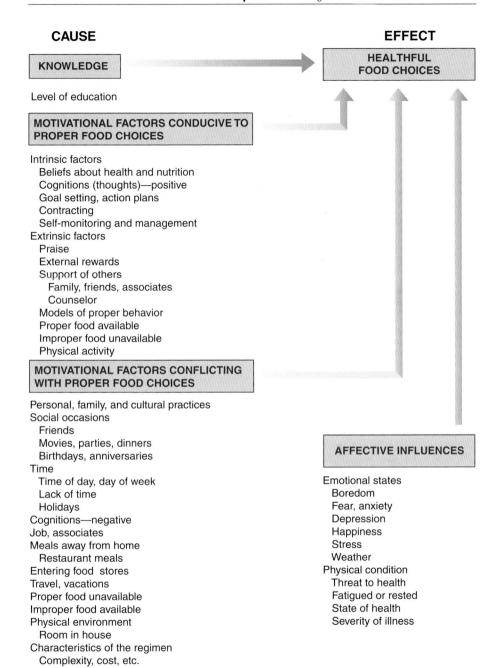

CAUSE

EFFECT

KNOWLEDGE

HEALTHFUL
FOOD CHOICES

Level of education

MOTIVATIONAL FACTORS CONDUCIVE TO
PROPER FOOD CHOICES

Intrinsic factors
   Beliefs about health and nutrition
   Cognitions (thoughts)—positive
   Goal setting, action plans
   Contracting
   Self-monitoring and management
Extrinsic factors
   Praise
   External rewards
   Support of others
     Family, friends, associates
     Counselor
   Models of proper behavior
   Proper food available
   Improper food unavailable
   Physical activity

MOTIVATIONAL FACTORS CONFLICTING
WITH PROPER FOOD CHOICES

Personal, family, and cultural practices
Social occasions
   Friends
   Movies, parties, dinners
   Birthdays, anniversaries
Time
   Time of day, day of week
   Lack of time
   Holidays
Cognitions—negative
Job, associates
Meals away from home
   Restaurant meals
Entering food stores
Travel, vacations
Proper food unavailable
Improper food available
Physical environment
   Room in house
Characteristics of the regimen
   Complexity, cost, etc.

AFFECTIVE INFLUENCES

Emotional states
   Boredom
   Fear, anxiety
   Depression
   Happiness
   Stress
   Weather
Physical condition
   Threat to health
   Fatigued or rested
   State of health
   Severity of illness

FIGURE **1-1**   Variables Motivating Change in Food Choices and Health Behavior.

ADHERENCE TO DIET CHANGES

Changing food choices may sound easy, but it is actually a very complex endeavor. The characteristics of the dietary regimen are the most important factors in adherence. Adherence is defined as the extent to which the individual's food choices and behaviors coincide with dietary recommendations. Research has shown that patients with diabetes and other diseases have difficulty adapting to lifestyle changes. Poor adherence is multifaceted and is linked to both educational level and patient perception, including self efficacy. One study showed that having greater trust in one's physician reduced the difficulty of lifestyle change for patients.[11] This finding is probably generalizable to dietetics professionals.

Dietary changes encompass many of the factors associated with a higher incidence of nonadherence. They include required changes in lifestyle, which tend to be restrictive, are of long duration or last a lifetime, and interfere with customary family habits and practices. If other barriers exist, such as high cost of the foods, lack of access to the proper foods, or extra effort, time, and skill required to prepare the meals, the likelihood of nonadherence increases.

To change food behaviors, the counselor and the client must have good rapport, with the counselor taking into consideration the person's lifestyle, concerns, and expectations. Adherence may be more satisfactory if the client sees the same counselor at each visit and if clear-cut communication occurs based on what the client is willing to do. The client should set the goals for change, or select from alternatives suggested by the counselor if the client is unable to define any. A warm and caring environment and prompt scheduling of appointments put the client in a good frame of mind. Long waiting periods at an appointment do not.

In patients with diabetes mellitus, dietitians reported the following barriers to dietary adherence: lack of time, lack of health symptoms, lack of education, poor self-esteem, lack of empowerment, and misinformation from family, friends, and others with the same disease. To overcome these barriers, dietitians recommend individualizing meal plans, teaching patients to plan ahead, teaching about medical complications from lack of adherence, and setting obtainable goals.[12]

Measures of dietary adherence are examined frequently. As clients return for follow-up appointments, discussions may focus on what worked and what went well, as well as what did not work, to define the extent to which the person's food choices and behaviors coincide with the goals developed or the physician's dietary prescription. This information is useful in setting additional goals for change with the client.

It is unrealistic to expect 100% adherence 24 hours a day, 7 days a week. Travel, parties, holidays, and other events may be times when people relax their diet for a limited period of time. The short-term pleasure of a piece of chocolate cake or apple pie, for example, may take precedence temporarily over the dietary regimen. In the Dietary Approaches to Stop Hypertension (DASH) trial, lack of food variety and unappetizing foods contributed to noncompliance with the DASH diet for hypertension.[13]

How is adherence measured? Adherence to diet is often evaluated based on oral and written self-reports of foods and beverages consumed, both subjective measures. Daily self-monitoring records of food intake, interviews such as diet histories and

24-hour recalls, and the professional's subjective judgment are used to collect data. These methods depend on the client's honesty and accuracy in reporting.[13]

The challenge for health professionals is to be sensitive cross-culturally in helping clients change their food choices without disturbing the sociocultural functions of food. For dietary changes to succeed, a combination of

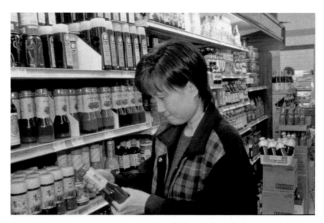

Counseling ethnic groups requires knowledge of their foods.
Source: United States Department of Agriculture.

approaches—including behavioral and cognitive interventions, self-efficacy, relapse prevention, self-monitoring, stages of change, social support, and educational strategies—may be necessary to assist people to make changes in food choices. Strategies for promoting change and for working with clients to improve adherence are found throughout the book.

NUTRITION CARE PROCESS

The Nutrition Care Process (NCP) is a framework for thinking and decision making that registered dietitians use to guide professional practice in providing high-quality nutrition care.[14] The NCP is a four-step process that includes (1) nutrition assessment, (2) nutrition diagnosis, (3) nutrition intervention, and (4) nutrition monitoring and evaluation. Nutrition education and nutrition counseling are fundamental interventions in step three of the NCP, along with coordination of nutrition care, food and/or nutrient delivery, and supplements.[15]

After completing step one, nutrition assessment, a new component of the NCP is nutrition diagnosis. Using standardized language and terminology, a framework outlines three domains within which 62 nutrition diagnoses or problems may fall. The domains are intake (diet, nutrition support), clinical (functional, biochemical, weight), and behavioral–environmental (knowledge and beliefs, physical activity and function, food safety and access).[15] Chapter 5 describes the nutrition care model in more detail. Communication is fundamental to each step in the process. Based on the nutrition assessment, clear documentation of the nutrition problem (diagnosis) and the treatment intervention will provide the means to document what dietetics professionals do. Some case studies in this book provide practice in following the new recommendations of using the standardized language for the NCP.[15] As this is a relatively new development in dietetics, the language will continue to evolve.

The NCP is one part of the Scope of Dietetics Practice Framework.[16] The three broad areas in the framework are the foundation knowledge of the profession, evaluation resources to gauge performance, and decision aids to define one's scope of practice.

This framework provides the practitioner with the analytical tools to determine whether an activity is within the typical Registered Dietitian (RD) or Dietetic Technician Registered (DTR) skill set and how to determine whether a particular activity fits within an individual's ability to practice safely.[16] The Scope of Dietetics Practice Framework takes into account the knowledge and skills set by the Commission on Accreditation for Dietetics Education, the Code of Ethics for the American Dietetic Association (ADA) and Commission on Dietetic Registration (CDR) members, the Standards of Practice and Standards of Professional Performance for ADA members, and numerous national and state regulations and research across the profession. As dietetics professionals refer to these materials, they guide practice, and the decision tree assists in personal assessment of competence.[16] For example, all of the preceding references concur that dietetics practitioners educate and counsel clients. However, a personal assessment of competence could identify that the practitioner is not competent with a particular ethnic culture and should learn more before counseling individuals in that culture.

The Scope of Dietetics Practice Framework is particularly helpful as practitioners diversify their practice into newer career options. Several of the developing careers are health coaching, supermarket tour guides, and virtual (online) diet counseling.[17]

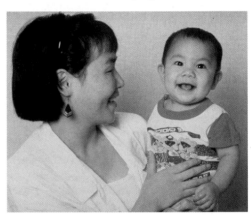

Basically health coaching is providing information to help clients lead healthy lifestyles. Dietetics professionals have the skills to provide this information. Generally the coach determines gaps in knowledge or skills and advises clients on how to fill them. Health coaching is not medical nutrition therapy. Medical nutrition therapy provides a systematic assessment, diagnosis, treatment, and intervention as described in the NCP,[14] whereas health coaches provide advice.[17] Health coaches may work independently or

Children learn food preferences at home.
Source: United States Department of Agriculture.

with the physician to improve disease management. Skills coaches include questioning, listening, and visioning.[18]

Other dietetics business ventures are built on counseling and education skills. Supermarket tours require that dietetics practitioners know the science of food and nutrition and translate it into terms, graphs, and languages that the consumer can understand and use.[19]

Of course, our traditional roles also rely on communication. Translating the science of nutrition into practical food preparation, and food and meal intake and patterns, is fundamental to dietetics whether this is applied to a community, group, family, or individual. The art of communication also is essential in the manager's role played by many dietetics professionals. All professionals need the ability to communicate and work effectively with their employees, with others on their same level, with superiors who are in authority, and with customers and clients. Dietetics professionals communicate to both individuals and to groups in meetings and classes. The basic principles of communication in the following chapters apply in all practice settings, although the details of application may differ.

Varying roles, varying settings, and the terminology of the moment all contribute to different names for practitioners and the individuals with whom they interact. For the purposes of this book, practitioners may be referred to as dietetics practitioners or professionals, food and nutrition practitioners or professionals, counselors, teachers, dietitians, or technicians. The receiver of the information may be the client, individual consumer, patient, or group. The authors intermixed these terms throughout the text based on what seemed to fit best. There is no correct terminology.

Knowledge of food, food habits, the cultural influences of food, and the factors influencing lifestyle behaviors are fundamental for dietetics professionals. The ability to communicate with others is essential to all dietetics practitioners independent of their type of position or practice setting. The use of the new standardized language and terminology for the profession of dietetics improves our communication in providing effective, quality nutrition care. The use of the Scope of Dietetics Practice Framework assists us in considering boundaries of practice and providing quality, safe care to those we serve.

CASE STUDY 1

Karen, a 35-year-old married woman, made an appointment with a registered dietitian in private practice to get counseling for weight loss and maintenance. Karen works full-time as a secretary at a bank, often going out to lunch with coworkers. Her husband is in computer sales. They have three children ranging in age from 6 to 10 years, and all are in school. Karen's mother comes to watch the children after school until she arrives home. Karen is 5'5" tall and weighs 170 pounds. She weighed 135 when she was married 12 years ago.

Karen described her daily schedule. She gets up early to make breakfast and help the children get ready for school. After work, she is tired and the children are hungry and clamoring for dinner, so she describes dinner as a "rush job" or something brought in. After cleaning up, she helps the children with homework, does laundry or other housework, attends evening activities at the school, runs errands, gets the children to bed, and then retires herself.

1. What lifestyle factors may help or hinder Karen in adhering to different food choices so that she can lose weight?
2. What suggestions or alternatives can you give Karen to overcome any problems identified in question one?

REVIEW AND DISCUSSION QUESTIONS

1. How do dietetics professionals use communication skills?
2. List five influences on people's food habits or behaviors.
3. What factors influence dietary adherence?

4. What strategies can be used to help people make dietary changes and promote better dietary adherence?
5. What are the major three components of the Standards of Dietetics Practice Framework?
6. Where in the Nutrition Care Process is education and communication incorporated?

SUGGESTED ACTIVITIES

1. With someone trying to make changes in food choices, discuss the changes and the factors influencing the changes, including any opportunities, challenges, or barriers. What are the factors influencing the person's adherence?
2. Select a dietary regimen, such as increased fiber, restricted sodium, reduced calorie, or reduced fat and cholesterol, and follow it yourself for 7 days. Keep a daily record of all foods eaten. How easy or difficult was it to comply with the dietary change for a week? What factors helped or hindered your adherence?
3. Write down what you would eat in these situations if you were following the same dietary regimen: birthday, wedding, holidays such as Christmas or Passover. How are decisions made regarding food choices for these events?
4. Think about your own food practices. What influences them? To what extent are social and cultural factors involved?
5. Discuss with peers the family and cultural origins of your food habits.
6. Watch three hours of television or examine three current magazines. What food products are advertised? What are the messages? How do these ads influence food choices? Compare with peers.
7. In your culture, what foods are served on special occasions, such as weddings and holidays. Compare with peers.
8. Interview a person from a different cultural or ethnic group to determine what is eaten on a daily basis and on holidays.
9. Visit the American Dietetic Association (ADA) web site at www.eatright.org and look at the standardized language textbook and the Dietetics Scope of Practice Framework. Discuss how they will be relevant to your professional education.

WEB SITES

http://culturedmed.sunyit.edu/bib/food/index.html   Bibliography on cultural issue and food
http://www.nal.usda.gov/fnic/pubs/bibs/gen/ethnic.html   Resource on food and culture

REFERENCES

1. Gabaccia DR. We Are What We Eat. Cambridge, MA: Harvard University Press, 1998.
2. Cultural globalization. Encyclopedia Britannica Online. Available at: http://www.britannica.com/eb/article-225002/globalization. Accessed August 27, 2007.
3. Rozin P. The meaning of food in our lives: a cross-cultural perspective on eating and well-being. J Nutr Educ Behav 2005;37(Suppl 2):S107–S112.

4. International Food and Information Council. 2007 Food & Health Survey: Consumer Attitudes Toward Food, Nutrition & Health. Available at: http://ific.org/research/foodandhealthsurvey. cfm. Accessed August 28, 2007.

5. USDA Economic Research Service. 2005 Food Consumption Available at: http://www.ers.usda.gov/Briefing/Consumption. Accessed September 5, 2007.

6. Lawn J. Ten trends for 2008 (part 1). Food Management July 2007. Available at: http://www.food-management.com/article/17352. Accessed September 4, 2007.

7. Fas in Fat: How Obesity Policies Are Failing in America, 2007. The Trust for America's Health. Available at: http://healthyamericans.org/reports/obesity2007. Accessed November 27, 2007.

8. Galloway RD. Health promotion: Causes, beliefs and measurements. Clin Med Res 2003;1:249–258.

9. Kennedy E, Davis CA. Dietary Guidelines 2000—the opportunity and challenges for reaching the consumer. J Am Diet Assoc 2000;100:1462.

10. Fine J. An integrated approach to nutrition counseling. Top Clin Nutr 2006;21:199–211.

11. Bonds DE, Camacho F, Bell RA, et al. The association of patient trust and self-care among patients with diabetes mellitus. BMC Fam Pract 2004;5:26. Available at: http://www.pubmed-central.nih.gov/articlerender.fcgi?artid = 535564. Accessed September 7, 2007.

12. Williamson AR, Hunt AE, Pope JF, et al. Recommendations of dietitians for overcoming barriers to dietary adherence in individuals with diabetes. Diabetes Educ 2000;26:272.

13. Windhauser MM, Evans MA, McCullough ML, et al. Dietary adherence in the dietary approaches to stop hypertension trial. J Am Diet Assoc 1999;99S:S76.

14. Lacy K, Pritchett E. Nutrition Care Process and Model: ADA adopts road map to quality care and outcomes management. J Am Diet Assoc 2003;103:1061–1072.

15. American Dietetic Association. Nutrition Diagnosis and Intervention: Standardized Language for the Nutrition Care Process. Chicago: American Dietetic Association, 2007.

16. American Dietetic Association. Scope of Dietetics Practice Framework. Available at: http://eatright.org. Accessed September 4, 2007.

17. Lipscomb R. Health coaching: A new opportunity for dietetics professionals. J Am Diet Assoc 2006;106:801–803.

18. Caton J. Dare to dream . . . a look at entrepreneurship. Nutrition Entrepreneurs. Available at: http://www.nedpg.org/pdfs/DaretoDreamvolume1.pdf. Accessed November 27, 2007.

19. Brown D. Unique careers for dietetics professionals. J Am Diet Assoc 2005;105:1358–1360.

Communication

OBJECTIVES

- Define operationally effective communication.
- List the components of the communication model.
- Discuss ways to make verbal communication effective.
- Relate ways to improve listening skills.
- List communication barriers and how to overcome them.
- Describe the communication process.
- List behaviors related to effective active listening.

"There is no pleasure to me without communication: there is not so much as a sprightly thought comes into my mind that it does not grieve me to have produced alone, and that I have no one to tell it to."
—MICHEL DE MONTAIGNE (1553–1592)

W ell-developed communication skills increase the likelihood of the dietetics professional's success with clients and staff. The American Dietetic Association (ADA) recognizes "communications," including interpersonal communication, as one of the content areas providing foundation knowledge and skills for competent professional practice. Communication with health care team members is important in identifying those in need of nutrition care and then in communicating with patients and clients about nutrition-related problems during the Nutrition Care Process (NCP).[1,2] Since managing human resources is also in the Scope of Dietetics Practice Framework, communication with one's staff is also frequent.

This chapter introduces the interpersonal communication process, including verbal and nonverbal communication, listening skills, and communicating with legislators. It discusses communication as a process, examines its components, and points out applications for practitioners. A model of the communication process is presented and discussed, followed by an explanation of the implications of the process for the verbal, nonverbal, and listening behaviors of the dietetics practitioner. The chapter concludes with a discussion of negotiating and communicating skills to use with legislators.

EFFECTIVE COMMUNICATION DEFINED

Effective communication can be operationally defined for dietetics practitioners as the ability to use language that is appropriate to the client's and staff's level of understanding, the ability to develop a relationship between themselves and their clients and staff, the ability to talk to them in a way that relieves anxiety, the ability to communicate to them in a way that ensures their being able to recall information, and the ability to provide them with feedback.

Communication is the heart of the provider–patient relationship.[3,4] Consumers have identified communication style as a key indicator of their perception of the quality of health providers and related care.[5] Among the new focus areas to bring better health to all citizens is the goal to "use communication strategically to improve health," both personal and public health.[6] Good communication contributes to health promotion as well as disease prevention efforts. Possessing only an intellectual appreciation of the various communication skills is of little use. Being able to pass a test by explaining how you ought to interact with clients and staff, how to defuse their hostility, and how to create a supportive communication climate is not the same as actually being able to do it. Putting the principles into practice requires a conscious effort, repeated attempts, and many trials. With practice, in a relatively short time, you will notice a difference in the way others respond to you. Honing the skills, however, is an ongoing process and begins with an understanding of the many elements included in the interpersonal communication exchange.

INTERPERSONAL COMMUNICATION MODEL

Complicated processes are easier to grasp when they can be visualized in a model. The model, of course, is not the same as the process, just as a map is not the same as the territory it depicts. A model, in short, is not the actual phenomenon; rather, it is a graphic depiction to aid understanding. Viewing the model allows students to grasp the entire process from beginning to end instantaneously; it also allows them to envision the individual components and to consider what might occur if any one component were eliminated or distorted. For this reason studying the communication model to examine and understand the role of each component is essential for professionals who are intent on expanding and improving their own communication repertoire.

Components of the Communication Model

The elements included in the human communication model are the following: sender, receiver, the message itself—verbal and nonverbal, feedback, and interference. They are depicted graphically in **Figure 2-1**.

Sender

Senders of the messages speak first. They initiate the communication.

Receiver

Receivers of the message—listeners—usually interpret and transmit simultaneously. They may be listening to what is being said and thinking about what they are going to say

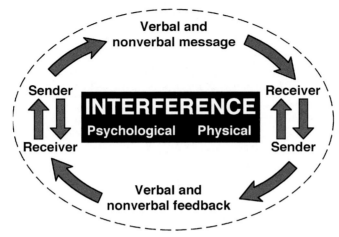

FIGURE **2-1** Communication Model.

when the senders stop talking. Even when silent, it is impossible for receivers in a two-way communication transaction not to communicate. They may be reacting physiologically with a flushed face or trembling hands, or in some other way, depending on their inferences from the message. Senders make inferences based on the receivers' appearance and demeanor and adjust subsequent communication accordingly.

Message

The receiver interprets two messages simultaneously: the actual verbal message and the nonverbal message inferred from the sender and the environment. Nonverbal inferences arise from the perceived emotional tone of the sender's voice, facial expression, dress, choice of words, diction, and pronunciation, as well as from the communication environment.

Feedback

The term "feedback" refers to the process of responding to messages after interpreting them for oneself. It is the key ingredient that distinguishes two-way from one-way communication. In two-way, face-to-face communication, the sender is talking while looking at the other person. The other person's reactions to the sender's message, whether agreement, surprise, boredom, or hostility, are examples of feedback. Unless the communication channel is kept clear for feedback, distortion occurs, leaving the sender unable to detect accurately how the message is received.[7]

In written communication, writers cannot clarify for readers because they do not see them. Even when writers carefully select words for the benefit of their intended readers, written communication is generally less effective than one-to-one verbal communication because of the inability to re-explain and adjust language in response to the feedback from receivers.

Interpersonal communication, after the first few seconds, becomes a simultaneous two-way sending-and-receiving process. While senders are talking, they are receiving nonverbal reactions from receivers. Based on these reactions they may change their tone, speak louder, use simpler language, or in some other way adjust their communication so that their message is better understood.

Interference

This term denotes the many factors inherent in the communicators (sender and receiver) and their environment that may affect the interpretation of messages. These factors include the unique attributes inherent in each of them; the room size, shape, and color; temperature; furniture arrangement; and the physiological state of each communicator at the moment. The sophisticated communicator needs to understand these dynamics and compensate or safeguard accordingly, so that the intended message is the one received.

A crying baby, the sound of thunder, and low-flying planes, for example, not only can hinder the receiver in hearing the sender's message, but also can generate messages and interpretations in the receiver that were never intended by the sender. Another source of interference is the physiological state of the communicators at the moment. No two bodies are exactly alike. Because no one has shared in the exact life experience of another, no two people understand language in precisely the same way.

Today's "Americans," more than ever, originate from a wide variety of cultural and ethic backgrounds. This increases the likelihood of a miscommunication in a verbal exchange with people from outside their group. Distortions can stem from psychological interference as well, including bias, prejudice, and closed-mindedness. Psychological interference in health care patients is often owing to fear of illness and its consequences. The job of senders is to generate in receivers those meanings for language that are closest to the senders' own. Because meanings are not universal, they can be affected by external as well as internal influences. Communication environment, cultural differences, the distance between speakers, lighting, temperature, and colors are a few of the variables that can affect meanings ascribed to a message. These variables can be sources of interference and account for the difficulty in generating in others the meanings people intend.

VERBAL AND NONVERBAL COMMUNICATION

Verbal communication includes the actual words selected by the sender and the way in which these symbols are arranged into thought units. Nonverbal communication includes the communication environment, the manner and style in which the communication is delivered, and the internal qualities inherent in the sender and receiver that influence their interpretation of external stimuli. Although both verbal communication and nonverbal communication occur simultaneously during interaction, they are discussed separately here in the context of their influence on the communication process. The salient point to remember is that the lack of clear communication, particularly regarding the work expectations used for appraisal by the dietetics practitioner may be the most common cause of poor employee performance. Conscious and clear communication is the key to a congruent relationship with both clients and staff.

Verbal Communication

To keep the communication channel open between the client or employee and the dietitian or dietetic technician, the professional needs to know how to create a supportive climate. A supportive climate is one in which as one person speaks, the other listens, attending to the message rather than to his or her own internal thoughts and feelings. A defensive climate, which occurs when the other person is feeling threatened, creates the opposite effect, with the listener "shutting down." When this happens, there is little point in continuing the interaction because the message is no longer penetrating. Although maintaining a supportive climate is always a concern, it becomes especially crucial when the professional is attempting either to discuss a topic viewed differently or to resolve conflict and defuse anger.

Although accurate communication exchanges have the best chance of being understood when the conditions of a supportive climate are present, sustaining a supportive climate is imperative when attempting to resolve conflict. Conflict can be positive and act as the catalyst to move a relationship forward. Contemporary organizational theory, in fact, states that conflict is essential for organizational development and even sometimes encouraged.[7]

The verbal guidelines for creating a supportive communication climate are to (1) discuss problems descriptively rather than evaluatively; (2) describe situations with a problem orientation rather than in a manipulative way; (3) offer alternatives provisionally rather than dogmatically; (4) treat clients as equals; and (5) be empathic rather than neutral or self-centered.

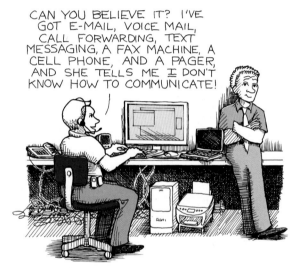

CAN YOU BELIEVE IT? I'VE GOT E-MAIL, VOICE MAIL, CALL FORWARDING, TEXT MESSAGING, A FAX MACHINE, A CELL PHONE, AND A PAGER, AND SHE TELLS ME I DON'T KNOW HOW TO COMMUNICATE!

Good communication skills must be developed.

Descriptive Rather Than Evaluative

Ordinarily, when approaching topics that tend to provoke defensiveness in clients, professionals should think through the discussion before engaging the client, so that the problem area is exposed descriptively rather than evaluatively. Whenever people feel as if others are judging their attitudes, behavior, or the quality of their work, they show an increased tendency to become defensive. Such comments as "You don't seem to be trying," "You don't care about cooperating," or "You are selfish" are based on inferences rather than facts. So when the other's response is "I do care," "I am too trying," or "I am not selfish," the framework for an argument is set, with no way of proving objectively who is right or wrong. Instead of making judgments regarding another's attitudes, the safest and least offensive way of dealing with a touchy issue is to describe the facts as objectively as possible. For example, when the professional tells a client descriptively that his or her continuing to eat chocolate several times each day is frustrating to her as the client's counselor, she is confronting the problem honestly and objectively without being evaluative. The client can then address the topic rather than argue about the professional's negative evaluation of his or her poor attitude, lack of concern, or uncooperativeness.

In a work-related situation, accusing an employee who has arrived late several mornings of being "irresponsible" and "uncaring" is likely to provoke a hostile refutation or cold silence. The employee may believe that being late does not warrant a reprimand. There may, in fact, be a reasonable explanation about which you should inquire. Describing how being late is causing problems to those who depend on him or her and causing work to back up is honest and descriptive and allows for nondefensive dialogue.

Problem-Oriented Rather Than Manipulative

Orienting a person to a problem rather than manipulating him or her promotes a supportive communication climate. Frequently, when people want others to appreciate their point of view, they lead them through a series of questions until the other reaches the "appropriate" insight. This is a form of manipulation and provokes defensiveness as soon as respondents realize they are being channeled to share the other's vision.

E X A M P L E : "Several weeks ago you agreed that you were going to stop eating chocolate; however, each week you continue to acknowledge eating chocolate candy bars. About a month ago, you agreed to switch to fresh fruit as a snack, but that has not occurred. Last week you suggested that you were willing to eat a high-fiber cereal for breakfast, and today you acknowledge that you haven't followed through on that. If you were dealing with a client like yourself, would you begin to get the feeling that this person is playing games with you?"

A discussion with the client would probably be more productive if the practitioner took a direct problem-oriented approach.

E X A M P L E : "In 6 weeks you have gained 3 pounds. With the diet planned, we anticipated a 4 to 5 lb weight loss. There seems to be a discrepancy here. Let's discuss what possibilities might explain the weight gain."

Employees and clients respect the professional when they believe the professional is being straightforward and authentic. A slick, manipulative style ordinarily can be seen through immediately and causes others to become disdainful.

Although as the practitioner you should plan opening remarks descriptively rather than evaluatively, after making such remarks you should allow for spontaneous problem solving without preplanned solutions. Creative, superior, and long-lasting solutions are more likely to occur when each person hears out the other fully and is heard in return and when the client initiates the solution. When a practitioner is intent on "selling" a solution, there is a natural disposition on the part of the other to block out conflicting opinions. The problem-solving process is discussed in detail in other chapters.

In the previous examples, the practitioner's subsequent remarks depend on how the client or employee responds to the directive to explain the underlying problem. The professional needs to give the client time to think; this often means waiting for an answer. Providing excuses or putting words into the other's mouth is a mistake. The practitioner needs to learn the discipline of sitting through the tension of silence supportively until the client or employee responds. Frequently, the first explanations are those that people believe will not upset or shock the professional. The "real" reasons, however, may not be revealed until the client or staff member feels secure enough to risk shocking the professional without fear of being humiliated or embarrassed. In other words, after the first explanations are offered, dietitians or dietetic technicians would do best simply to repeat in their own words what they have understood. Only when the clients or employees are comfortable enough, will they be able to express their authentic reactions, questions, or answers, these ordinarily being less logical, more emotional, and more risky to expose.

Provisional Rather Than Dogmatic

When offering advice to clients or helping them to solve problems, the professional should give advice provisionally rather than dogmatically. "Provisionally" implies the possibility of the practitioner changing his or her options, provided that additional facts emerge. It keeps the door open for clients to add information. When advice is offered in a dogmatic way, it becomes threatening for clients or employees to challenge or to add their own information. A dogmatic prescription might be, "This is what you must do. I know this is the way to solve your problem." A provisional prescription might be, "Here are several alternative things you might consider," or "There may be other ways of handling this problem; perhaps you have some ideas too, but here are things you might consider."

Egalitarian Rather Than Superior

In discussing issues, clients and professionals should regard each other as equals. Whenever the possibility of defensiveness exists, even between persons of equal rank, any verbal or nonverbal behavior that the other interprets as an attempt to emphasize superiority generates a defensive response. In the relationship between professionals and clients or managers and employees, the dietetics practitioners' tendencies to emphasize status or rank may arise unconsciously from a desire to convince the other to accept their recommendations. Comments such as the following may cause the other to feel inferior, hurt, or angry: "As a consumer, you may find this difficult to understand, but it works," or "Just do what I recommend; I've been doing this for 10 years." Certainly, there is nothing wrong with professionals letting clients know that they are educated and competent. In fact, clients often need and appreciate the reassurance. However, the manner in which it is done is crucial. A more effective and subtle way to solve problems with a client is to say, "I have studied this problem and dealt with other clients who have similar symptoms. I am interested, however, in incorporating your own insights and plans into the solution. You must be satisfied and willing to try new eating habits, so please express your views, too. We will continue to modify over time."

An employee making a recommendation to a manager that the manager had tried unsuccessfully many years ago, might be told, "If I were in your shoes, I would think the same thing. Someday when you are more experienced, you'll know why it won't work." The subtle underscoring of the inferior relative status of the subordinate could be enough to cause a defensive battle. The professional would have done far better with a comment such as "I can understand why you say that. I have thought the same myself, but when I tried, it was not successful." Here, the employee is left feeling reinforced and appreciated rather than humiliated. Showing respect for the client's and employee's intelligence and life experiences and recognizing their human dignity facilitates cooperation.

In conflict resolution, problem solving, and the discussion of any issues that may be threatening to the client or employee, collaboration is far more effective than trying to persuade the person to act according to the dictates of the professional. Collaboration has other virtues as well. People feel more of an obligation to uphold solutions that they themselves have participated in designing. If clients are trying the professional's solution, they may feel little satisfaction in proving that he or she was right; however, if the solution is one that was arrived at through collaboration, there is genuine satisfaction in proving its validity. An additional reason for practitioners to involve others in problem solving is that often a valid solution that is superior to any that the individual or professional would have discovered alone can be arrived at through collaboration. Two people sharing insights, knowledge, experience, and feelings can generate creative thought processes in each other, which in turn generate other ideas that would not otherwise have emerged.

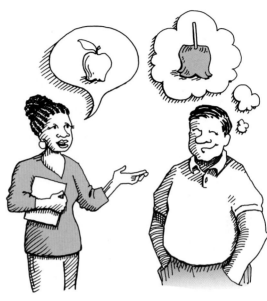

To determine whether or not the receiver has the correct message, feedback is necessary.

Empathic Rather Than "Neutral"

Another verbal skill essential to maintaining a supportive climate is the ability to put oneself in the other's shoes. For a helping professional, however, this is not enough. To be effective in working with clients and employees, dietetics practitioners must be able to demonstrate in some way their desire to understand what it is those they are helping are feeling. This "demonstration" might be an empathic response to their comments. In an empathic response, the listener tells the other that he or she is attempting to understand not only the speaker's content, but also the underlying feelings. For example, a client might say, "For my entire life I have eaten spicy foods; they are a part of my culture. I don't know what my life will be like without them." The professional might then respond, "You seem to be worried that the quality of your life will change because of the dietary changes."

If the professional is accurate in his or her empathic remarks, the client will acknowledge it and probably go on talking, assured that the helper listens. If the professional is wrong, however, the client will clarify the judgment and continue to talk, assured that the helper cares. Thus, the dietetics practitioner need not be accurate in inferring the other's feelings as long as he or she is willing to try to understand them. In addition, empathic responses allow the professional to respond without giving advice, focusing instead on the individual's need to talk and to express feelings and concerns. Before clients or employees can listen to the professional, they must express their concerns; otherwise, while the practitioner is talking, the clients or employees are thinking about what they will say when the practitioner stops talking.

An employee who has asked to be released from work on a busy weekend to attend a family gathering out of town might receive the following neutral response: "No offense, but a rule is a rule. If I make an exception for you, others will expect it too." Alternatively, the employee would still feel sad about working but would feel less antagonistic toward the supervisor if he or she were to receive the following empathic response: "I realize how badly you feel about not being able to attend the family gathering. I feel terrible myself having to refuse your request. I am truly sorry, but I can't afford to let you off." The supervisor, by letting the subordinate know that he or she has understood the subordinate's underlying feelings and is sympathetic, uses the most effective means of defusing the subordinate's anger or antagonism.

Paraphrasing, a Critical Skill for Dietetics Professionals

Most people have not incorporated the skill of paraphrasing into their communication repertoire. Even after people realize how vital this step is and begin to practice it, they may feel uncomfortable. Often the person just beginning to use paraphrasing in interactions feels self-conscious and fears others may be insulted or think he is "showing off" professional communication skills. A hint for the professional feeling awkward about asking clients and staff to paraphrase would be to ask for the paraphrase by acknowledging your own need to verify that what was heard is what the other intended.

> E X A M P L E: "I know that I don't always explain as well as I should, and that frequently, people have questions. The topic is complicated. Just to be sure I clearly covered the instructions, would you mind explaining in your own words how you will plan your meals?"

Of course, it takes less time to ask, "Do you understand?" However, asking this question is less effective. Because of the perceived status distinction between the helper and the person being helped, the latter may be ashamed to admit that he or she has not understood. Perhaps the person being helped is thinking that he or she can read about it later or ask the patient in the next bed for an explanation after the professional leaves the room. When persons of perceived higher status ask others if they "understand," almost always the answer is, "yes." This phenomenon is particularly likely when working within certain ethnic groups, such as the Japanese. Another possibility is that the client or staff member honestly believes that he or she has understood, and for that reason has answered, "yes." The understanding, however, may include some alteration of the original message, in the form of substitution, distortion, addition, or subtraction. The skill of paraphrasing needs to become second nature and automatic for the dietetics practitioner to verify important instructions and significant client or staff disclosures.

Because of the anxiety attached to being in the presence of another of perceived higher status, the client or staff member may be less articulate than usual when describing symptoms or explaining a problem. The dietetics practitioner should paraphrase to verify that he or she understands the message as the "sender" intends. The professional should try to avoid sounding too clinical with such comments as "What I hear you saying is . . ." or "Let me repeat what you just said"; rather, keep the language clear, simple, and natural. A comment such as "I want to make sure I am understanding this; let me repeat what you are saying in my own words" is more natural.

Two points need to be emphasized regarding paraphrasing: (1) Not everything the other person says needs paraphrasing. It would become a distraction if, after every

SELF-ASSESSMENT

Paraphrase the following:

1. Client: "I've been overweight most of my life. I've tried many different diets: I lose a few pounds, and gain it all back."
2. Employee: "I don't know why you want to keep changing things around here. Our old manager was satisfied with our procedures."

sentence, the professional interrupted with a request to paraphrase. Paraphrasing is essential only when the discussion is centered on critical information that must be understood. (2) Paraphrasing often leads to additional disclosure and therefore tends to cause longer interaction sessions. People are so accustomed to being with others who do not really listen that when they are with someone who proves he or she has been paying attention by repeating the content of what has been said, they usually want to talk more. For the dietetics professional, this additional information can be valuable. Another benefit is that after the client or staff member has expressed all questions and concerns and has cleared his or her mental agenda, he or she is psychologically ready to sit back and listen or to solve problems. By talking too much or too soon, the professional may not be able to convey all of the message to the other, who may be using the difference in time between how fast the professional speaks and how fast the professional's own mind processes information (the human mind operates five to eight times faster than human speech) to rehearse what he is going to say next.

Nonverbal Communication and Image Management

Of the two messages received simultaneously by receivers—verbal and nonverbal—ordinarily the nonverbal is more influential. As receivers of messages, people learn to trust their interpretations of nonverbal behavior more than the verbal word choices consciously selected by the sender. Intuitively, they know that control of nonverbal behavior is generally unconscious, whereas control of verbal messages is usually deliberate.

Communication experts and social scientists feel that the image that a person projects accounts for over half of the total message conveyed to another person at a first meeting.[7] Personal appearance, including clothing, hairstyle, and accessories, is one of the most important elements of the image. Personal space variables should be experimented with to determine where a person feels most comfortable and how that distance makes others feel. Research has shown that when it comes to health care, there has been a documented "strong association between the professional's physical appearance and clients' initial perceptions of competence."[8]

The chief nonverbal vehicles inherent in communicators are facial expression, tone of voice, eye contact, gesture, and touch, with meanings varying across cultures. Receivers of communication perceive nonverbal behavior in clusters. Ordinarily, people do not notice posture, eye contact, or facial expression isolated from the other nonverbal channels. For this reason, professionals need to monitor all nonverbal communication vehicles so that together the clusters are congruent with one another as well as with the verbal messages.

Facial expression is usually the first nonverbal trait noticed in interaction. A relaxed face with pleasant expression is congruent with a supportive climate. A supportive tone of voice is one that is calm, controlled, energetic, and enthusiastic. Supportive eye contact includes gazing at the other person in a way that allows the communicator to encounter the other visually—to the extent of being able to notice the other's facial and bodily messages. Besides being an excellent vehicle for feedback, eye contact also ensures the other person of the dietetics professional's interest and desire to communicate. Attending to the other visually allows inferences of interest, concern, and respect. The professional's posture is best when leaning somewhat toward the person rather than away from the person. Large expansive gestures may be interpreted as a show of power and generally should be avoided.

Like eye contact, touch can work positively in two ways: (1) Through a gentle touch, a pat, or a squeeze of the hand, one can communicate instantly a desire to solve a problem without offending the other. Touch can communicate affection, concern, and interest faster than these messages can be generated verbally. (2) Like eye contact, touch is a vehicle for feedback. Although an individual may look calm, controlled, and totally at ease, a touch can reveal nervousness and insecurity. These clues, when monitored by the dietetics practitioner, often provide insight. The practitioner reacts to them by spending more time putting the person at ease; he or she has the individual paraphrase to make sure information is being understood and makes an effort to alter the communication style to be more overt in support. People usually respond positively to touch, whether or not they are consciously aware of it.

Although the preceding content is valid for most of the contemporary American public, remember that variations among ethnic groups may require professionals to adapt their nonverbal behavior (see **Box 2-1**). If the client shows any sign of resisting or objecting to the professional's eye contact or touch, for example, the professional should immediately desist.

Dietetics Professionals Must Be Alert to Nonverbal Signals From Others

Besides the professional's concerns with the environment and his or her own verbal and nonverbal behavior in an attempt to create a trusting climate, the professional must also be sensitive to nonverbal cues in other people. Even though the practitioner is being open, natural, caring, and attending to his or her own behavior and the environment, the internal anxiety, confusion, nervousness, or fear in people may be causing them to misunderstand or to react inappropriately.[4] Two requirements for effective interpersonal communication are to observe the nonverbal cues in others and then respond to them in an affirming way.

If the client or employee is nodding the head to suggest understanding but looks puzzled, the professional needs to verify understanding by having the person paraphrase important instructions or dietary recommendations. If the patient is flushed, has trembling hands, or tears rolling down the cheeks, the professional may need to deal directly with relieving anxiety before communicating instructions or explanations. Until the patient is relaxed enough to concentrate, optimal two-way communication is unlikely.

After talking with one another for only a few minutes, both the dietetics practitioner and the client can sense the "warmness" or "coldness" of the other, as well as the degree of the other's concern. Each person tends to generalize these impressions, while inferring

Box **2-1**

Inappropriate Nonverbal Messages According to Some Cultural or Ethnic Traditions

Australia	Winking at women is improper.
Brazil	A-OK means the same as flipping the middle finger in the United States.
	Thumb between index and middle finger is an obscenity.
Bulgaria	A nod means "no;" a shake of the head, "yes."
China	A formal, dark suit with beige loafers at an important meeting is taboo.
Egypt	Tapping fingers together means, "Would you like to sleep together?"
England	Shouting in public is frowned on.
Fiji	Folding one's arms shows disrespect.
Finland	Folding one's arms shows arrogance and pride.
Greece	Waving is an insult.
Hungary	Saying "bus" means fornication.
Japan	Only an occasional glance into the other person's face is polite. An uncovered neck in women is considered sensuous; keep covered.
Parts of Europe	Gucci loafers are considered bedroom slippers.
Phillippines	Women dressed in trousers, blouse, and braless is taboo.
Romania	Eating with your napkin on your lap is taboo.

additional traits. If the speaker has a gentle touch, pleasant expression, and looks directly into the eyes of the listener as he or she talks, he or she might be generating inferences in the listener of being a caring spouse, supportive community member, or loving parent. After the initial positive impression has been created, the impression tends to spread into other areas not directly related to the behavior originally observed. The process can work in reverse as well. If the professional does not look at the client as he or she talks or touches the client too firmly and has an unpleasant facial expression, the inferences being created now may be negative—arrogance, lack of concern, indifference, and "coldness." Even though these initial reactions, both positive and negative, may be inaccurate, faulty first impressions are common. The helping professional might not be given a second chance to win the client's trust and cooperation; the client's inferences regarding the professional's concern and positive regard need to be anticipated and begun at the initial encounter.

Positive Affect Must Be Consistent

Seeing clients or employees regularly gives practitioners (or managers) an opportunity to reinforce or alter the perceptions the other person has of them. If you are cold, aloof, and uncaring on a daily basis, and, suddenly, because it is time to conduct a performance appraisal or counseling session with an employee, you act differently, you will not be believed. Practitioners need to be consistent in adding positive inferences to the impressions of their staff and clients. Dietetics professionals must make a total commitment to the word-of-mouth process by listening and questioning effectively, taking appropriate action, focusing on a subordinate or client orientation, delivering on promises, and teaching people—both employees and clients—how to seek information efficiently.

Not only is it important to attempt to generate concern through your own nonverbal behavior, manner, and disposition, it is also essential to control, whenever possible, the communication environment so that it, too, leads to positive inferences with a minimum of "interference." Attractive offices, pastel-colored rooms, soft lighting, comfortable and private space for counseling, and comfortable furniture all can add to the client's or staff member's collective perception, promoting inferences that you as a professional are concerned. Empirical studies, for example, reported that because so much of the professional's counseling takes place in a clinical setting, more attention must be given to creating an inviting educational atmosphere within this environment and attending closely to nonverbal cues.[9,10]

Related indirectly to effective communication are the actual dress and physical appearance of the professional. Dress and appearance are usually consciously selected, and they are nonverbal communication vehicles. The female dietetics practitioner who is overly made up or too strongly scented or the male practitioner who is wearing a nose ring or open shirt revealing a hairy chest may be well-meaning and competent. However, by their dress they risk offending a more conservative person. Professionals communicate their image best when they are clean and wearing clean and pressed clothing and only mildly scented cologne. Because any ostentatious show of

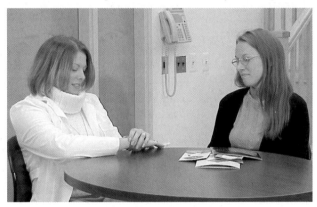

Clients are aware of the professional's nonverbal behavior.

material wealth or status tends to provoke a defensive reaction in others, items such as expensive jewelry and other valuable possessions should not be worn.

Another aspect of effective communication is conflict management. In the workplace, the way to win an argument is to stop it as quickly as possible by settling the dispute rationally. This is not easy to do because generally people are programmed to respond to aggression in one of three ways: fighting back, running away, or becoming immobilized. Sometimes, when dealing with a hostile client or employee, the professional may want to remain calm and supportive, but the body may refuse to cooperate. The face may turn red, hands may begin to shake, and voices may become loud and threatening. If this occurs, acknowledge that although you had wished to resolve the problem with the individual, you are feeling defensive and realize that this might be upsetting the person. Because the individual sees the physical manifestations of the professional's defensiveness, the dietetics professional should acknowledge the reaction rather than attempt to feign control. Under these circumstances, avoid further immediate communication and schedule another appointment after regaining composure.

Among the requirements for effective interpersonal communication is the need for the dietetics practitioner to send verbal and nonverbal messages that are congruent with one another. A client may hear a practitioner say, "I want to help you; I'm concerned about your health and the possible recurrence of your heart problem as a result of your food choices." But if, at the same time, the client sees the practitioner making no attempt to connect physically through handshake and looking down at notes or checking his or her watch rather than looking at the client, the contradictory second message of impersonality or impatience will be more intense than the stated message of concern. The professional may have said all the "right" words but is judged as insincere.

Helping professionals and managers who do not genuinely like working with people are destined ultimately to fail; often, however, professionals who do like people and care for their clients and employees fail as well. To be successful in working with others, the professional must develop congruent verbal and nonverbal communication skills. A person can develop all the appropriate verbal skills and still be unsuccessful in calming a hostile employee or in securing a client's agreement to the dietary plan. Only when the professional treats others with respect, soliciting their opinions and responding to them, can an environment of trust and openness be created.

> *"Communication is a continual balancing act, juggling the conflicting needs for intimacy and independence. To survive in the world, we have to act in concert with others, but to survive as ourselves, rather than simply as cogs in a wheel, we have to act alone."*
> DEBORAH TANNEN (20TH CENTURY)

LISTENING SKILLS

Well-developed listening skills are an essential requirement for effective interpersonal communication between health practitioners and their clients and staff.[11-15] An individual with average intelligence can process information at speeds of approximately five times that of human speech. The higher the intelligence, the faster the mind tends to process information. Some individuals can think at speeds of eight to ten times the rate of human speech. Thus, while practitioners are listening to their clients or staff members talk, they have time to be thinking about other things simultaneously. Everyone has had the experience of listening to a speaker and thinking about what that person might be like at home or of letting the mind wander to other topics. From the speaker's clothes, shoes, jewelry, diction, and speech patterns, people tend to fill in details and develop an elaborate scenario while they listen, more or less, to the presentation. The process of good listening involves learning to harness your attention so that you are able to concentrate totally on the speaker's message, both verbal and nonverbal. Development of these skills is not difficult, but it does require a conscious effort and perseverance.

Listening is taught as an academic subject in the department of communication studies in most colleges and universities; in fact, people have earned PhD degrees studying the subject. The bottom line, however, is that listening ability can be enriched only when the person desires such enrichment and is willing to follow the training with practice. The following list of four of the most common issues related to poor listening is an excellent starting place for readers who desire to practice improving listening skills:

1. Most people have a limited and undeveloped attention span.
2. People tend to stop listening when they have decided that the material is uninteresting and tend to pay attention only to material they "like" or see an immediate benefit in knowing.
3. Listeners tend to trust their intuition regarding the speaker's credibility, basing their judgments more on the speaker's nonverbal behavior than on the content of the message.
4. Listeners tend to attach too much credibility to messages heard on electronic media, such as radio, television, movies, tapes, and so forth.

Listening can be improved with practice. The most important step in such improvement is resolving to listen more efficiently. Simply being motivated to listen causes one to be more alert and active as a receiver. The following are specific suggestions for improving listening:

- *Remember to listen carefully.* Before engaging in the communication transaction, listeners should remind themselves of their intent to listen carefully.
- *Be objective.* The communication situation should be approached with the attitude of objectivity, with an open mind, and with a spirit of inquiry.
- *Watch for clues.* Just as one uses bold type and italics in writing, speakers use physical arrangement, program outlines, voice inflection, rate, emphasis, voice quality, and bodily actions as aids to help the listener determine the meaning of what is being said and what the speaker believes is most important.
- *Take your time.* Listeners need to make use of the thinking–speaking time difference and to remind themselves to concentrate on the speaker's message. They must use the extra time to think critically about the message, to relate it to what they already know, to consider the logic of the arguments, and to notice the accompanying nonverbal behavior—all simultaneously.
- *Find the real meaning.* Listeners need to look beyond the actual words to determine what the speaker means, and to determine whether the clusters of accompanying nonverbal behavior are congruent with the verbal message.
- *Respond to confirm your understanding.* Listeners need to provide feedback to the speaker, either indirectly through nonverbal reactions or directly through paraphrasing, to verify that what is being understood by the listener is what the speaker intends.

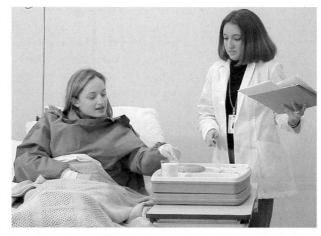

Listening is an essential skill.

Giving accurate feedback is the best way to prove that another person's message has been heard and understood. Ultimately, the most valuable listening skill is ongoing practice. Those who want to improve their listening must put themselves in difficult listening situations, must concentrate, and must practice good listening.

NEGOTIATION

Negotiation permeates human interaction; everyone needs to negotiate. Negotiation can be defined as a process in which two or more parties exchange goods or services and attempt to agree on the exchange rate for them. Negotiating with clients refers to the exchange of alternatives for dietary change between the dietetics professional and the client. The purpose of this section of text is to introduce dietetics practitioners to the concept and to reference them to more detailed accounts.[16–21]

Before actually engaging in the negotiating process, people need to take time to assess their own goals, consider the other party's goals and interests, and develop a strategy. Generally, the process is considered to consist of five stages: preparation and planning, definition of ground rules, clarification and justification of one another's positions, the actual bargaining and problem-solving discussion, and, finally, closure and implementation. Negotiating with clients involves discussing several alternative dietary changes, involving the client in the selection of the alternative being considered, and modifying the options until they are acceptable.

The following suggestions can improve your negotiating skills in the workplace:

- *Begin with a positive overture.* Concessions tend to be reciprocated and lead to agreements. Even a small concession is perceived as a positive overture and stimulates a reciprocal give-and-take climate.
- *Address problems, not personalities.* There is little value in focusing on the personal characteristics of the other. Negotiators understand that what is important is the other's ideas or position (which can be disagreed with), not the individual personally. Separating the people from the problem and not personalizing differences characterize the seasoned negotiator.
- *Pay attention to initial discussions and offers.* Everyone has to have an initial position, and it should be thought of as merely a point of departure. When initial offers are extreme and idealistic, the sophisticated negotiator remains calm and nonjudgmental and counters with a more realistic option or options.
- *Emphasize win–win solutions.* Inexperienced negotiators often assume that any gain must come at the expense of the other party. When a person is patient and willing to tolerate the uncertainty and ambiguity that accompanies what seems like a deadlocked situation, creative thinking is most likely to occur, along with solutions that allow both people to be satisfied and conclude with win–win solutions. When you enter into the process assuming a zero-sum game in which one can only win if the other loses, missed opportunities for trade-offs that could benefit both sides occur. When conditions are supportive and options are framed in terms of the opponent's interests, synergetic solutions are most likely to surface in negotiations.
- *Create an open and trusting climate.* To negotiate well, the negotiator needs well-honed communication skills, especially the skill of listening. Skilled negotiators ask more

questions, focus their alternatives more directly, are less defensive, and have learned to avoid words and phrases that can irritate others. They know how to create an open and trusting climate, the kind of climate so critical for an integrative settlement.

Although there appears to be no significant direct relationship between an individual's personality and negotiation style, cultural background is relevant. The contemporary practitioner or negotiator benefits from an understanding of the other's cultural context. For example, the French tend to like conflict and tend to take a long time in negotiating agreement, not being particularly concerned about whether their opponents like or dislike them. The Chinese, too, tend to draw out negotiations, but they believe negotiations never end and are always willing to start over. Americans, however, are known for their impatience and desire to be liked. Many astute international negotiators turn these characteristics to their advantage with Americans by dragging out negotiations and withholding friendship as conditional on the final settlement.

Negotiating skills improve with time and experience. You need to understand the principles and look for opportunities to practice them. Dietetics practitioners need not wait for differences to begin learning. Practicing in your personal life is often less threatening and can provide an excellent training field.

COMMUNICATING WITH LEGISLATORS

Knowledge of how to communicate with legislators has become another skill critical for health care professionals generally and dietetics professionals specifically. Thousands of voices compete for congressional attention as laws are written and money is provided for everything from health care to weapons.[22–24]

Lobbying can be both effective and ethical. In a democratic society, where government is designed to represent and protect the interests of all citizens and all parties, talking with legislators is exactly what people should do to ensure that decisions and legislation reflect a consensus and take into consideration the interests of all parties affected. Besides using the services of professional lobbyists, organizations such as the ADA benefit from the networking and contacts made by the members of the profession. One of the most effective ways to make legislators aware of issues is at the grassroots level. It is naive to assume that government officials know everything they need to know about the dietetics profession. It becomes the members' responsibility to talk with elected representatives, get to know them and their staff, get on a first-name basis with them, and earn their trust and respect. The time to become networked with public officials, making sure they appreciate the point of view from the perspective of dietetics practitioners, is before they start considering legislation that might be of interest to the dietetics profession. Some of the ways to get the message across include working with the profession's national association, writing letters, making phone calls, meeting with congressional representatives or senators in the home district, developing a relationship with the district administrative assistant, and developing a relationship with health staffers who handle the issues relating to the dietetics profession.

Individuals, organizations, and professional associations can influence the way laws are made and enforced. The contemporary dietetics professional should consider the task of communicating with legislators as another professional responsibility. The professional who learns how to communicate with legislators and develops a network of political connections becomes invaluable to the organization and develops increased power and prestige as a result.

This chapter has presented numerous suggestions for improving the dietitian's and dietetic technician's communication competence with clients and staff. One can, however, read and reread this chapter, pass a quiz on the material with a grade of A+, and still be ineffective in practicing communication skills. To develop communication skills, readers must begin immediately to put into practice what has been read. Do not be discouraged because practice is necessary. Generally, months of conscious attention to these skills are needed before they become a part of your natural approach to clients and staff.

Nothing is as frightening to humans as the fear of uncertainty and ambiguity. When people have the opportunity to try out new communication behavior, forces within them tend to pull them toward their past behavior. Even when the old strategies are unsuccessful, they generally tend to be repeated because the probable outcomes are predictable.

The professional who is serious about increasing communication competence needs to swallow hard and stretch, forcing himself or herself to attempt the new behavior. The time to begin is now. You do not need to have access to clients or staff. You can exercise these skills just as effectively in your personal as in your professional life. Despite all the problems, improved communication is possible, and the professional who is aware of the problems and the recommended safeguards to minimize them is going to be more effective.

CASE STUDY 1

Joan Stivers, RD, noted on the medical record that her patient, John Jones, age 63, was 5'11" tall and weighed 250 pounds. A retiree, he was just diagnosed with type 2 diabetes mellitus. Joan stopped by his hospital room, introduced herself, and told him that the purpose of her visit was to discuss his current food intake. During the conversation, Mr. Jones and his roommate were watching a baseball game on television and periodically commented briefly on the plays and players. Finally, Mr. Jones said, "You need to talk to my wife, not me. She does the cooking." Just then, the physician came by to make rounds.

1. Identify the barriers to communication.
2. What should the dietetics professional do to overcome the barriers?

CASE STUDY 2

John is a new employee in the kitchen. He was hired as an assistant cook 2 months ago. Although his skills are good, the manager noticed that his attendance could be better. In the past 2 weeks, he has been late for work three times, ranging from 10 to 35 minutes. Today he is late again, and the manager asks him to come into the office.

1. What should the manager do to create a supportive communication climate?
2. What should the manager say to John?

REVIEW AND DISCUSSION QUESTIONS

1. In the helping professions, what conveys the professional's effectiveness with clients and staff?
2. What are the common elements of the definition of communication?
3. What are the components of the communication model?
4. What are the verbal guidelines for creating a supportive communication climate?
5. Of the two messages received simultaneously by receivers, which is more influential, verbal or nonverbal?
6. What are the four most common poor listening habits?
7. Describe an empathic response.
8. What are some specific suggestions for improving listening?
9. Why are verbal and nonverbal communications linked?
10. Distinguish between a dogmatic and a provisional prescription in dietetics.

SUGGESTED ACTIVITIES

1. After filling out the questions below, join with classmates in groups of three to share and discuss your responses with one another.
    A. What types of nonverbal signals from your instructor or supervisor indicate to you that he or she is unhappy?
        (1)
        (2)
        (3)
    B. What nonverbal cues indicate that you are getting angry?
        (1)
        (2)
        (3)
    C. List some of the nonverbal signals that you send when you are talking and someone interrupts you.
        (1)
        (2)
        (3)
    D. List some of the nonverbal signals you send when you want to signal confidence or approval of the other person.
        (1)
        (2)
        (3)
    E. List changes you might make in the room where you are reading to alter its climate positively.
        (1)
        (2)
        (3)
2. Write a two-paragraph description of a current interpersonal conflict you are experiencing. Be sure to indicate: (1) the behavior on the part of the other that has caused

you a problem and (2) what "feelings" you are experiencing as a result of that behavior. Do not sign your name unless you want to be acknowledged. After the instructor has collected the descriptions, he or she may read them and either invite students to participate in role-playing of the situations using the guidelines for supportive verbal and nonverbal behavior or engage the class in a case study discussion of how the communication skills might be used to resolve the conflict.

3. You can increase your knowledge of nonverbal behavior by viewing others talking but not hearing what they are saying. Turn the television to a soap opera or talk show; turn off the volume, watch the nonverbal behavior, and try to interpret it. After 3 to 5 minutes, turn the volume up. Then again, turn off the volume. Do this several times and attempt to grasp the verbal messages without the sound by merely interpreting the nonverbal behavior. Take notes and be prepared to share your experience in class.

4. As an in-class exercise, silently jot down the general "meanings" you derive from the nonverbal behaviors listed below. Compare answers with classmates. Is there general agreement on all, or is there a range of answers? Where answers vary, discuss the possible reasons why.
   A. Lack of sustained eye contact
   B. Lowering of eyes or looking away
   C. Furrow on brow
   D. Tight lips
   E. Biting lip or quivering of lower lip
   F. Nodding head up and down
   G. Hanging head down
   H. Shaking head right to left
   I. Folding arms across chest
   J. Unfolded arms
   K. Leaning forward
   L. Slouching, leaning back
   M. Trembling hands
   N. Flushed face
   O. Holding hands tightly
   P. Tapping foot continuously
   Q. Sitting behind a desk
   R. Sitting nearby without any intervening objects

5. The following is an exercise that you might try with friends. The first person expresses the message to the second person, who in turn expresses it to the third, and so on, until six people have heard it. Ordinarily, the message is audiotaped and played back. This allows the participants to see the many ways in which messages are altered as they pass from person to person.

   MESSAGE: A child has hurt herself at the pool, and I must report it to the police. It is necessary, however, for me to get to the hospital as soon as possible. She was walking up the diving board and getting reading to jump, when someone in a blue bathing suit pushed ahead. A boy in a red suit tried to stop her, but she fell off and landed on her back. The boy claims it was the young girl's fault, but she blames him.

WEB SITES

COMMUNICATING WITH LEGISLATORS

http://www.house.gov/writerep/

http://www.ncsl.org/programs/pubs/onlinedirectory.htm

http://www.nocall.org/legadvocacy/legcommunications.html

http://www.senate.gov/general/contract_information/senators_cfm.cfm

LISTENING SKILLS

http://www.listen.org/Templates/facts.htm

http:www.mindtools.com/CommSkll/ActiveListening.htm

VERBAL AND NONVERBAL COMMUNICATION

http://www.faculty.ucr.edu/%7Efriedman/nonverbal.html

http://members.aol.com/nonverbal2index.htm

MOTIVATION AND SELF ESTEEM

http://www.humanlinks.com/manres/articles/self_esteem.html

REFERENCES

1. Commission on Accreditation for Dietetics Education. Eligibility requirements and accreditation standards. Chicago: American Dietetic Association, 2006.
2. Lacey K, Pritchett E. Nutrition care process and model: ADA adopts road map to quality care and outcomes management. J Am Diet Assoc 2003;103:1061–1072.
3. Visocan B, Switt J; Scope of Dietetics Framework Committee, ADA. Understanding and using the Scope of Dietetics Practice Framework: A step-wise approach. J Am Diet Assoc 2006;106:459–463.
4. Stein K. Communication is the heart of provider-patient relationship. J Am Diet Assoc 2006; 106:508–512.
5. Consumer Bill of Rights and Responsibilities: Chapter 5, Respect and Nondiscrimination. Available at: http://www.hcqualitycommission.gov/cborr/chap5.html. Accessed January 5, 2006.
6. U.S. Dept. of Health and Human Services: Healthy People 2010. McLean VA, International Medical Pub, 2001:2801.
7. Robbins S, Judge T. Organizational Behavior, 12th ed. Englewood Cliffs, NJ: Prentice Hall, 2006.
8. Stein K. Good or bad: what you see isn't always what you get. J Am Diet Assoc 2006;106: 1022–1024.
9. Giannini A. Measurement of nonverbal receptive abilities in medical students. Perceptual and Motor Skills 2000;90:1145–1159.
10. Langton S. The mutual influence of gaze and head orientation in the analysis of social attention direction. Quart J Exp Psych 2000;53:825–832.
11. Wachs J. Listening. AAOHN J 1995;43:590–592.
12. Mechanic D, Meyer S. Concepts of trust among patients with serious illness. Soc Sci Med 2000;51:657–668.
13. Doescher M, Saver B, Franks P, et al. Racial and ethnic disparities in perceptions of physician style and trust. Arch Fam Med 2000;9:1156–1163.
14. Hagevik S. Just listening. J Environ Health 2001;62:46–47.

15. Giordano J. Effective communication and counseling with older adults. Int J Aging Hum Dev 2000;51:315–324.

16. Bragg T. The manager as negotiator. Occup Haz 2000;62:53.

17. Frings C. How to negotiate effectively. Med Lab Observer 2000;32:38.

18. Allen DW, Ch'ien A, et al. Employment contracts, negotiation strategies, and the nurse practitioner. Nurs Pract 2000;25:18.

19. Mangan D. Shape a contract you'll be glad you signed. Med Econ 2000;78:79–80, 83–84.

20. Hagevick S. Negotiating your way to success. J Environ Health 2000;62:34–36.

21. Mandel J. Top 10 tips for negotiation. Med Meetings 2000;27:106.

22. White J, Hughes B. If dietetics is your profession, public policy is your business. J Am Diet Assoc 2001;101:172–173.

23. Landers S. Ashwini S. How do physicians lobby their members of Congress? Arch Intern Med 2000;160:3248–3251.

24. Hofford R. Seven tips for effecting legislative change. Fam Pract Manage 2001;8:35–38.

Interviewing

OBJECTIVES

- Discuss the purposes of different kinds of interviews, such as a nutrition interview and a preemployment interview.
- Explain the conditions necessary for effective interviewing.
- Identify the parts of an interview and what should be included in each.
- Discuss the advantages and disadvantages of various types of questions.
- Develop a list of appropriate questions for a nutrition interview and sequence them.
- Identify the different types of responses to an interviewee's remarks.
- Use techniques of interviewing and conduct a nutrition interview.

Professional: "What did you have to eat yesterday?"
Client: "Yesterday? I don't remember."

Effective interviews depend on the client's memory and cooperation as well as the skill of the interviewer. Although the client may not be able to answer the preceding question on the spur of the moment, short-term memory can be improved with some prompting. The client may be reminded of the day of the week, where he or she spent the day, whether meals were eaten at home or at a restaurant, whether others were present, and so on.

Diet is a factor in several causes of death in the United States, such as heart disease, diabetes mellitus, and some cancers, making nutrition interventions important in health promotion, disease prevention, and treatment. As part of assessment, the practitioner often starts with a diet or nutrition interview. Thus, the American Dietetic Association (ADA) recognizes "interviewing techniques," the subject of this chapter, as required competencies for professional practice.[1]

Before beginning to counsel people about their nutritional needs or food choices, it is important to understand their lifestyle, cultural issues, and dietary practices. Using interviewing techniques, the practitioner questions the client to complete an assessment of current eating practices and nutritional adequacy, and to plan an intervention appropriate to the individual and the health problem.

Interviewing skills are equally important in management positions. They are used to screen potential new employees, to obtain information from current employees, and to explore solutions to problems.

A common misperception is that an interview involves two people having a conversation, with one person asking questions and the other answering. Nothing could be further from the truth. Interviewing may be defined as a guided communication process between two people with the predetermined purpose of exchanging or obtaining specific information by questioning. The goal of the interview is to collect specific, accurate information from the respondent while maintaining an interpersonal environment conducive to full disclosure.

This chapter covers the basics of interviewing skills. Included are the principles and process of interviews, the conditions facilitating interviews, the three parts of an interview, the use of different types of questions, and the types of interviewer responses. The interview is a complex process with many interacting variables. One must be aware of the impact of the environment, culture, verbal and nonverbal communication interactions, perceptions and roles of the two parties, needs and interests, personalities, attitudes, beliefs and values, and feedback. To become a skilled interviewer takes time and practice until the principles and techniques come naturally.

An effective interviewer must be a good listener. The interviewer concentrates on both the verbal responses and the nonverbal behavior, or body language, of the respondent. To discover what is important to the client, listen not only for facts, but also for emotions, attitudes, feelings, and values. A person newly diagnosed with diabetes mellitus, for example, may be upset, anxious, or fearful. These emotions need to be recognized and dealt with before counseling begins.

To illustrate the interviewing principles and process, two examples of interviews are presented in this chapter—the nutrition interview and the preemployment interview. Although a full explanation of the content of these types of interviews is beyond the scope of this book, a brief explanation of each follows. For more detailed information on content, other sources should be examined.[2–10]

NUTRITION INTERVIEWS

A food and nutrition interview or diet history is an account of a person's food habits, preferences, eating behaviors, and other factors influencing food choices. An initial nutrition assessment interview is the first step in the Nutrition Care Process (NCP)[9] and serves one or more purposes:

- Makes the counselor and client aware of current dietary practices and their origins, influential lifestyle factors, and related information.
- Identifies any nutrition-related problems and screens for malnutrition so that an appropriate nutrition diagnosis and intervention is planned.
- Contributes to accurately defining the nutritional status of the client in conjunction with other data.
- Defines problems and issues so that realistic goals for change can be set.
- Helps the counselor identify possible alternatives so changes can be suggested.
- Provides baseline data against which to monitor changes.
- Enables the counselor to continue to develop rapport and a good relationship with the client.

In completing the food and nutrition history, you may collect specific information to identify nutrition-related problems:[9,10]

1. The consumption of food (i.e., intake of foods, patterns of meals and snacks, food portions, cues to eating, nutritional and herbal supplements, and current diets).
2. Knowledge of nutrition and health (i.e., knowledge and beliefs about nutrition, self-monitoring and self-care practices, previous nutrition counseling and education, readiness to learn, and stage of change).
3. Physical activity and exercise (i.e., activity patterns, sedentary time, and exercise frequency, intensity, and duration).
4. Food availability (i.e., family food planning, purchasing, and preparation abilities, food safety, food and nutrition program utilization, and food insecurity).

Currently, there is no gold standard method for obtaining information about a person's dietary intake, but approaches used frequently are the 24-hour recall, the record of usual daily food intake, and the food frequency checklist; the situation guides the selection. Motivational interviewing is discussed in Chapters 4 and 5. In the 24-hour recall, the interviewer asks the client to recount the types and amounts of foods and beverages consumed in the previous 24-hour period. To enhance memory, one may need to ask the individual to recall where the meal was eaten (home, work, restaurant), other events that happened during the day (watching television, exercising, e-mail, shopping), and others who were present (family, friends). The second method, the usual daily food intake, asks clients to explain the types and amounts of foods and beverages that they usually consume during one day's time. Responses show what the person typically eats during meals and snacks. In both approaches, the portion sizes, the methods of food preparation (frying versus baking), the between-meal snacks, the time and place food is consumed, the condiments, the use of vitamin and mineral supplements or alternative nutrition therapies, and any alcoholic beverages consumed require consideration.

No method is considered to have a high degree of accuracy in assessing the nutritional status of the client, and each has potential deficiencies and inherent inaccuracies.[5,8,11–15] For example:

- The previous 24-hour period may not have been typical.
- Weekends may differ from weekdays.
- There are seasonal variations.
- The person may be unable to judge portion sizes.
- The person may have memory lapses.
- There is underreporting, especially among the overweight.
- Certain foods may be considered socially undesirable or unhealthy by clients, so they prefer not to reveal eating them.

To overcome the problem of judging portion sizes, counselors may use three-dimensional food models, food pictures, serving utensils, dishes, and various sizes of beverage glasses. An 8-ounce glass is small, for example, compared with the large servings at convenience stores and fast-food restaurants. Clients may be confused, because the Food and Drug Administration (FDA) and U.S. Department of Agriculture (USDA) portion sizes differ and restaurants serve larger portions than either of them. Consumers have difficulty recognizing portions appropriate for their weight and activity level.[16] Portions of foods such as potato chips, French fries, and popcorn may be difficult to visualize. A deck of cards, a baseball, or pieces of foam of various sizes can help visualization. A selection of food packages and food labels may also be helpful.

Reports indicate that clients do not volunteer information about foods they consider that others think are less desirable. Examples of sensitive topics may include chocolate, alcoholic beverages, certain snacks, butter or margarine, take-out foods, and others.[8,11] A skilled interviewer needs to inquire about these.

One way to increase the accuracy of the information is also to use a food frequency checklist. This checklist identifies the daily, weekly, or monthly frequency of a client's consumption of basic foods, such as milk and dairy products, meats–fish–poultry, eggs, fruits and fruit juices, vegetables and salads, breads and cereals, desserts and sweets, butter–margarine–fats–oils, between-meal snacks, and beverages, including coffee, tea, colas, and alcoholic beverages. If the client responds about consumption of orange juice during the food frequency checklist, for example, and it was not mentioned during the usual daily intake, the interviewer can prompt the client to recall where it fits into the daily pattern and in what amount. This improves the assessment of energy and nutrient intake.[5] Extensive food frequency questionnaires containing 120 or more food items are used in nutrition research studies.

To save time, the diet history and food frequency checklist can be narrowed to focus only on the health problem, such as emphasizing dietary sources of fat in heart disease, foods high in sodium in hypertension, or calcium and vitamin D in osteoporosis. An example is the MEDFICTS (**M**eats, **E**ggs, **D**airy, **F**ried foods, **I**n baked goods, **C**onvenience foods, **T**able fats, and **S**nacks) instrument used to evaluate adherence to Step 1 and 2 diets of the National Cholesterol Education Program. It concentrates on recording foods and portions contributing total fat, cholesterol, and saturated fat.[17,18]

PREEMPLOYMENT INTERVIEWS

Managing human resources is part of the scope of dietetics practice.[19] An example of an interview used by a manager is the preemployment interview with prospective employees. Several applicants may be interviewed for a position. A structured interview in which all questions are preplanned and each applicant is asked the same questions is recommended.[4,7] The same interviewing principles and techniques are used, but for a different purpose. In this case, the interviewer wants to find the individual with the capability of performing the duties and responsibilities of the job according to the job-related knowledge, skills, and abilities in the job description. Because federal legislation outlaws discrimination based on race, color, religion, gender, national origin, age over 40, and disability, questions about any of these are avoided as they may lead to costly lawsuits. Those who need more information should consult additional resources.[4,7]

CONDITIONS FACILITATING INTERVIEWS

For best results, you need to increase your effectiveness as an interviewer[6,20] by doing the following:

- Clearly define the purpose of the interview to the interviewee.
- Attend to verbal and nonverbal behavior by listening.

- Build rapport.
- Provide freedom from interruptions.
- Provide psychological privacy.
- Have appropriate physical surroundings.
- Have emotional objectivity.
- Consider the personal context of the respondent.
- Limit note taking or explain why notes are needed.

Purpose

When an interviewer is asking questions, the respondent may be wondering why the questions are necessary. Without knowing the answer, a person may be unwilling to respond. For these reasons, the interviewer needs to explain the purpose of the interview. With clients, you can stress that the interview is necessary to provide better assistance with problems, services, or health care recommendations. For example: "Let's do a careful evaluation of the food you eat and see if we find any ways to enhance your choices." With job applicants, note that it is important to find an employee who will be satisfied with the company and the position. If the purpose is clear and understood, better cooperation from the interviewee may be expected.

Attentiveness

Listening attentively helps to create a climate in which the interviewee can communicate easily. Professionals need to develop skills in listening—an active, not a passive, process that requires a great deal of concentration. Many interviewers tend to talk too much. Instead, the interviewer should listen carefully and assist respondents in communicating their thoughts, feelings, and information. The message includes both verbal and nonverbal behaviors. Periodically paraphrasing or summarizing confirms that you are listening and trying to understand.

Keep in mind that the interviewee is also observing you. Frequent looking at one's watch, failure to maintain eye contact, sitting back in too relaxed a posture, frowning, yawning, and tone of voice all may convey a negative message and inhibit effective interviews. Attentiveness can be shown, for example, by appropriate nonverbal behaviors such as friendly eye contact, interested facial expression, good posture, smiling, and nodding.

Building Rapport

Rapport should be established early in the interview and continue to be developed. Rapport is the personal relationship established between the interviewer and the respondent. It is important to build a warm and supportive climate, to release stress, to put the person at ease, and to provide nonjudgmental verbal and nonverbal responses no matter what the person says. The client's self-disclosure should not be labeled "right" or "wrong."

The relationship between the two parties develops over time. The interviewer strives to create an environment of respect and trust by arranging conditions in which individuals perceive themselves as accepted, warmly received, valued, and understood. Trust must be earned; without it vital self-disclosure on the part of the respondent may be limited. People will not give personal information unless they trust the other person.

Setting yourself up as the "expert" and the respondent as the "receiver of one's expertise" will inhibit the relationship. "I've had a lot of experience with this and will be able to tell you what to do," is not a helpful approach. Respondents may be overwhelmed by the professional's expertise and position, replying with information they think is being sought or is acceptable instead of what is useful.

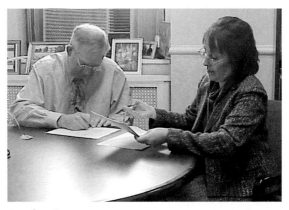

An informal setting improves an interview.

Rapport may be inhibited by addressing people by their first names, a practice common with close friends and family. This may be interpreted as too informal or a lack of respect by some people and in some cultures. A woman 72 years of age, for example, may not like being called "Martha" by someone who is 25 years old. When in doubt, use both names, such as "Martha Smith," "Mrs. Smith," or a query "would you prefer to be addressed as Mrs. Smith or Martha?" The custom of the workplace is a guide. Also tell how you wish to be addressed. Addressing yourself by your surname and the client by the first name creates a superior–subordinate relationship.

Freedom From Interruptions

To devote full attention to the interviewee, freedom from interruptions is needed.[6] The professional should arrange to have phone calls held; if a call must be answered, the phone conversation should be brief, with apologies given to the interviewee. In the hospital setting, asking to turn off the television, closing the door, and selecting a time when staff and visitors are less likely to interrupt is advisable.

Psychological Privacy

Since private matters will be discussed, the interviewer and interviewee should be alone. A quiet office without interruption is preferable. At the patient's bedside in a hospital setting, however, others may be present in the room. Whenever possible, arrange the setting so that the interview cannot be overheard and is not interrupted; this promotes the giving of undivided attention and that adheres to Health Insurance Portability and Accountability Act (HIPAA) requirements.[6]

Assure the interviewee that information revealed will be treated confidentially and shared only with pertinent health care providers. Anecdotes and stories should not be shared with others over coffee breaks, lunch, or social gatherings.

Physical Surroundings

A comfortable environment with proper furniture, lighting, temperature, ventilation, and pleasant surroundings can enhance an interview. A setting should be arranged in which eye contact can be maintained. Since standing over a patient lying in hospital bed may trigger deferential behavior, it is preferable to be at the same head level. The optimum distance between people involved in an interview is 2 to 4 feet—about an arm's length—but cultural practices differ.[20]

The most formal seating arrangement is for one person to sit across the desk from another, whereas a chair alongside the desk is less formal and makes people feel more equal in status.[6] Two parties seated without a table is informal, but when viewing materials, a round table is less formal than a square or rectangle because it eliminates the head-of-the table position. In general, the fewer barriers to the line of sight, the better. A desk top with a computer, telephone, books, plants, and other materials between you and the client is a psychological barrier.

Emotional Objectivity

The interviewer's personal feelings and preferences should be controlled and not revealed to the interviewee. The client should feel free to express all feelings, attitudes, and values and, in the process, may express some that are contrary to those of the professional. An attitude of acceptance and concern for the interviewee should be maintained, with a desire to understand behavior rather than pass judgment. A raised eyebrow, look of shock, surprise, or amusement, or an incredulous follow-up question (e.g., "You had three beers for lunch?" or "All you had for lunch was a box of cookies?") may cause an client to change or end the story.

The professional relationship is most easily established with persons similar to ourselves whereas barriers may arise if there are differences. People from all socioeconomic groups, various cultural and ethnic groups, and ages from young to elderly participate differently in the professional relationship. A thorough understanding of the food choices and practices of other groups is helpful.

Interviewers should develop an awareness of their own conscious and unconscious values and prejudices. These include not only racial, ethnic, and religious preferences, but also exaggerated dislikes of people and their characteristics. Examples may include the poorly or weirdly dressed, the uneducated, aggressive women, meek men, highly pitched voices, or weak handshakes. Identifying your own intolerances may help to control any expression of them through nonverbal behaviors.

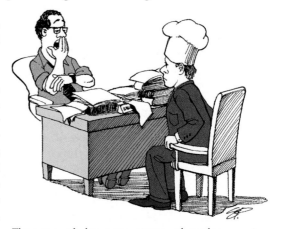

Things to avoid when communicating with another.

Personal Context

Interviewees bring with them their own personal contexts or systems of beliefs, attitudes, feelings, and values that must be recognized. Concerns about perceived threats to health can be so frightening, for example, that they preoccupy thoughts and block conversation. Interviewers need to recognize the respondent's situation and the subjective and objective aspects of it. After a heart attack, for example, a man may feel fear, resentment, anger, anxiety, dependence, or regression, which may interfere with concentration and cooperation. An understanding of the psychological reactions to illness and ways of dealing with them is necessary.

You may need to facilitate the venting of feelings and to acknowledge them before proceeding with the interview. A job applicant, for example, may have been laid off recently from a long-time position. The subjective way the person feels about the situation, however, is as important as the facts. Anxiety, nervousness, and depression may be evident. The manager should be alert to verbal and nonverbal clues as they give a frame of reference for understanding. Although the professional is focused on the task, to be effective the personal context of the respondent should not be ignored. The interviewee's thoughts and feelings come first.

Usually, the practitioner has some background information about the person in advance. In the hospital setting, the medical record is the source of information on the social, cultural, and economic circumstances that may influence the goals for change and treatment: marital status, number in the household, age, employment, religion, level of education, physical health, medications, weight and height, medical history, and results of lab tests and X-rays. In preemployment interviews, the application form should be examined before the interview, since it contains information on education and previous work experience.

Cognitive approaches conceptualize four distinct stages that a person goes through in response to another's questions, each of which may lead to errors in responses—comprehension, retrieval, estimation/judgment, and response. Comprehension is the first stage in which the interviewee interprets the meaning of the question asked. In retrieval, the second stage, the respondent searches short-and long-term memory for an appropriate answer. Third, in estimation/judgment, the interviewee evaluates the relevance of the information from memory, decides whether or not it is appropriate, and possibly combines various bits of information. In the fourth and final stage, response, other factors may be weighed, such as how sensitive the information is, whether or not the answer is socially expected or desirable, the amount of accuracy to provide, and so forth. The person then provides a response to the question.[21]

Note Taking

Taking too many notes may hamper the flow of conversation, inhibit rapport between the two parties, and prevent the interviewer's concentration on the verbal and nonverbal answers of the respondent. In addition, the interviewee may be distracted or apprehensive about what is being written.[6]

An inexperienced interviewer, however, may find it necessary to take some notes. If so, they should be as brief as possible. To avoid concern, the individual should ask the interviewee's permission to jot down a few notes and should explain why they are necessary and how they will be used. The practitioner may say, for example: "Is it all right if I take a few notes so that later, I can review what we said?"

While writing, try to maintain eye contact as much as possible. You need to develop a few key words, phrases, or abbreviations to use. A breakfast of orange juice, cereal, toast, and coffee with cream and sugar, for example, may be abbreviated, "OJ, cer, tst, C-C-S," while a pineapple–cottage cheese salad may be noted as "P/A-CC sld."

Comprehensive notes should be dictated or recorded immediately after the person has departed. Waiting 15 minutes or longer, seeing another client or job applicant, or accepting phone calls may cause the interviewer to forget essential information.

PARTS OF THE INTERVIEW

Each interview can be divided into three parts.

- Opening
- Exploration
- Closing

The beginning of the interview, or opening, involves introductions and establishing rapport, a process of creating trust and good will between the parties.[20] The exploration phase includes the use of questions to obtain information while maintaining the personal relationship, as the interviewer guides and directs the interview with responses. In the final phase, the interview is closed and any future contacts are planned. **Table 3-1** summarizes the interview process.

Opening

The opening sets the tone of the interview—friendly or unfriendly, professional or informal, relaxed or tense, leisurely or rushed—and influences how the interviewee perceives you. Practitioners should greet the client and state their name and job title, for example, "Good morning. I'm Judy Jones, a registered dietitian." A smile, eye contact, a handshake or placing a hand on the other's hand or arm, and a friendly face and tone of voice are supporting nonverbal behaviors.

In the hospital setting, the interviewer may ask, "Are you Mary Johnson?" If answered affirmatively, you may respond, "I'm glad to meet you. Do you prefer to be addressed as Mrs. Johnson or as Mary?" The professional may add how she prefers to be addressed, such as "Please call me Judy."

If the patient's physician has requested the contact, the interviewer may mention this. "Did Dr. Smith tell you that he asked me to visit you?" If the person answers "no," explain about the physician's request. A discussion of the nature and purpose of the interview may follow, along with how the individual will benefit from the interview. For example:

T A B L E **3-1** | The Interview Process

Phases	Tasks
Opening	Introductions
	Establish rapport
	Discuss purpose
Exploration	Gather information with questions
	Explore problems
	Explore both thoughts and feelings
	Continue building rapport
Closing	Express appreciation
	Review purpose; ask for comments or questions
	Plan future contacts

"Dr. Smith mentioned that you have high blood pressure. He asked me to talk with you and see whether we can find a way to reduce the amount of salt and sodium in the foods you eat. This will help you control your blood pressure."

Before unleashing a barrage of questions, a few minutes may be spent on other topics to develop some rapport. A dialogue, not a monologue, is appropriate. Discussion of known information from the medical record or from the application form of job applicants may be appropriate. Alternatively, the weather, sporting events, holidays, a national or international event, traffic, parking, or any topic of joint interest may be helpful in opening the discussion. Although you have a task to complete, small talk is important in developing and building the relationship. It should not be prolonged, however, or the interviewee may be wondering when you will get to the purpose of the discussion. A time frame for the interview may be mentioned.

When interviewees initiate the appointment, it is preferable to let them state in their own words their problem or purpose for coming. The manager may ask, "What brought you to the Friendly Company to seek employment, Mr. Smithfield?" or "How have things been going since your last appointment when we talked about your goals for change?" or "When we talked on the phone, Mrs. Jones, you mentioned that your doctor told you that you have borderline diabetes. How can I help?" When interviewees are given the chance to express themselves first, the interview begins with their agenda, or what they think is important.

Although it may be time-consuming for a busy person, the opening exchange of either information or pleasantries is important and should not be omitted. Rapport, a degree of warmth, a supportive atmosphere, and a sense of mutual involvement are critical components in the interview. Willingness to disclose information about oneself is influenced by the level of trust established in the relationship, and cooperation and disclosure are crucial to the success of interviews. Interviewees quickly develop perceptions of the situation and make decisions about the amount and kind of information they will share. They form impressions of the interviewer just as the professional does of them. Before directing the conversation to the second stage, the purpose or nature of the interview should be clearly stated and understood so the person knows what to expect.

SELF-ASSESSMENT

How satisfactory are the following openings? How can they be improved?

Employment Interview:

1. "Come on in. I'm very busy today, but need to hire a new employee. Do you have any work experience?"
2. "Hi, I'm Steve Johnson (shaking hands). We're looking for a cook for early shift. Do you prefer early hours or late?"

Patient/Client Interview:

1. "Hi, Mr. Jones. I'm Mary, a registered dietitian. Have you been on a diabetic diet before?"
2. Entering patient room: "Good morning, Julia. What's up? How are you guys doing today? I'm here to tell you what to eat on a sodium-restricted diet."

Exploration

In the second stage, the interviewee is asked a series of questions; these are the tools used by the practitioner to obtain information. They are not spur of the moment. A good interviewer has carefully preplanned these questions in a prepared "interview guide," an outline of the information desired or topics to be covered that are relevant to the purpose of the interview. The guide should tell not only what questions will be asked, but also how questions will be phrased to gain the most information in the limited time available. With practice, a natural flow will occur.

Topics should be arranged in a definite sequence. In a nutrition or diet history, for example, the interviewer may desire information about beverages consumed, eating in restaurants, portion sizes, meals, methods of food preparation, and snacks. Put in sequence, the list includes meals, portion sizes, methods of food preparation, snacks, beverages, and eating in restaurants. See **Box 3-1** for questions and directives for diet histories.

B ox 3-1

Examples of Questions and Directives for Diet Histories

1. "Who plans and prepares the meals at home? Who does the grocery shopping?"
2. "Are you currently restricting your food choices in any way?" (because of allergy, religion, intolerance, etc.)
3. "Please tell me about any questions or issues you have in making food choices; about the people in your family who eat together and any dietary problems they have."
4. "How physically active are you?"
5. "Now I am going to ask you to think of all the foods and beverages you consume in a typical day. Please tell me about the first food or drink you have after arising and the portion size of that food."
6. "That's good. Now tell me about what you eat and drink next including the amount."
7. "And then, what would you eat or drink next?"
8. "What types of seasonings do you use in cooking? Tell me about them."
9. "Snacks and beverages are often forgotten. What do you have between each of your meals and during the evening or before bed?"
10. "You haven't mentioned alcoholic beverages, including beer and wine. Please tell me about them?"
11. "How often do you take a vitamin–mineral supplement or use herbs or alternative therapies? Please describe the kinds and amounts."
12. "What time of day are your meals?"
13. "How many times a week do you eat a meal away from home? What would you have?"
14. "Would you say that the amounts of foods you have described are typical, more than usual, or less than usual?"
15. "To summarize what you have told me, can you tell me how many servings you eat daily or weekly of these foods?" (continue with a food frequency checklist)

In a preemployment interview, the sequence may be previous work experience, career goals, education, present activities and interests that are job-related, and personal qualifications. Specific questions intended to gain information about the applicant's qualifications, compared with those in the job description, should be planned in advance.

Although it ensures that information is gathered in a systematic manner, the interview guide should not be followed strictly. Never read from the list of questions or try to follow a predetermined sequence. The interviewer should be thoroughly familiar with the questions and not have to refer to them constantly. When the interviewee brings up a topic or asks a question, this shows interest and should be pursued. Knowing the purpose and significance of each question is important so that questions are not asked in a perfunctory manner and so the interviewer does not accept superficial or inadequate answers.

Asking a job applicant about offices held in organizations, for example, is an attempt to seek information about leadership ability and the acceptance of responsibility. The technique of inquiring about career plans over the next 3 to 5 years attempts to learn about short- and long-range goals. See **Box 3-2** for preemployment interview questions. To answer fully, interviewees must see how the questions are relevant. With clients, the professional can explain that the answers are a basis for nutrition assessment, counseling, or education.

Using Questions

Questions play a major role in interviews as tools of the trade. The wording of questions is as important as one's manner and tone of voice. A friendly approach in asking the questions communicates the desire to understand and be of assistance. The kind of questions asked should require the other person to talk 60 to 70% of the time. Questions that are highly specific or may be answered with one word, such as "yes" or "no," should be avoided initially but may be necessary later to follow up on specific information.

Questions may be classified in three ways: open or closed, primary or secondary, and neutral or leading.[20]

Open and closed questions

Open questions are broad and give the interviewee great freedom in deciding what to say while giving the professional an opportunity to listen and observe. The following are examples of open questions:

"Will you tell me a little about yourself?"
"What are some foods you like to eat?"
"What have you done in the past to try to lose weight?"

At the beginning of an interview, open questions are less threatening and communicate more interest and trust; answers reveal what the interviewee thinks is most important. Disadvantages are that they may involve a greater amount of time, the collection of unnecessary information, and lengthy, disorganized answers.[6,20]

The following are examples of open questions with moderate restrictions:

"Can you tell me about the types of meals you eat?"
"What did the doctor tell you about your health and diet?"
"What were your job responsibilities in your previous position?"
"How did you become interested in this position?"
"What skills do you have that are important for this job?"

BOX 3-2

Sample Preemployment Interview Questions

Permissible Questions and Their Significance

In general, questions asked in preemployment interviews should be job related or predictive of success on the job. They should elicit information to compare the individual's qualifications and interests with those of the job description for the vacant position. Depending on the applicant and the job opening, the following are examples with their significance:

1. "Now I would like to ask you some questions about yourself and your previous work experience." Introduces the line of questioning.
2. "Tell me about your previous work experience and how it relates to the job you are interested in." Gives general impressions of whether the person is qualified.
3. "Please describe for me one or two important accomplishments in your previous job." Gives abilities.
4. "What were your responsibilities on your previous job?" Gives knowledge, skills, and abilities.
5. "What would you say are your greatest strengths as a worker? Areas to improve?" Gives skills and abilities.
6. "What kind of work interests you?" Tells interest and motivation.
7. "What subjects in school did you like most and least?" Shows interests.
8. "What was your grade point average and class rank?" Shows mental ability and motivation.
9. "While in school, what extracurricular activities did you participate in that have a bearing on this job?" Shows diversity of interest, interpersonal skills, and teamwork.
10. "What organizations do you belong to that are relevant to the job you are applying for?" Shows interests and interpersonal skills.
11. "What offices have you held?" Shows leadership ability and acceptance of responsibility.
12. "What are your career goals? Where do you see yourself in 3 to 5 years?" Shows whether or not the person plans ahead and what their plans are, as well as whether or not they are congruent with those of the company.
13. "What hours do you prefer to work? How much flexibility do you have with your schedule?" Tells availability during various hours of the day and days of the week.
14. "What brought you to our company to apply for work? Why would you like to work for us?" Tells whether the person is knowledgeable about the company and interests.
15. "Do you prefer to work alone or in a group?" Tells if the person would work well in a team environment.
16. "Tell me about a time at your last job when teamwork was important."
17. "How would you describe yourself as an employee?"
18. "What questions do you have?"

Questions That Should Not Be Asked

Certain subjects can be the basis for complaints of discrimination on the basis of race, color, gender, marital status, national origin, religion, age, and disability. For this reason, the following questions are examples of ones that should be avoided in pre-employment interviews. If the questions are not job related, do not ask.

1. "What is your nationality and native language?"
2. "What is your religious faith?"
3. "What is your marital status?"
4. "What is your maiden name?"
5. "Where does your spouse work? What does he (she) think of your working?"
6. "Who will baby-sit for you?"
7. "Do you have a family or plans to start a family?"
8. "What is your date of birth? Date of graduation from school?"
9. "Do you have any health problems or disabilities?"

In follow-up visits, open questions should be broad to allow the client to determine the focus of the interview. Examples are, "How are your food goals progressing?" or "What progress have you made since we last talked?" The professional should begin discussion with whatever is of current concern to the client. For opening questions, the interviewer should also refer to the records regarding the client's background, problems, and previous counseling goals.

Closed questions are more restrictive; that is, they limit answers. Some closed questions are more limiting than others, such as:

"Who cooks the food at home?"
"Do you salt your food?"
"Tell me about any snacks you eat between meals."
"What special diet or food restrictions, if any, do you follow?"

Closed questions give the interviewer more control, require less effort from the interviewee, and are less time consuming, which is of value when only a short screening is needed. Disadvantages include the inhibition of communication, which might result if the interviewer shows little interest in the answers, the need for additional questions to obtain information, and getting answers that may not reveal why the respondent feels as he or she does. Table 3-2 summarizes the advantages and disadvantages of the different kinds of questions.

Primary and secondary questions

Questions may also be classified as primary or secondary. Primary questions or requests are used to introduce topics or new areas of discussion. The following are examples:

"Now that we have discussed your most recent position, please tell me about your former job with Smith & Company."
"Now that we have discussed the foods you eat at home, tell me about what you eat when you go to restaurants."

Note that mentioning what was just said shows that you have been listening.

T A B L E **3-2** | **Advantages and Disadvantages of Questions**

Type of Question	Advantages	Disadvantages
Open	Gives interviewee control	Time consuming
	Communicates trust/interest	Supplies unneeded information
	Less threatening	
	Tells what the person thinks is important	
Closed	Gives interviewer control	Provides incomplete answers
	Provides quick answers	Short answers force more questions
	Verifies information	
Primary	Introduces new topics	
Secondary	Elicits further information	
Leading		Directs person's answer
		Reveals bias of interviewer
Neutral	More accurate answers	

Secondary questions or requests attempt to obtain further information or explanation that primary questions have failed to elicit. They are also referred to as "follow-up" questions. Interviewees may have given an inadequate response for many reasons, including poor memory, misunderstanding of the question or amount of detail needed, and the feeling that the question is too personal or irrelevant, or that the professional would not understand the response. Specific follow-up questions, such as the following, may be asked:

"How much orange juice do you drink?"
"What do you put in your coffee?"
"In your previous position, how many people did you supervise?"

Neutral and leading questions

Neutral questions are preferred to leading questions.[6,20] Neutral questions do not suggest an answer, whereas leading questions direct the respondent toward one answer, an effect that may be unintentional on the part of an inexperienced interviewer. Leading questions reveal a suggested or expected answer, as in the following examples:

"You drink milk, don't you?" "Yes, of course." Instead, ask: "What beverages do you drink?"
"You aren't going to eat desserts anymore, are you?" "No." Instead ask: "What will you have for dessert?"
"Breakfast is *so* important. What do you have? Cereal?" Instead ask: "What do you have to eat and drink first after you wake up?"

One of these questions assumes the client eats breakfast, and in these instances people probably answer as they think they are expected to, even if they usually omit the meal. Clients may change their answers on the basis of a nonverbal appearance of the practitioner of surprise, disgust, dislike, or disagreement with what clients are saying. To receive uninhibited responses from clients, the interviewer needs to avoid these appearances.

SELF-ASSESSMENT

Identify the following questions as open, closed, primary, secondary, or leading.

1. "You mentioned that the only meal you eat at home is dinner. Can you tell me where you eat your breakfast and lunch and what you are likely to have?"
2. "Do you put catsup on your hamburger?"
3. "What do you put on your salad?"
4. "How do you cook your meats?"

You do not need to impress people with medical and dietetics vocabulary. Complex terminology should be avoided or used sparingly, and only when you are sure that the client understands. The following is a statement likely to be misunderstood in a conversation: "People with hyperlipidemia should avoid eating foods containing saturated and trans-fatty acids and emphasize monounsaturates and polyunsaturates instead. This can help lower levels of low-density lipoproteins." Instead say: "People with high blood cholesterol need to eat fewer foods that contain large amounts of saturated and trans-fat. We can discuss what they are and other substitutes."

Directives

When you as the interviewer sense that too many questions are being asked and the respondent may be developing a feeling of interrogation, you may introduce some questions as a statement or directive. For example: "How has your diet been going?" may be changed to "I'd be interested in hearing how your diet has been going." "How did you become interested in this position?" may be changed to "I'd be interested in some of the reasons you decided to apply for this position." This makes the interview more conversational. Questions should be asked one at a time and the interviewer should concentrate on listening carefully to the answers rather than thinking ahead to the next questions to be asked.

Sequencing Questions

Questions can be arranged in a "funnel," "inverted funnel," or "tunnel" sequence.[20] A funnel sequence begins with broad, open questions and proceeds to more restrictive ones.

EXAMPLE: "Tell me about the foods you eat during a day's time."
"What do you have for snacks between meals?"
"We haven't discussed alcoholic beverages—what do you like to drink?"

Beginning the interview with open-ended questions poses the least threat to the client and encourages a response. The person then volunteers much information, making it unnecessary to ask additional questions.

At times, an inverted funnel sequence may be preferable. In preemployment interviews, for example, applicants may feel more comfortable dealing with a specific question than with a broad, open one, such as "Tell me about yourself," when they are apprehensive and unsure of what to say or what the interviewer expects.

The funnel sequence is a series of questions, each covering a different topic to gain specific information. It may be an appropriate choice in a nutrition interview.

In taking a diet history, questions or statements starting with "What" or "Tell me about" elicit better responses than "Do you . . .?" See diet history examples. Questions that do not require a sufficient answer or may be answered with one word or "yes" or "no" are less productive, as in the following examples:

EXAMPLE: "Do you eat breakfast?" "Yes."
"Do you like milk?" "No."
"How often do you eat meat?" "Every day."

A series of short, sequential, dead-end questions from the professional's list of information to be gathered prevents people from telling their stories their way, and information may be omitted as a result. Instead, gather this information using a broad opening question or directive, as follows:

EXAMPLE: "Please tell me about the first foods and drinks you have most days, what you eat, and the amount."

"Why" Questions

Some professionals recommend avoiding questions beginning with "why."[12] "Why" may indicate one's disapproval, displeasure, or mistrust, and it appears to ask the person to justify or explain his or her behavior, for example:

"Why don't you follow your diet more closely?"
"Why don't you eat breakfast?"
"Why did you resign from your job?"
"Why don't you exercise more often?"

Clients may react defensively or explain their behavior in a manner they believe is acceptable.

"I don't follow my diet because I don't like it. You wouldn't like it either."
"I can eat breakfast if you think I should."
"I resigned because there was no chance for advancement."
"I don't exercise because I don't have time. Do you exercise?"

If threatened by a "why" question and unwilling to reveal the answer, the individual may answer in an evasive manner, in which case nothing is gained.

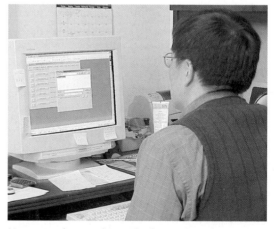

Nutrient analysis may be completed on a computer.

RESPONSES

After the client answers, the interviewer may respond in one of several ways, some of which are recommended and others, less helpful.

1. Understanding responses
2. Probing responses
3. Confrontation responses
4. Evaluative responses
5. Hostile responses
6. Reassuring responses

Understanding Responses

The understanding response is one of the best choices. With it, practitioners try to understand the person's message and recreate it within their own frame of reference. People have more rapport with those who try to understand them rather than judge them. This may lead to more cooperation on the part of the client.

> **EXAMPLE:** Mrs. Jones: "I haven't lost any weight this week. I ate just a few cookies. The diet doesn't work."
> Counselor, paraphrasing a feeling rather than a fact: "You are feeling concerned because you haven't lost any weight, Mrs. Jones, and you are wondering if it was something you ate, or a problem with the diet?"

The paraphrase in this understanding response helps the person feel accepted even if her behavior has not been perfect. The client will feel safe in expressing her sentiments and exploring them further.

Note that the professional should focus on Mrs. Jones's feelings and attitudes, rather than only on the content of what she said. She may be feeling concerned or disappointed with the diet or with herself. She may feel guilty. She may be frustrated with trying to change her food choices. The counselor has guessed "concerned," and if this is not correct, Mrs. Jones will correct the mistaken impression. This gives even more information.

The understanding response is most helpful in assisting clients to recognize problems and to devise their own solutions. The client may progress from initial negative feelings to more neutral ones and finally to more positive attitudes and solutions.

It is necessary to differentiate and understand both the content and the feelings of the client's remarks. To determine the content, you may ask yourself, "What is this person telling me or thinking?" Feelings may be classified as positive, negative, or ambivalent, and these may change as the interview progresses.[12] In identifying feelings, ask, "What is this person feeling, and why is he or she feeling that way?"

You may use the following sentence in paraphrasing the person's statement to verify your understanding. The answer may be inserted into a format.

> **EXAMPLE:** "I think I hear you saying that you feel. . . because. . ."

Although one may have an incorrect impression, such as a feeling that a person is concerned when the person actually is tired, the interviewee usually provides the correct interpretation, thereby furthering the interviewer's understanding. This process demonstrates that one is trying to understand.

To avoid overuse of the same phrase or sounding mechanistic, the phrase can be varied.

> **EXAMPLE:** "Do I understand correctly that you feel. . .?"
> "You seem to be saying that you are feeling. . ."
> "I gather that. . ."

"You sound. . ."

"In other words, you are feeling. . . "

Interviewee responses that suggest feelings about an event may provide an important key to the person's behavior. How clients feel about their lifestyles, food habits or choices, or their health is critical to dietary adherence. Food behaviors may be influenced by psychological, cultural, and environmental variables that are important to understand.

Job applicants may also express feelings about previous work experience, relationships with superiors and subordinates, and activities and interests. Preceding a statement with "I think. . .," "I feel. . .," or "I believe. . ." gives a signal that the statement expresses opinions, beliefs, attitudes, or values. Possible follow-up probes are included in the following examples:

EXAMPLE: "Can you explain more about your feelings?"

"What do *you* think about that?"

"What do you think causes that?"

Some men may find exploring feelings and emotions difficult and some cultures may value restraint of feelings.[22]

Probing Responses

The probing response is helpful in clarifying or in gaining additional information as respondents recall details. In dietary interviews, for example, details about food quantities, added ingredients, food preparation methods, and snacks are probed frequently. Probing implies that the person should give more information so that the counselor can understand.

EXAMPLE: Mrs. Jones: "I haven't lost any weight this week. I ate just a few cookies. The diet doesn't work."

Counselor: "Mrs. Jones you seem to think the diet doesn't work. I wonder if you could tell me a little more about that."

Rather than giving your advice, this response helps the person to tell her story, and further information can be obtained.

There are many probing techniques, which may be used in addition to secondary or follow-up questions. They should be nonthreatening, nonjudgmental, and nondirective to avoid leading people to specific answers. A brief silence may be effective, as may repetition of the last phrase spoken by the client or a summary sentence. Probing further in the case of superficial and vague responses, as well as probing for feelings about events, is suggested in the following paragraphs.

When a more detailed response is desired in the case of superficial answers, the following may be asked:

EXAMPLE: "Can you tell me more about that?"

"What do you do next?"

"Please explain a little more about . . ."

"What else?"

To obtain clarification if the answer is vague, you may respond:

EXAMPLE: "Could you clarify for me what you meant by . . .?" "I don't think I quite understand . . ."

Paraphrasing is another technique to ensure that the information is clear and correct. By repeating, summarizing, or rewording what was said, interviewers show that they are trying to understand.

When the person seems hesitant to go on, the interviewer may remain silent, pausing for the respondent to gather his or her thoughts and continue. The professional should appear attentive, with perhaps a thoughtful or expectant look, but should avoid eye contact for the moment. The inexperienced interviewer may find silence uncomfortable and embarrassing and push on too quickly, but a more experienced person realizes that too hasty a response may cause part of the story to remain untold or change what is disclosed. If the respondent does not go on within 30 to 60 seconds, however, he or she may perceive the silence as disinterest or disapproval; the interviewer should commence before such an impression occurs.

A technique useful in breaking a silence is to repeat or echo the last phrase or sentence the person has said, raising the tone of voice to a question.

EXAMPLE: "I follow my diet except when I eat out."
"Except when you eat out?"
"I especially enjoy doing special projects with coworkers."
"Special projects with coworkers?"

Repetition, however, should not be overdone, or it has a parrotlike effect. If this is noticed by the client, it will inhibit conversation.

A summary sentence stated as a question also elicits further elaboration.

EXAMPLE: "You say that you already know how to plan a diabetic diet?"
"You think this company is the one you want to work for?"

Other probes are the following:

EXAMPLE:
"Go on."
"I see."
"I understand, Mrs. Jones. Please continue."
"Uh huh."
"Hmmm."
"And next."
"Oh?" or "Oh!"
"Really?"
"Very good!"
"That's interesting."

"I see," "I understand," and "that's interesting" may give a feeling of acceptance and encourage conversation or elaboration of a point of view. "Very good" gives the person a pat on the back and is another kind of acceptance. Nonverbal probes include giving a quizzical look, leaning forward in the chair, and nodding of the head occasionally.

Confrontation Responses

Confrontation is an authority-laden response in which the interviewer tactfully and tentatively calls to the person's attention some inconsistency in his or her story, words, or actions, pointing out the discrepancy to the client.[22]

E X A M P L E : Mrs. Jones: "I haven't lost any weight this week. I ate just a few cookies. The diet doesn't work."

Counselor: "I'm a bit concerned. You say you want to lose weight and yet you have not lost any weight for a month. What do *you* think is the problem?

This response challenges and encourages the person to recognize and cope psychologically with some aspect of behavior that is self-defeating or to examine the consequences of some behavior. It should be said nonjudgmentally as discussion centers on resolution of problems.

Confrontation is an advanced level skill that should seldom be used by an inexperienced interviewer or when good rapport and a supportive atmosphere are missing. Otherwise, such responses can become threatening or appear punitive and will inhibit conversation.

During the interview, you can examine not only what the person says, but also what is not said. Are there gaps that the interviewer should be trying to fill? Also note nonverbal behaviors, such as tension, inability to maintain eye contact, hand movements, fidgeting, and facial expressions of discomfort, nervousness, anger, or lack of understanding. The nonverbal behaviors may be inconsistent with the verbal message, or may add to it.

Although practitioners adjust the pace of the interview to that of the respondent, they are also responsible for the direction of the interview. When the topics for discussion are inappropriate, the skilled interviewer brings the conversation back to appropriate topics. The client talking about his wife or children, for example, must be brought gently back to the nutrition history. A job applicant discussing a recent visit to Spain must be brought back to relevant topics. People who are especially talkative may ramble frequently, requiring more direction and leadership on the part of the interviewer. In these cases, restating or emphasizing the last thing said that was pertinent to the interview and asking a related question can be helpful.

Evaluative Responses

In the evaluative response, the interviewer makes a judgment about the person's feelings or responses or implies how the person ought to feel. The evaluative response leads to the offering of advice by the professional for the solution to the client's problem and is seldom helpful.

E X A M P L E : Mrs. Jones: "I haven't lost any weight this week. I ate just a few cookies. The diet doesn't work."

Counselor: "I suggest that you stop buying those cookies, Mrs. Jones."

Note that the evaluative response leads to giving advice, not to problem solving. Little attempt is made to understand the psychological needs of the client or the reasons that the cookies were eaten. The recipient of the advice has the choice of following the advice or not. At times, some people ignore advice as a means of maintaining their independence.

Hostile Responses

In the hostile response, the professional's anger or frustration is uncontrolled, and the response may lead to antagonism or humiliation of the client.

E X A M P L E : Mrs. Jones: "I haven't lost any weight this week. I ate just a few cookies. The diet doesn't work."

Counselor: "You're not acting very mature, Mrs. Jones. I've *told* you before to avoid all sweets and desserts if you want to lose weight. You haven't lost any weight for a month! Why are you *still* buying cookies?"

SELF-ASSESSMENT

Identify the following types of responses as understanding, probing, confrontation, evaluative, hostile, and reassuring.

1. "The food does taste different without salt. Let's see if we can find some substitutes that you can try."
2. "I know you can do it. It just takes time."
3. "How do you expect to lose weight if you continue to eat fast foods every day?"
4. "That's interesting. Tell me more about that."
5. "You say that you watch your food choices weekdays, but eat whatever you want on weekends. Do you think that's why you haven't lost any weight?"
6. "When you're at a party, try to find someone to talk to instead of eating."

The hostile response may lead the client to a reply that retaliates.

EXAMPLE: Mrs. Jones: "How would you know about dieting? Look how thin you are."

A vicious cycle of angry, hostile responses results, thus destroying the professional–client relationship. This type of response should be avoided. The fact that the client is anxious about the inability to follow the diet has been ignored.

Reassuring Responses

With a reassuring response, the client is prevented from working through her feelings because the interviewer suggests that there is nothing to worry about. Too frequently, a client's expressions of anxiety are followed by the counselor's reassuring response that things will improve and that the person should not worry.

EXAMPLE: Mrs. Jones: "I haven't lost any weight this week even though I am trying."
Counselor: "Don't worry, Mrs. Jones. It takes time to adjust to new eating patterns. You'll do better next week."

This response suggests that the problem does not exist, or that the counselor does not want to discuss it. Such responses make it difficult to solve the client's problem or to discuss it further. Admission of failure with the diet may have been difficult for the client, but it indicated a desire to discuss the problem.

CLOSING THE INTERVIEW

The third part or closing of the interview takes the shortest amount of time but should not be rushed or taken lightly. During the closing, a word of appreciation sincerely expressed, such as thanking the person for his or her time and cooperation, is appropriate. Another suggestion is to review the purpose of the interview and declare its completion. "That's all the questions I have. Thank you for your time and information." You may ask if there are any questions the client would like to ask or any other comments he or she wants to make, which may elicit important new information for which adequate time

SELF-ASSESSMENT

How satisfactory are these closings? How can they be improved?

Employment Interview:
Standing up, "I have another applicant waiting, so our time is up. Thanks for coming today." Shakes hands.

Client Interview:
"Well I have all the information I need. Thank you for coming."

should be available. For example: "What else would you like to ask or tell me about?" You may ask the client to summarize points, goals, or next steps agreed on.

The time, place, and purpose of future contacts should be mentioned. To a hospitalized patient, the professional may say, "I'll stop by to see you tomorrow to discuss your food choices with you." With a client, arrangements for a future appointment may be made: "When can we meet again to discuss your progress and answer questions?" To make sure that each has understood the other, plans may be paraphrased. People tend to remember the last thing said.

As a courtesy to job applicants, they should be told approximately when the employment decision will be made and how they will be notified if selected, as, for example, "We are interviewing additional candidates for this position, but if you are selected, you'll hear from human resources in about a week or two. Thank you for coming and for your interest in our company." For those not selected, a letter may be sent thanking them for their applications and interest in the company and telling them the position has been filled. This letter is a public relations effort that may be handled by the human resources department.[6] The applicant who hears nothing after an interview may react negatively or telephone again for information.

You may signal the close of the interview nonverbally by breaking eye contact, pushing back the chair, placing hands on the arms of the chair, standing up, offering to shake hands, smiling, and walking the interviewee to the door.

The interview session should be followed by a self-evaluation to determine areas that went well, as well as those that could be improved for the next interview. Questions you may ask include the following:

- How effective was the atmosphere? Was it relaxed and informal with good rapport?
- How effective was my interview opening?
- How effective were my questions in obtaining information I needed?
- How effective were my responses to the person's statements?
- How nonjudgmental and empathic was I?
- How effective was my interview closing?
- How much time did I listen versus talk?

Figure 3-1 presents a sample client interviewing/counseling evaluation form.

In summary, interviewing is a skill. As with other skills, it takes practice to develop. The inexperienced interviewer needs to plan in writing what topics need to be covered. Various types of questions can be prepared in advance in an appropriate sequence for the three parts of the interview. Physical surroundings and freedom from interruption should be planned.

EVALUATION OF CLIENT INTERVIEWING/COUNSELING TECHNIQUES FORM

COMPETENCY: *Utilizes effective communication skills in the practice of dietetics.*

CLINICAL AREA: _____

NAME OF INTERN: _____

EVALUATED BY: _____

INTERVIEW SKILLS OR BEHAVIOUR — Date:	3	2	1	COMMENTS
CLIMATE OF INTERVIEW				
1. Observes initial social amenities.				
2. Indicates mutual respect.				
3. Responds positively to signs of anxiety.				
4. Shows empathy.				
5. Elicits comments about self and concerns about diet, medical condition, etc.				
USE OF QUESTIONS				
6. Uses non-leading (gives no clues to desired answer)				
7. Uses nondirective (avoids yes/no, single word answers)				
8. Uses open-ended (allows for elaboration)				
9. Questions are easily understood				
10. Demonstrates the use of clarification (e.g. paraphrasing)				
LISTENING ABILITY				
11. Identifies "clues" for further probing				
12. Utilizes and understands information offered				
13. Uses appropriate verbal & nonverbal clues to engage client response				
14. Avoids unnecessary interruptions				
15. Separates interviewing activies from counseling				
16. Shows a nonjudgmental, noncritical attitude toward client's eating pattern and chosen lifestyle				
LANGUAGE				
17. Uses language appropriate to the situation				
18. Provides explanation for each step in the process				

COUNSELING SKILLS OR BEHAVIOUR — Date:	3	2	1	COMMENTS
1. Elicits client's statement of purpose and objectives				
2. States purposes and objectives of diet modification/counseling.				
3. Provides accurate explanations and rationale including diet: health relationship				
4. Answers client's questions about diet and/or disease clearly and accurately				
5. Adjusts explanations to learning abilities, constraints of time, etc.				
6. Accesses client's understanding by having client restate information in his/her own words				
7. Enlists active participation of client in formulating goals and planning of diet				
8. Encourages client indentification of obstacles and helps client develop strategies				
9. Uses visual and other teaching aids appropriately and provides educational resources				
10. Demonstrates correct use of self-disclosure				
11. Maintains rapport with client throughout				
12. Summarizes principles of diet				
13. Re-states client goals				
14. Explains goals for next visit and establishes plan for follow-up				
15. Presents counseling within reasonable time frame				

EVALUATION KEY:
3 = Consistently demonstrates skill
2 = Adequately progressing with skill development
1 = Needs greater emphasis

FIGURE 3-1 Client Interviewing/Counseling Evaluation Form. (Courtesy of School of Health Related Professions, University of Medicine and Dentistry of New Jersey.)

These conditions put the professional in a better position to concentrate on the interviewee and on the process of developing rapport, noting the verbal and nonverbal responses, and providing understanding responses with empathy.

CASE STUDY 1

Josephine Brown is an applicant for a job as assistant cook at a school lunch program at Willard High School, which has an enrollment of 200 students. According to her application, her address is in the high school district, she is a high school graduate, and she has worked for the past year as a cook at a nursing home.

On greeting her, the manager notices that she appears to be 35 to 40 years old and wears a wedding ring.

1. How would you develop rapport with Mrs. Brown?
2. What is the purpose of the interview?
3. Make a list of questions you would ask her. Explain why each question is relevant.

CASE STUDY 2

Delores Maynard is a 55-year-old woman who works in a corporate office. She visits the corporate wellness center and makes an appointment with Joan Stivers, a registered dietitian. D.M. is 5'2" tall and weighs 190 pounds. She has mild hypertension. She is married with two grown children.

Joan: "What brings you to this appointment? How can I help?"
D.M.: "Well, I need to lose some weight to help control my blood pressure."
Joan: "Can you tell me about any other times you have tried to lose weight?"
D.M.: "I wasn't overweight until after I was married and bringing up two kids. Then I gradually gained weight. Over the years, I've tried many different diets. I lose weight but gain it all back, and sometimes more."

1. What questions would you ask in obtaining D.M.'s nutrition history? Put them in sequence. Discuss the reason why each questions is important in assisting the client.
2. What related questions would you like to ask, such as questions about meal preparation, food shopping, vitamin–mineral supplements, family meal practices, snacks, eating in restaurants, and weekend meals?
3. What other questions would you explore related to D.M.'s family and lifestyle?

REVIEW AND DISCUSSION QUESTIONS

1. What are the possible purposes of a diet history or nutrition interview? Of a preemployment interview?
2. What conditions facilitate an interview?
3. Explain the three parts of an interview. What occurs in each part?
4. Differentiate between the following types of questions: open and closed; primary and secondary; and neutral and leading.
5. Explain the six types of responses.

SUGGESTED ACTIVITIES

1. Watch an interview on television noting the parts of the interview, techniques used, and verbal and nonverbal responses. Write up your reactions and analysis.
2. Observe a television interview show, such as *Larry King Live,* the *Tonight Show* with Jay Leno, the *Oprah Winfrey Show,* or others. What types of questions are asked? What kinds of responses does the interviewer obtain? What was the level of rapport between the two parties? Construct an interview guide from the questions asked and their sequence.
3. Plan an interview guide specifying the content and sequence of questions. Write examples of various kinds of questions, such as open and closed, primary and secondary, neutral and leading. Which kinds of questions do you prefer to answer?
4. Divide into groups of two for role-playing using the 24-hour recall, with each person interviewing the other in turn. Use various types of responses, such as probing, paraphrasing, and understanding. If three people are available, the third may serve as evaluator.
5. Using an interview guide, make an audiotape of a simulated or actual interview using the usual daily food intake, if the participant's permission is granted. Complete an evaluation.
6. Using an interview guide, make a videotape of a simulated or actual interview, if the participant's permission is granted. This will show both the verbal and nonverbal behaviors as well as any personal idiosyncrasies. Complete an evaluation
7. Turn on the television set without the sound. Try to interpret the nonverbal behavior you are seeing.
8. Visit three offices and observe the physical surroundings. Which is most comfortable and conducive to communication? Why? Which is least comfortable? Why? Arrange the furniture in a room or office for an optimum interviewing setting.
9. Change the following technical words that are used by professionals into terms that will help a client to understand their meanings: fiber, nutrients, sodium, lipids, protein, serum glucose, carbohydrates, low-density lipoproteins, polyunsaturated fatty acids, saturated fatty acids, colitis, gastric ulcer, hypertension, fluid intake, osteoporosis.
10. Directions: Read the lettered statements below. Identify both the thought the person is expressing and the feelings the person may be experiencing. Write a paraphrased statement reflecting the thought or content of the message:
    A. "I've had diabetes for 6 years. They put me on a diet and insulin injections when I first found out about it, and I check my blood sugar sometimes. The diet isn't too bad."
    B. "I'm expecting my second baby. I never paid any attention to what I ate during my first pregnancy and my baby was healthy."
    C. "The doctor told me that I can go home tomorrow, but I live alone so I have no one to help me with a diet, and I'm in no hurry to leave."
    D. "Joan talks to people all day long and doesn't get her work done. The rest of us have to finish for her or we get yelled at."
    E. "I've been working here for 10 years. Now you come in as a new supervisor and want to change everything around. What's wrong with keeping things the way they are?"
    F. "How do you expect me to get all this work done? First, you tell me to do one thing, and then you tell me to do another."

Directions: Write a second paraphrased statement reflecting the feelings in the preceding examples, such as:

"You seem to be feeling (angry, depressed, lonely etc.) because. . . ."
"It sounds like you feel. . . ."
"I hear you saying that you feel. . . . Tell me if I'm understanding you accurately."

E X A M P L E : Client: "My friend and I are both dieting. She has lost weight, but I haven't even though I have been trying."
Counselor: "You seem to be feeling upset because your friend has lost weight and you haven't."

Discuss your paraphrases with others.

11. Obtain a copy of the MEDFICTS questionnaire, available online at http://www.limipc. com/medical%20info/cholest/medficts.htm. Use it to obtain information from a person who is seeking to limit the intake of fat and evaluate the result.
12. Obtain a copy the mini nutrition assessment (available in 12 languages), available online (http://www.mna-elderly.com). Use it with an elderly person and evaluate the result.
13. Identify which of these preemployment questions are permissible and which are not.
    A. "Our floors are slippery when wet. Do you limp?"
    B. "Can you work weekends?"
    C. "Are you planning to have children?"
    D. "Can you work on religious holidays?"
    E. "What is your computer knowledge?"
    F. "What were your responsibilities on your previous job?"
14. Interview an experienced human resources recruiter about the questions asked, the degree of structure in the interview, and Equal Employment Opportunity (EEO) concerns.

WEB SITES

http://www.cdc.gov/brfss/   Behavioral Risk Factor Surveillance System, a telephone health survey system, including nutrition and physical activity

http://www.cdc.gov/nchs/   National Center for Health Statistics; includes data on the National Health and Nutrition Examination Survey (NHANES)

http://courses.washington.edu/theralab/winter/week2lipids/fat.pdf /   Northwest Lipid Research Clinic Fat Intake Scale

http://www.eeoc.gov/abouteeo/overview-laws.html/   Information about federal laws prohibiting job discrimination

http://www.hr-guide.com/   Information on employee interviews

http://www.job-interview.net/   General information on employee interview questions

http://www.limipc.com/medical%20info/cholest/medficts.htm/   Copy of the MEDFICTS (Meat, Eggs, Dairy, Frying foods, In baked goods, Convenience foods, Table fats, Snacks) questionnaire used in assessing diets of patients with heart disease

http://www.med.upenn.edu/weight/nighteatingform   Questionnaire on night eating

http://www.mna-elderly.com/   A nutritional assessment tool to identify elderly people at risk of malnutrition, available in 12 languages from Nestle Nutrition

http://riskfactor.cancer.gov/DHQ /forms/   National Cancer Institute site with a 124-item self-administered diet history questionnaire

REFERENCES

1. Commission on Accreditation for Dietetics Education. Eligibility Requirements and Accreditation Standards. Chicago: American Dietetic Association, 2006.
2. Arthur D. Recruiting, Interviewing, Selecting & Orienting New Employees, 4th ed. New York: American Management Association, 2006.
3. Dessler G. Human Resource Management, 10th ed. Englewood Cliffs, NJ: Prentice-Hall, 2004.
4. Bohlander GW, Snell SA. Managing Human Resources, 14th ed. Cincinnati: Thomson/South-Western, 2007.
5. Lee RD, Nieman DC. Nutritional Assessment, 3rd ed. Boston: McGraw-Hill, 2003.
6. Hudson NR. Management Practice in Dietetics, 2nd ed. Belmont, CA: Thomson/Brooks/Cole, 2005.
7. Losyk B. How to hire the right people. Public Mgt 2003;85:24–26.
8. Thompson FE, Suber AF. Dietary assessment methodology. In: Coulston AM, Rock CL, Monsen ER, eds. Nutrition in the Prevention and Treatment of Disease. San Diego: Academic Press, 2001.
9. Lacey K, Pritchett E. Nutrition care process and model: ADA adopts road map to quality care and outcomes management. J Am Diet Assoc 2003;103:1061–1071.
10. American Dietetic Association. Nutrition diagnosis: a critical step in the nutrition care process. Available at: http://www.eatright.org/ada/files/Final_Draft_publication1_2_smallest.pdf. Accessed September 29, 2006.
11. Amend A, Melkus GD, Chyun DA, et al. Validation of the dietary intake data in black women with type 2 diabetes. J Am Diet Assoc 2007;107:112–117.
12. Tapsell LC, Brenninger V, Barnard J. Applying conversation analysis to foster accurate reporting in the diet history interview. J Am Diet Assoc 2000;100:818–824.
13. Yon BA, Johnson RK, Harvey-Berino J, et al. The use of a personal digital assistant for dietary self-monitoring does not improve the validity of self-reports of energy intake. J Am Diet Assoc 2006;106:1256–1259.
14. Johnson RK, Friedman AB, Harvey-Berino J, et al. Participation in a behavioral weight-loss program worsens the prevalence and severity of underreporting among obese and overweight women. J Am Diet Assoc 2005;105:1948–1251.
15. Novotny JA, Rumpler WV, Riddick H, et al. Personality characteristics as predictors of under-reporting of energy intake on 24-hour dietary recall interviews. J Am Diet Assoc 2003;103:1146–1151.
16. Young LR, Nestle M. Expanding portion sizes in the US marketplace: implications for nutrition counseling. J Am Diet Assoc 2003;103:231–234.
17. Holmes AL, Sanderson B, Maisiak R, et al. Dietitian services are associated with improved patient outcomes and the MEDFICTS dietary assessment questionnaire is a suitable outcome measure in cardiac rehabilitation. J Am Diet Assoc 2005;105:1533–1540.
18. Kris-Etherton P, Eissenstat B, Jaax S, et al. Validation for MEDFICTS, a dietary assessment instrument for evaluating adherence to total and saturated fat recommendations of the National Cholesterol Education Program Step 1 and Step 2 diets. J Am Diet Assoc 2001;101:81–86.

19. Understanding and using the scope of dietetics practice framework: a step-wise approach. J Am Diet Assoc 2006;106:459–463.

20. Stewart CJ, Cash WB. Interviewing Principles and Practices, 11th ed. Boston: McGraw-Hill, 2006.

21. Jobe JB, Mingay DJ. Cognitive research improves questionnaires. Am J Public Health 1989;79:1053–1055.

22. Evans DR, Hearn MT, Uhlemann MR, et al. Essential Interviewing: A Programmed Approach to Effective Communication, 6th ed. Belmont, CA: Thomson/BrooksCole, 2004.

CHAPTER 4

Counseling

OBJECTIVES

- Discuss the dietetics practitioner's role in counseling clients and staff.
- Define counseling, its role, and the process of counseling.
- Identify the attributes of a successful counselor.
- Describe various theories of counseling.
- Describe the stages of the Transtheoretical Model.
- Describe motivational interviewing as a form of counseling.
- Differentiate between directive and nondirective counseling approaches and their uses.

Counseling—the art of providing listening, advice, guidance, or direction regarding an action or decision to help a person change

One of the key roles of the dietetics professional is to promote the optimal health of the public. The practitioner translates the science of nutrition into healthful food and nutrient intake for the individual or group. To achieve appropriate food intake, often behaviors and lifestyles must change. Nutrition counseling focuses on helping clients accomplish these changes. Counseling also comes into play in the managerial aspects of dietetics in the form of staff counseling for development or remediation.

The Commission on Accreditation for Dietetics Education of the American Dietetic Association requires that dietetics students have a working knowledge of counseling theories and methods and that they be able to counsel individuals on nutrition. Counseling is essential to the success of the food and nutrition professional, whether as a manager, a clinical or community care practitioner, or a counselor in private practice. As health care intensifies its emphasis on outcomes, the results of counseling will be examined more fully. If the intervention, whether assessment, education, or counseling, does not produce a change in knowledge, skills, behavior, or health outcome, the continuation of the intervention will be questioned. However, it is not always easy to measure the impact of an intervention on behavior.

Counseling may be defined as a process that assists people in learning about themselves, their environment, and the methods of handling their roles and relationships.

It involves problem solving, identifying goals, and change. Counselors assist individuals with the decision-making process, resolving interpersonal concerns, and helping them learn new ways of dealing with and adjusting to life situations. Counseling is a science with a body of literature that assesses techniques and their effectiveness. It is also an art; the skills of the counselor allow the counselor to customize the counseling to the individual client.

This chapter is an overview of the counseling process; Chapter 5 describes nutrition counseling in more detail. Counseling is a process that involves the development of a trusting, helping relationship between counselor and client, evaluation of the client issues, and various techniques of problem solving. The approaches to counseling may be classified as nondirective or directive. The nondirective or "client-centered" approach is often applied to the nutrition counseling of clients. It includes listening and helping the person determine how to proceed. Directive counseling is often applied to staff regarding job-related issues; it includes the counselor providing advice, reassurance, and clarity.

NONDIRECTIVE COUNSELING

The nondirective approach to counseling is often called "client-centered" and is best represented by the writings of its originator, Carl Ransom Rogers. Dr. Rogers' theory was first presented in his book, *Counseling and Psychotherapy* (1942) and was further refined in subsequent publications.[1,2] The theory is constantly developing, changing with experience and research; however, the fundamental assumptions have not changed. The theory is one of the more detailed, integrated, and consistent theories currently existing and has led to, and is supported by, a greater amount of research than any other approach to counseling.[3]

A basic assumption in the Rogerian client-centered point of view is that humans are basically rational, socialized, and realistic. Individuals, if their needs for positive regard from others and for positive self-regard are satisfied, possess an inherent tendency toward realizing their potential for growth and self-actualization. Counseling releases the potentials and capacities of the individual.

One of the most important characteristics of the Rogerian theory is the relationship it suggests between the counselor and the client. The underlying assumption is that the client cannot be helped simply by listening to the knowledge the counselor possesses or to the counselor's explanation of the client's personality or behavior. Prescribing "cures" and corrective behaviors are seen as being of little lasting value. The relationship that is most helpful to clients and that enables them to discover within themselves the capacity to use the relationship to change and grow is not a cognitive, intellectual one. "One of the phrases that Rogers used to describe his therapy is 'supportive, not reconstructive,' and he uses the analogy of learning to ride a bicycle to explain: When you help a child to learn to ride a bike, you can't just tell them how. They have to try it for themselves. And you can't hold them up the whole time either. There comes a point when you have to let them go. If they fall, they fall, but if you hang on, they never learn."[4] Rogers suggests that the counselor possess four specific characteristics for the therapy relationship: acceptance, congruence, understanding, and the ability to communicate these to the client.

The counselor needs to be accepting of and respect the clients as individuals as they are, with their good and bad points, their conflicts and inconsistencies. Only after clients are convinced that they are accepted unconditionally and nonjudgmentally can they begin to trust the counselor.

Exceptional counselors are characterized by congruence within the counseling relationship. They are unified, integrated, and consistent, with no contradictions between what they are and what they say. These counselors are able to express outwardly to their clients what they are feeling within themselves. Their verbal and nonverbal behaviors are consistent.

The counselor must experience an accurate, empathic understanding of the client's world as seen from the inside, sensing the client's world as if it were his or her own, but without losing the "as if" quality. This empathy is essential to Rogerian therapy. This understanding enables clients to explore freely and deeply and develop a better comprehension of themselves.

It is of no value for the counselor to be accepting, congruent, and understanding if the client does not perceive or experience this. The acceptance, congruence, and understanding need to be communicated to the client verbally and nonverbally. Rogers is definite in his belief that these not be "techniques," but a genuine and spontaneous expression of the counselor's inner attitudes, having contact with people.[3]

If the counselor has these characteristics and attitudes and is able to communicate them to the client, then a relationship develops that is experienced by the client as safe, secure, free from threat, and supportive. The counselor is perceived as dependable, trustworthy, and consistent. This outcome requires being a good listener, having intuition, providing feedback on both data and feelings, and providing inspiration.[5] This is the type of relationship that supports behavioral change, whether you are working with clients or with staff. Central to the Rogerian approach is reflection on what the client said, the mirroring back to the client of what he or she is saying.[4]

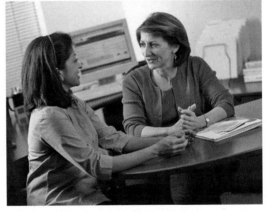

The relationship is key to successful counseling.
Source: United States Department of Agriculture.

COUNSELING PROCESSES

Various models describe the counseling process. Many have a Rogerian foundation and incorporate the client's readiness for change and transforming a behavior. Counseling is an individualized process that does not involve giving ready-made advice, but suggesting constructive alternatives based on what is important to and manageable for the client.[6] Counseling is an interactive process that goes well beyond education of the client. Several approaches are described next, including the Transtheoretical Model, also called the Stages of Change Model, and motivational interviewing. The Transtheoretical Model identifies stages of change that individuals pass through before actualizing a change.[7] Motivational interviewing is an approach designed to "help clients build commitment and reach a decision to change."[8] Chapters 6 and 7 expand this discussion to behavioral therapy and social cognitive theory.

Assessing Stages of Change

Prochaska and colleagues have developed a Transtheoretical Model or Stages of Change Model **(Figure 4-1)**. It is a framework for understanding clients' readiness to change to healthier eating practices. Change is *not* viewed as a single event, such as "I will eat less sodium starting today." People who need to make changes progress through six identified stages: precontemplation (no intention of changing in the next 6 months), contemplation (intending to change but not soon), preparation (intending to change in the next month), action (recent changes in food choices), maintenance (changes maintained for 6 months), and termination (changes maintained for 5 years).[7]

People do not change their food choices just because we tell them to or because they know they should. The key to successful nutrition counseling and education is to assess and identify the person's stage or readiness for change and match the intervention to it. Different counseling strategies are needed, for example, for those unaware of a problem, for those resisting efforts to change, and for those intending to change at a future time. This should increase the effectiveness of the intervention, assist the client in progressing to the next stage because of enhanced motivation and readiness, and reduce the likelihood of dropping out of treatment because the intervention was not appropriate.

Many health interventions and educational programs are action oriented, assuming that people are making changes or are ready to do so. However, about 40 to 50% of people are in the precontemplation stage, in denial, or resistant to change; 20% are in the preparation stage; and only about 20 to 25% are in the action stage.[7,9] Assuming that the client is at the action stage can be counterproductive and lead to failure and dropout. Determining readiness to change is crucial in deciding on the approach to intervention. Practitioners need to provide skills and support change at every stage and help people move to the next stage and eventually to action.

Precontemplation

In stage 1, precontemplation, a person is unaware or under-aware that a problem exists, denies that there is a problem or is not interested in change, and thus has no plans to change eating practices or start exercising in the near future.[7,9] The person may have previously tried a change such as weight loss, and failed, and he or she may be resistant to the health professional's efforts to suggest possible changes. Perhaps a visit to the doctor initiated a referral to see the dietitian for weight loss, even if the patient was satisfied with his or her weight. To identify this stage, you may ask: "Are you seriously intending to change (name the problem behavior) in the next 6 months?" For example, for people ignoring the relationship between a high-fat diet and coronary heart disease, you may ask: "Have you thought about eating less fat (or more fruits and vegetables) in the next 6 months?" At this stage, a person with high levels of low-density lipoprotein cholesterol may need to know the benefits of a lower blood level, for example, and the risks of not addressing the problem. An attempt to focus instead on making dietary changes may not be effective in precontemplation. **Table 4-1** lists sample questions and interventions at each stage.

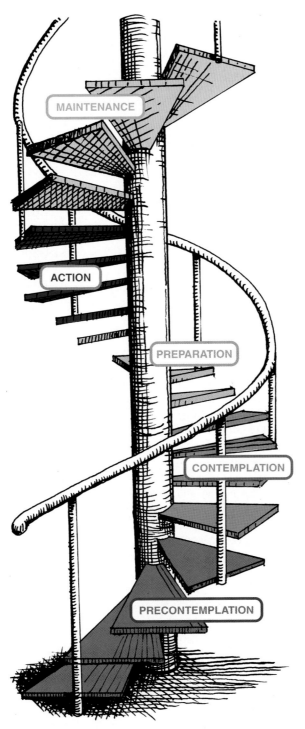

FIGURE **4-1**   Clients Progress Through Stages of Change.

TABLE **4-1** | Stages of Change

Stage	Question for Client	Intervention
Precontemplation	"What can I do to help?"	Consciousness raising
	"Do you ever read articles about . . .?"	Assess knowledge
	"What do you know about the relationship between . . ."	Increase self-awareness, give information
	"Does anyone in your family have this problem?"	Assess values, beliefs
	"Are you aware of the consequences?"	Cognitive restructuring
	"How do you feel about making a change?"	Discuss risks and benefits
Contemplation	"What changes have you been thinking about?"	Assess knowledge
	"What are the pros and cons?"	Assess values, beliefs
	"How do you feel about it?"	Assess thoughts, feelings
	"What would make it easier or harder?"	Decrease barriers
	"What would be the results of the change?"	Self-evaluation
	"How can I help?"	Cognitive restructuring
Preparation	"Are you intending to act in the next 1–6 months?"	Self-efficacy, commitment
	"How will you do it?"	Decision making
	"What changes have you made already?"	Discuss beliefs about ability
	"How will your life be improved?"	Plan goals
Action	"What are you doing differently?"	Stimulus control
	"What problems are you having?"	Self-reinforcement
	"Who can help you?"	Social support
	"How can I help?"	Self-management
	"What do you do instead of(former behavior)?"	Goal setting, group sessions, self-monitoring, relapse prevention
Maintenance	"How do you handle times when you slip up?"	Coping responses
	"What obstacles are you facing?"	Relapse prevention
	"What are your future plans?"	Self-management
	"What issues have you solved?"	Commitment, goal setting, control environment
Termination		Self-management, self-efficacy

Contemplation

In stage 2, contemplation, a person is aware that a problem exists and intends to do better eventually, such as eating differently or exercising more. He or she has no serious thought or commitment, however, to making a change and keeps putting it off.[7,9] The person may be mentally struggling with the amount of energy, effort, and cost of overcoming a problem and may be discouraged by previous failures. You may ask:

"What have you been thinking about in terms of making a change?"
"What are the pros and cons of doing it?"
"How can you change your environment?"
"What do you think about eating less fat? What are the barriers or obstacles to doing it?"

The balance between pros and cons can result in ambivalence that keeps people at this stage for long periods of time, even months or years.[10,11]

Preparation

In stage 3, preparation, a person is more determined to change and intends to take initial action soon, perhaps in about 30 days, but not today.[7,9] He or she may report small changes in the problem behavior, such as reading a few food labels or buying fat-free ice cream.

Action

In stage 4, action, a person attempts to overcome the problem by actively modifying food choices, behaviors, environments, or experiences.[8,9] Remember that most clients are *not* in the action stage when referred for counseling. Considerable commitment of time and energy is required in the action stage when people are trying to change. You may ask: "What are you doing differently?"

Maintenance

In stage 5, maintenance, a person consolidates and stabilizes gains made over several months to maintain the new, healthier habits and works to prevent relapse.[7,9,11] Maintaining weight loss, for example, takes continuing effort. For some people, this stage continues for months, years, or a lifetime, or until the behavior becomes a pattern and is incorporated into their lifestyle. You may ask: "How do you handle small lapses?" (Additional information on counseling about lapses and relapse is provided in Chapter 7.)

The ultimate goal is the termination stage in which changes have been maintained for 5 years. However, some types of problems, such as weight management, may require a lifetime of maintenance instead. People, for example, tend to become more sedentary and overweight as they age, thus contributing to continual problems.

Prochaska proposed that people proceed through the stages in a spiral, rather than a linear, fashion.[7,9] Because lapses and relapse are common problems, recycling to an earlier stage, such as from action to preparation or from preparation to contemplation, may be expected several times as people struggle to modify or cease behaviors. People may avoid high-fat foods, for example, and then start eating them again. Lapse and relapse and the negative emotional reactions (guilt, shame, failure) that may result are discussed in more detail in Chapter 7. It is hoped that people learn from their mistakes with the help of the counselor and continue trying.

A second dimension of the model examines the processes of change or activities people use to progress through the stages of change when there are shifts in behaviors, attitudes, and intentions.[11] The processes of change should be integrated into the stages of change so that the treatment intervention matches the client's stage of change.

In the early stages, focusing on the benefits of making a change and how that change can improve the individual's life or health is suggested. The goal is for the client to think about the problem. Clients may, however, doubt their ability to change and have decreased self-efficacy at this point. In precontemplation (consciousness raising), providing nutritional information (oral, written, web addresses) about the benefits of healthy choices and about the individual's risk for chronic disease based on dietary habits with the advantages of change is suggested. Self-reevaluation of thoughts, feelings, values, problems, self, and environment is appropriate. The client needs to weigh the pros and cons of change, with the pros ("I'll see my grandchildren grow up.") outweighing the cons ("I can't eat whatever I want."). Cons outweigh the pros at this stage.

Cognitive and affective self-reevaluation, in addition to raising awareness, is suggested in the contemplation stage. Self-liberation (a belief that one can change and the actual making of a commitment to it) and behavioral goals (discussed in Chapter 5) are important in the preparation stage. In the client's assessment, the benefits or pros must outweigh the cons or costs. In the action and maintenance stages, behavioral techniques (see Chapter 6) of stimulus control, reinforcement management, self-monitoring, recipe modification, coping responses during conditions when relapse is likely, and developing a social support system of significant others are useful. Keep in mind that the client may be at an early stage for one change, such as increasing fruit and vegetable intake, while at another stage for a different behavior, such as increasing exercise or decreasing portion size.

Motivational Interviewing

Motivational interviewing was originally developed from work with "addictive behaviors," but the intervention approach can be used in a variety of situations. It offers an approach for increasing the client's readiness to change eating behaviors. Even if people are aware of damaging consequences of their behavior, such as overeating or nonnutritious choices, they may use "short-term gratification at the expense of long-term harm."[8]

This motivational approach draws on client-centered counseling; it guides rather than directs or advises the client. It can be integrated into Prochaska and colleagues' Stages of Change Model in which people move from being unaware or unwilling to do anything about a problem, called *precontemplation*, to considering the possibility of change or contemplation, preparing to make a change, or determination and finally taking action.[7] The client may be at any of several stages; thus, the initial step is to assess where the client is.

Motivational interviewing strategies draw on principles of social, cognitive, and motivational psychology; on ambivalence, or the conflict between restraint and indulgence, which can be immobilizing; and on the theory of self-regulation. The approach works well with people who are reluctant to change. These people are the "precontemplators" and "contemplators."[7] The concept of the "importance" of the change to the person and the "confidence" in the ability to make the change are importance to the determination of readiness to change.[12] Rollnick suggests that you can assess readiness for change by asking two questions: How important is the change to you? How successful do you think you will

BOX **4-1**

Assessing Importance and Confidence of the Patient

Useful Questions to Explore Importance

What would have to happen for it to become more important for you to change?

What would have to happen before you seriously considered changing?

How important is this change on a scale of 1 to 10?

What would need to happen for your importance score to move up from . . . to . . .?

What stops you moving up from . . . to . . .?

What are the motivators to retain your [current behavior]?

What are some of the concerns you have (or things you dislike) about . . . [current behavior]?

What concerns do you have about . . . [current behavior]?

If you were to change, what would itbe like?

Where does this leave you now? (When you want to ask about change in a neutral way).

Useful Questions to Build Confidence

What would make you more confident about making these changes?

How confident are you about accomplishing this change?

How could you move up higher, so that your score goes from . . . to . . .?

How can I help you succeed?

What have you found helpful in any previous attempts to change?

What have you learned from the last time you tried this type of change?

If you were to decide to change, what might your options be? Are there any ways you know about that have worked for other people?

What are some of the practical issues you would need to address in order to achieve this goal? Do any of them sound achievable?

Is there anything you can think of that would help you feel more confident?

Adapted from Rollnick S, Mason P, Butler C. Health Behavior Change—A Guide for Practitioners. New York: Churchill Livingston, 1999.

be regarding the change?[5] **Box 4-1** gives you a series of questions to use in assessing these two areas with clients.[5] These questions assist in determining the stage of change.

What is motivational interviewing? It is "a particular way to help people recognize and do something about their present or potential problem."[8] It is especially useful with clients who are ambivalent about or reluctant to change. It helps to resolve the ambivalence and move them toward change. Once people become unstuck from the conflicting motivations of whether or not to change that immobilize them, they can move toward a decision and a commitment to take action.

What is the role of the counselor? An authoritarian role that sends the message "I'm an expert and will tell you what to do" is counterproductive. The responsibility for change lies with the client: "It's up to you to decide what to do. It's your choice." The goal is to "increase the client's motivation, so that change arises from within rather than imposed from without."[8] The client, not the counselor, needs to develop and speak aloud the arguments for change. One image of the counselor is that of a helper accompanying a person on a journey. The guide "needs the qualities of a companion and the skills of someone who knows the route," but acknowledges the client's personal responsibility for change and freedom of choice.[8] Individuals who successfully conduct motivational interviewing focus on reflection, including reinforcing positive statements about change, rather than responding with questions and advice.[13]

Motivational interviewing is described as having an "'elicit–provide–elicit' framework."[13] The counselor elicits what the person understands or needs about the situation, provides information in a neutral manner, and then elicits what the client thinks about the provided information. In this way, the counselor directs the client toward motivation to change. Once the client is motivated to change, behavioral motivation or cognitive counseling strategies are often started.

Principles of Motivational Interviewing

Five general principles underlie this approach:

1. Express empathy.
2. Develop discrepancy.
3. Avoid arguments.
4. Roll with resistance.
5. Support self-efficacy.[8]

Express empathy

Empathy suggests acceptance. The counselor seeks to understand the client's feelings and beliefs in a noncritical, nonjudgmental manner. The counselor listens carefully and respectfully. Empathy involves the counselor verbally reflecting what the client says to clarify and amplify the client's experience, feelings, and meanings, even if the counselor has not had a similar experience. Sharp attention to each client statement allows the counselor to hypothesize as to the meaning. The best guess as to the meaning is then reflected back to the client for verification. Ambivalence is considered normal. The client often considers continuing the current behavior desirable. The reasons must be explored, so attempts can be made to decrease or counterbalance them.

Develop discrepancy

The counselor seeks to *develop discrepancy* between present behavior and a new behavior, that is, where the person is and where he or she wants to be. One approach is to examine the implications and benefits of the current course of behavior as well as the benefits and implications of change, determining the relative importance of each (see **Table 4-2**). If the person has a conflict with an important goal, such as better health, self-image, or happiness, change is more likely. An individual's motivation to change increases when people see a discrepancy between present behavior and goals that are important to him or her.

People who come for counseling on their own, as opposed to those referred by a health care provider, can be expected to perceive some discrepancy already. But they may be ambivalent, stuck between the conflict of whether or not to change. Then it is necessary to clarify the client's important goals and explore how present behavior conflicts

T A B L E **4-2** | **Cost–Benefit Analysis for Change**

Continue to Eat as Before		Change Eating Behavior	
Pros	**Cons**	**Pros**	**Cons**
Pleasurable	Damages health	Better health	Change is difficult
Comfortable	Bad example for family	Feels better	Can't party with friends
Easy		Loses weight	Requires effort
Decreases loneliness			

with them. The goal is to increase the discrepancy until it overrides the attachment to the current behavior. Eventually, clients may see and articulate the arguments for change as their own. The client has more commitment to change when he or she makes the decision, thus increasing motivation.

Avoid arguments

A third principle is that the counselor *avoids arguments* and confrontation. When a counselor argues that the client needs to change, the client defends the opposite view and resists change. People assert their ability to do as they please and make their own decisions. Although the purpose of motivational interviewing is to increase awareness of a problem and the need to change, the counselor does not want to confront and thus increase resistance to change.

Roll with resistance

If the client is *resistant*, the counselor can acknowledge that reluctance to change and ambivalence are natural and understandable. The client may be offered new information or alternatives to consider. Or, rather than generating solutions, the counselor can ask the client for solutions to his or her problems. This involves the client in problem solving.

Support self-efficacy

Self-efficacy refers to a person's belief in his or her ability to succeed with a specific task. It is a key to motivation for change. If a person does not believe he or she can change, little or no effort will be made. A client may be encouraged by the counselor's offer of help or by seeing the success of others in the same or similar situations (role models). The counselor needs to reinforce the client's hope, optimism, and self-efficacy.

Reflective Listening

How the counselor responds to what the client says is an important element of reflective listening. Reflective listening may be one of several types. The counselor may repeat part of what the person said or may rephrase slightly using different words. Paraphrasing is a more major restatement in which the counselor tries to determine the meaning in the statement and reflects back in new words adding to or extending the meaning. Finally, the deepest form of reflection is to reflect feelings in a paraphrase that searches for the client's emotions behind the statement. Thinking up a response to what the client is saying and offering it is *not* reflective listening. Nor is giving advice, making suggestions, criticizing, consoling, reassuring, sympathizing, probing, or telling clients what they "should" do.

EXAMPLE: *Client:"I just don't know if I can lose weight, but I need to."(ambivalence)*
Counselor:"Of course you can."(reassuring)
Client:"But it is so difficult."
Counselor:"Yes, it is."(sympathizing)
Client:"I never have eaten breakfast, because I don't have time."
Counselor:"Just have some cereal and milk."(giving advice)

In the above example, the counselor is not really listening or giving the client a chance to explore the problem. Instead, the reflective listener hears and decodes the message, makes a reasonable guess as to the meaning, and puts the guess into a responding statement. The statement is a declarative one and not phrased as a question, as follows:

EXAMPLE: *Client:"I just don't know if I can lose weight, but I need to."(ambivalence)*
Counselor:"It sounds as if you are pulled in two ways. You want to lose weight. At the same time, you wonder if you can do it successfully." [Avoid:"You are concerned about losing weight?" as a question.]
Client:"But it is so difficult."
Counselor:"You found that your past efforts to change what you eat and lose weight were difficult. I think it's great that you want to try again."
Client:"I never have eaten breakfast, because I don't have time."
Counselor:"Your morning schedule must be a busy one."

Reflective listening and responding is a way of checking the meaning rather than assuming that you know exactly what is meant. It is a guess or hypothesis. This allows the client to keep moving in thought. Not every comment is reflected, however. The counselor decides what to emphasize and what to ignore.

In the early stage of the interview, open-ended questions allow individuals to explore the problems and help establish an atmosphere of trust and acceptance. The counselor may say: "In the time we have together, I want to get an understanding of any issues you have with your choices of foods. I'll be listening so I can understand your concerns. I'll also need to get some specific information from you. What do you see as the issues? What would you like to discuss first? What concerns you about your food intake?"

The client does most of the talking. The counselor may ask what problems concern the person or do the benefit analysis for change. Follow up with the reflective listening. Periodic summaries move the interview along. You may summarize the client's statements about the problem, the client's ambivalence, self-motivational statements made by the client, and your assessment of the situation. Draw together the reasons for change. This helps clients make up their minds. It reinforces what they may already know to be true, but may be avoiding. Reflection is especially important after answers to open-ended questions and after self-motivational statements.

Motivation may be defined as "the probability that a person will enter into, continue, and adhere to a specific change strategy."[8] The counselor needs to increase the likelihood that the person will move toward change. The counselor wants to note and facilitate any self-motivational statements on the part of the client. There are several possible examples. First, the client recognizes that a problem exists. ("I guess my weight is a problem affecting my blood pressure.") Second, the client may express concern about the problem nonverbally, for example, by facial expression, sighing, tone of voice, or verbally ("I've got to make changes now and eat better for the sake of my health.") Finally, the client may feel positive about the change, thus reflecting self-efficacy. ("I'm sure I can start exercising this week.") Reflecting back these types of statements allows the client to hear the message for the second time and enhances self-motivation. The counselor can reinforce nonverbally, such as by nodding the head.

The counselor may question the client to evoke self-motivational statements.

E X A M P L E : *For problem recognition:"What difficulties have you had in relation to your choices of foods?"*
For concern:"In what ways does choosing different foods or eating differently concern you?"
For intention to change:"What are the reasons you see for making a change?"
For optimism:"What encourages you to think that you can make this change?"

When clients reach the action stage of change, their questions can still be met with reflections. Here are possible questions to ask:

"What is the next step?"
"What do you plan to do?"
"Where do we go from here?"
"What good results will occur from this change?"

If the client asks the counselor for advice or information, one approach is to offer several alternatives rather than only one. For example: "I can give you several alternatives. Then you can tell me what you think will work for you." When the client selects an alternative, he or she is more likely to try it and adhere to it than if the counselor provides only one option. The client takes responsibility for a personal choice. In the case of only one alternative, the client may say: "That sounds good, but it won't work for me," thus rejecting the solution.[8]

Goal Setting

Reaching a final plan requires setting clear goals. Having goals can facilitate change. Goals have been found to motivate because they set a standard against which the client can compare a current with a new behavior. They should be clearly stated, reasonable, and attainable. Selecting goals enhances personal choice and control, making it more likely that the person will succeed. Goals motivate change.

Effective counseling helps clients to identify and overcome any barriers to change and acknowledges that lapses and

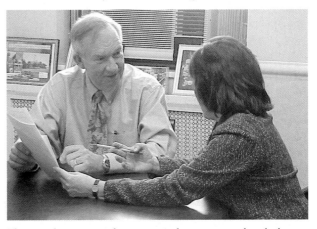

The counselor may use a directive or nondirective approach, or both.

relapses are a normal part of the change process. These may include, for example, lack of time, cost, family environment, lack of social support, nonsupportive friends, fear of adverse psychological or physiological consequences, and so forth.

Clients need feedback about the change to enhance motivation. It can be provided in many ways. Examples are self-monitoring records; results of improved medical laboratory tests; positive comments from friends, family, and the counselor; and the client's own positive self-talk ("I'm doing better").

FRAMES

When time is limited, brief interventions have been found to be effective. They commonly include six elements, summarized by the acronym FRAMES.

Feedback
Responsibility
Advice
Menu
Empathy
Self-efficacy[14]

After the counselor's initial assessment, *feedback* about relevant health information is given by the counselor. Personal *responsibility* for change is emphasized. "It's up to you to decide. You're the one who has to make changes in your food choices." Choices must be made freely and decisions to change are made only by the client. The client decides what, if anything to do with the feedback. Clear *advice* to change or make changes may be given as a *menu* of the variety of alternative ways that changes could be accomplished. Motivation can be enhanced when a person freely makes a decision and feels responsibility for the change. *Empathy* for the client is emphasized and expressed. Finally, attempts are included to strengthen the person's *self-efficacy* for change, to reinforce positive thoughts, and to reinforce the ability to succeed.

Motivational interviewing can overcome ambivalence and move the client from precontemplation to contemplation. It promotes the client's readiness to change and to try various courses of action. The client elaborates and the counselor reflects back again. Rollnick and colleagues consider motivational interviewing a form of guiding rather than directive of giving advice.[15] Rollnick is suggesting that all consultations be based on a guiding style even if full motivational interviewing is not done.[15]

What variables promote or cause behavioral change is subject to much discussion and much-needed research. Resnicow and Vaughan are proposing that we need to look at health behavior change as a complex system, and borrowing from Chaos Theory the concept of fractal patterns. In this view, there are common patterns of behavioral change but "infinite combinations of knowledge, attitude, efficacy, and intention." They suggest that the goal of education or counseling is to create "motivational storms." Their example is that changes in knowledge, attitude, efficacy, and intention are like "the spinning ping pong balls (the interventions) in a lottery machine." The more the balls spin the greater the potential adherence to the receptor of change; periodic interventions keep the balls spinning, and tailored interventions increase the possibility of a motivational change. The beauty of this theory is that it is nonlinear and may expand our understanding of why and when interventions work.[16]

DIRECTIVE COUNSELING

The remainder of this chapter focuses on the general applications of directive counseling strategies as they might be used in nutrition counseling and in employee counseling. The discussion of nutrition counseling in Chapter 5 focuses on the application of nondirective counseling. Directive counseling tends to be most appropriate when the counselor is aware of the problem or is concerned about the behavior of the client, or both, but the client is unaware of the problem or is avoiding acknowledging it. Nondirective counseling tends to be most appropriate when the client has insight and calls on the counselor to assist in the problem solving. In practice, many counseling sessions use a composite of the two approaches such as in motivational interviewing.

In directive counseling, the counselor initiates discussion or approaches the client or staff member based on a direct referral from another practitioner or an employee situation. In nondirective counseling, the client or staff member is aware of the problem and seeks help from the counselor. Clients or staff tend to be far more likely to become defensive and resist problem solving under the conditions of directive counseling. For this reason, counselors using this method need to be especially sensitive to all verbal and nonverbal behaviors and to be supportive while attempting to explore the issue at hand.

Directive counseling is most common in the manager–employee relationship rather than in the dietetics practitioner–client relationship. Directive counseling techniques are used for remedial counseling sessions to address poor employee performance when employees are unaware or unwilling to address it themselves. Nondirective counseling is ordinarily the preferred counseling method when dealing with clients who need to plan and set wellness goals or with employees who have sought out the help of their manager or supervisor.[17]

Applications of Directive Counseling

Managers have a skill set that is different from a clinician's skill set. Often, individuals who are extraordinary in their professional expertise or ability to perform a professional task are selected to manage others. Promoting technical professionals into management without first providing them with adequate training for the job is like sending individuals to bat with two strikes against them. Although all dietetics practitioners have a strong foundation regarding the competencies for being a supervisor or manager, additional continuing professional education in directive counseling or conflict resolution is often desirable.

The use of directive counseling is for discussing unsatisfactory job performance. Counseling occurs after the manager has assessed that the employee knows his or her job description, has been trained for the position, and knows the performance expectation.[17] Directive counseling of employees is a form of discipline, and those administering it need to understand the concept. The root of the word "discipline" comes from Latin and means "to train" or "to mold." The attitude of the counselor needs to be that of a caring teacher who wishes to assist the other in improving. The objective of employee counseling is to change behaviors and develop productive members of the organization. After a manager has assembled and reviewed the facts surrounding a problem with sufficient detail, these must be shared and discussed with the employee. Next, the employee should be given options on how to correct the behavior and the consequences of failing to improve the behavior.

As pointed out earlier, clients or staff are far more likely to become hostile and defensive in directive counseling than in nondirective counseling, because they are "called in" rather than doing the "calling," and they may be more concerned with exonerating themselves of blame than with collaborating to solve the problem.

Employee Counseling

Employee counseling includes the discussion of a work-related problem. Unless dietetics practitioners have advanced degrees with appropriate clinical counseling experience, counseling staff should be limited to the job-related concerns and should not include probing into personal problems such as depression, drug abuse, alcoholism, and mid-life crisis. For such personal problems, the dietetics practitioner should provide referrals to professional therapists or employee assistance programs. When employee counseling loses its problem-performance orientation, it runs the risk of being interpreted as meddling or an invasion of privacy.

Managers have an obligation to conduct work-related counseling sessions with employees. These should be held as often as necessary, assisting the staff in their professional development as well as dealing with career problems as they occur. The manager should not postpone employee counseling until the annual or semi-annual performance appraisal interviews. Allowing problems to accumulate and handling them all at one time is generally ineffective. Employee counseling should occur as close to the incident as possible.

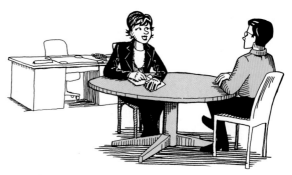

A casual setting creates a better rapport.

Guidelines for Directive Counseling

There are several stages in the counseling interview. They include involving, exploring, resolving, and concluding stages.

Involving Stage

In opening the discussion with the staff member, the counselor must be explicit in the desire to solve a problem rather than to punish. The aim is to improve the staff member's performance. One way of keeping the conversation from becoming threatening is to keep remarks performance-centered rather than to make judgments about the staff member. It is more supportive and factual to say, "You have been late six times in the past 2 weeks," than to say, for example, "Lately you don't seem to care about your job; your attitude is poor." Inferences are not facts. The manager could not possibly know the quality of the employee's "caring" for his job or the condition of his "attitude," but she does know the objective facts—that the employee has been late six times in 2 weeks.

Exploring Stage

Throughout the interview, the counselor focuses on objective facts, being specific about what has been seen, about what behaviors need to be improved, and about the consequences of not changing the behavior. If the complaint is from others, and the supervisor or manager is unable to document the examples from personal observation, discuss the situation with the individual with an emphasis on clarifying the issues and hearing the staff member's vantage point.

Resolving Stage

As in nondirective counseling, the counselor should provide adequate opportunity for employees to tell their side of the story, and their remarks should be paraphrased as well. Not only do people not know what they do not know, but they easily fall into traps of seeing, hearing, and selectively perceiving what they expect to see and hear. Giving employees an opportunity to tell their side of the story and then paraphrasing it and empathizing with what the employee is feeling usually leads to collaboration in the conflict-resolution process. There may be extenuating circumstances that no one on the staff is aware of, which account for the dysfunctional behavior of the employee. Having employees explain the problem from their own perspective may add significant insight and understanding.

Concluding Stage

After an agreement on a solution has been reached, the counselor should describe as specifically as possible what the consequences will be if the agreed-upon changes in the employee's behavior are not actualized. You might say, for example, "If you are absent without notice again, I am going to file a warning notice with human resources." The manager needs to remember at this point not to exaggerate the consequences or to mention consequences that will not be carried out. If the employee does continue the problematic behavior, the manager must go to the next level of the disciplinary process.

Although verifying understanding is important in nondirective counseling, it is even more important in directive counseling. The tendency for employees to experience physiological stress symptoms from the threat of being called in by the manager heightens the possibility of their misunderstanding some of the communication. Both the manager and the staff member need to paraphrase one another to verify that each has understood the other and that they agree on the final solution. An expression of confidence and support by the manager can help ensure successful implementation of an action plan that both parties have agreed on. Rather than saying, "Well, let's see what will happen," the manager provides more motivation by saying, "I think these are the kinds of ideas that can make a difference." Employees should be reminded that they are an important part of the team, that the manager does indeed care for them personally, and that their contributions to the staff are valued. If the action plan includes a multistep process for improvement, it would be wise to set follow-up meeting dates. Doing so not only confirms commitment, but adds incentive to begin the performance changes.

As in nondirective counseling, managers must attend to the supporting nonverbal behavior throughout the directive counseling interview. They should select a private place free of interruptions. The spatial dynamics of the location should allow the two people to feel close and intimate, since feelings are being shared and help is being given to solve the problem. The manager needs to act, talk, look, and gesture in a manner that allows the subordinate to infer that the purpose of the counseling session is to change dysfunctional behavior, not to reject or punish. Finally, the manager has to remember to allow adequate time for full expression of thoughts and schedule multiple sessions when appropriate.

Measuring the Outcomes of Counseling

The outcome of successful counseling is attaining the desired goals. These goals may be those of the employer, primary care provider, counselor and, most important, the clients or employees. The measurement may be short-term or long-term. Chapter 5 identifies many nutrition outcomes that can be measured. Beyond individual client or staff outcomes, dietetics practitioners need systematically to assess the results of their counseling to determine effectiveness. Questions such as the number of counseling sessions generally needed to create client change are essential to determine recommendations for care and reimbursement norms. Self- and periodic client evaluation of your counseling skills will assist in your professional counseling skill development.

Communication effectiveness is enhanced when the food and nutrition professional uses appropriate theories and strategies that promote behavioral change. This chapter examined several theories and models used in counseling. These include directive and nondirective counseling, the Transtheoretical Model (Stages of Change), and motivational interviewing.

CASE STUDY 1

The dietetics counselor is employed at a WIC (women, infants, and children) clinic. Her client is a 16-year-old who has just learned she is 4 months pregnant with her first child. Her older sister, 18, is accompanying her. Her diet history reveals the following:

Breakfast: None or soda and potato chips
Lunch: French fries, soda, and cookies
Dinner: Meat such as ham, potatoes, bread and butter, and soda
Snacks: Soda, snack foods, crackers, and cookies

Using the motivational interviewing process, respond to the following client's statements reflectively.

1. "My sister says I need to eat differently now that I am pregnant, but I like the foods I eat now."
2. "I'm not hungry in the morning. I have to leave for school at 7:15."
3. "I spend a lot of time with my friends. They can eat whatever they want."

CASE STUDY   2

John Miller, age 48 years, was referred by his physician to Joan Stivers, RD, as a result of a serum cholesterol level of 320 mg/dL. He is 6'0" and weighs 250 pounds.

Mr. Miller has a family history of heart disease. His older brother died of a heart attack. He is married with two children, aged 20 and 24 years. His wife is employed full-time and so did not come to the appointment with him.

During the interview Mr. Miller stated: "I know I have a bad family history. I also know that I have put on a few pounds in recent years and should try to lose them. But after a day at work, I enjoy my dinner."

1. What stage of change is Mr. Miller in?
2. How would you match your nutrition intervention to his stage of change? What strategies would you use?

REVIEW AND DISCUSSION QUESTIONS

1. Why is counseling important to most dietetics practitioners?
2. What are potential key outcomes from a counseling session, or a series of sessions?
3. Identify three differences between nondirective and directive counseling.
4. Describe the four characteristics of a quality counselor–client relationship and why they are important.
5. How is motivational interviewing different from the Transtheoretical Model of counseling?
6. List and explain the stages and processes of change.
7. Why is it important to know the person's stage of change when counseling a client?
8. What are the five principles underlying motivational interviewing?
9. Define and give two examples of reflective listening.
10. Why is it better to give the client more than one suggestion when he or she asks for suggestions?
11. Explain the four-stage process of counseling used in the directive counseling section. Provide an example of how this would work with an employee absenteeism issue.

SUGGESTED ACTIVITIES

1. To practice reflective listening statements, form groups of two, one playing the role of a client and one a counselor. Each client should think of two or three things about himself or herself that he or she would like to change (e.g., get more sleep, eat better, lose weight, get more organized and use time better, overcome procrastination, be happier, watch less television, make more friends). This can be stated as: "One thing I would like to change about myself is. . . ." The counselor develops one or two hypotheses of what the person means and puts one of them into a reflective statement rather than a

question. A reflection may be started with the following: "You are feeling. . . ." "It sounds like you. . . ." "You are saying that. . . ." "So you think. . . ."

2. During the next week, practice paraphrasing what others say. What reactions do you get? Does your paraphrasing tend to cause the other to go on talking?

3. Write both a paraphrase and an emphatic comment to the following comments made by a counselee:
   A. "I feel awkward discussing my eating habits. I feel embarrassed about my diet."
   B. "With working all day and a hungry family when I get home, I don't have time to cook."
   C. "I am at a point now where I don't believe I will ever lose the weight."

4. Form triads consisting of a counselor, counselee, and observer. Each individual should take a turn in each of the roles for 5 to 7 minutes. Try three approaches to counseling, the motivational interview, the Rollnick approach, and the four-stage approach. The counselee should play the role of a client interested in healthy eating. After each round, the observer should share reactions to the counselor's approach and encourage feedback from the counselee to the counselor. From the counselee's perspective, what did the counselor do that helped their interaction; what did the counselor do that hindered it? At the end, discuss how each approach helped you.

5. Repeat the activity in number 4. The counselee is a staff member who is not completing his work in a timely manner. Which approach was most helpful here and why?

6. During the next week, make arrangements to view a dietitian's counseling session, noting particularly what occurs during each stage of the process. What behavior on the part of the dietitian facilitates the building of rapport and trust? What techniques did you see that were reflected in the chapter? Discuss which characteristics of a successful counselor were expressed.

7. After each of the statements below, use the FRAME acronym approach to consider the comment.
   A. "My work situation is impossible. It seems that I'm the scapegoat for everybody. I'm beginning to wonder if I should consider looking for another job."
   B. "It doesn't seem fair to me that I should have to work weekends when the staff members who have been here only 2 years longer don't have to."
   C. "It seems easy every morning to promise myself that today I will stick to the program we designed. By noon, however, I begin thinking that I'll never be able to comply with the dietary changes for the rest of my life, so why bother?"

8. To practice developing understanding and using reflective listening, divide into pairs. Ask each person to prepare to discuss a personal experience that would be difficult for someone else to understand. The counselor can use open-ended questions but primarily reflections. The task is to use verbal and nonverbal skills to seek to understand the experience being described by the other. After 10 to 15 minutes, the pair may switch roles. At the conclusion, the instructor may wish to answer questions and ask for reactions to the activity.

9. Count the F's in the following statement:

FASCINATING FAIRYTALES ARE THE RESULT OF YEARS OF SCIENTIFIC STUDY COMBINED WITH THE EXPERIENCE OF CREATIVE MINDS.

Compare answers with several people. Why did you get different answers. How does this relate to issues as a counselor?

WEB SITES

http://www.motivationalinterview.org/   Information about motivational interviewing
http://www.oprf.com/Rogers/   Information about Carl Rogers

REFERENCES

1. Rogers C. Client-Centered Therapy. Boston: Houghton Mifflin, 1951.
2. Rogers C. On Becoming A Person. Boston: Houghton Mifflin, 1961.
3. Patterson CH. Theories of Counseling and Psychotherapy. New York: Harper & Row, 1966.
4. Carl Rogers, 1902–1987, by Dr. C George Boeree. Available at: http://www.ship.edu/~cgboeree/rogers.html. Accessed December 22, 2006.
5. Rollinick S, Mason P, Butler C. Health Behavior Change—A Guide for Practitioners. New York: Churchill Livingstone, 1999.
6. Fine J. An integrated approach to nutrition counseling. Top Clin Nutr 2006;21:199.
7. Prochaska JO, DiClemente CC, Norcross JC. In search of how people change: applications to addictive behaviors. Am Psychol 1992;47:1102–1114.
8. Miller WR, Rollnick S. Motivational Interviewing: Preparing People to Change Addictive Behavior. New York: Guilford Press, 1991.
9. Prochaska JO, Norcross JC, DiClemente CC. Changing for Good. New York: Avon Books, 1994.
10. Summerfield LM. Nutrition, Exercise, and Behavior: An Integrated Approach to Weight Management. Belmont, CA: Wadsworth, 2001.
11. Prochaska JO, Velicer WF. The Transtheoretical Model of health behavior change. Am J Health Promot 1997;12:38–48.
12. Hoy MK, Lubin MP, Grosvenor MB, et al. Development and use of a motivational action plan for dietary change using a patient-centered counseling approach. Top Clin Nutr 2005;20:118.
13. Resnicow K, Davis R, Rollnick S. Motivational interviewing for pediatric obesity: conceptual issues and evidence review. J Am Diet Assoc 2006;12:2024–2033.
14. Miller WR. Motivational interviewing: research, practice and puzzles. Addict Behav 1996;21:835–842.
15. Rollnick S, Butler CC, Kinnersley P, et al. Consultations about changing behavior. BMJ 2005;331: 961–963.
16. Resnicow K, Vaughan R. A chaotic view of behavioral change: a quantum leap for health promotion. Int J Behav Nutr Phys Act 2006;3:25.
17. Sperry L. Becoming an Effective Health Care Manager: The Essential Skills of Leadership. Baltimore: Health Professions Press, 2003.

Nutrition Counseling

OBJECTIVES

- Explain the steps in the Nutrition Care Process.
- Identify the information needed in a nutrition assessment.
- Consider appropriate nutrition diagnoses.
- Explain and practice the steps in goal setting with a client.
- List ways to evaluate the outcomes of nutrition intervention, including how to follow up.
- Describe several studies evaluating counseling techniques.
- Explain some of the expanding roles for professionals.

"I've experienced several different healing methodologies over the years—counseling, self-help seminars, and I'd read a lot—but none of them will work unless you really want to heal."

—LINDSAY WAGNER, ACTRESS

There is no single gold standard method or unifying theory of counseling patients and clients that ensures success in changing food choices and eating behaviors. Instead, dietetics professionals need to be proficient in using several different approaches and strategies while adapting them to the people they are counseling.

The previous chapter examined general counseling approaches and theories. This chapter explores a basic nutrition counseling process using a model as an outline. It emphasizes the patient-centered counseling model and process, matching the counseling intervention strategies to the stage of change, and using the goal-setting process. Later chapters emphasize other counseling approaches, including counseling with behavior modification, counseling for cognitive change (because thoughts may influence eating practices), the role of self-efficacy in making lifestyle changes, and preventing or dealing with lapses and relapse.

NUTRITION COUNSELING

Dietetics professionals, whether working in hospitals, academic health science centers, long-term care, corporate wellness programs, sports nutrition, public health agencies, private practice, or other settings, are responsible for assessing the nutritional status of patients and clients, selecting diagnoses, and intervening through counseling about what they are doing successfully and what they may need to change. The goal is to change people's eating behaviors and attitudes for the improvement of their health and reduction in the risk of chronic disease, such as cardiovascular disease, diabetes mellitus, hypertension, and renal disease. Nutrition counseling is a supportive process, characterized by a collaborative counselor–patient (or client) relationship, in which to set priorities, establish goals, and create individualized action plans that acknowledge and foster responsibility for self-care to treat an existing condition and promote health.[1]

Patient-Centered Counseling

The patient-centered counseling model provides an effective process for dietary change and long-term adherence in clients. The objectives of patient-centered counseling for dietary change are to (1) increase awareness of diet-related risks, (2) provide nutrition knowledge, (3) increase confidence to make dietary changes, and (4) enhance skills to promote long term changes in intake.[2]

These objectives underlie the four steps of the patient-centered counseling model:[2] assess, advise, assist, and follow-up.

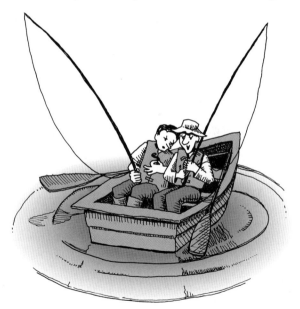

Assess

Assessment is an important component in the total approach to a patient-centered counseling approach. This involves obtaining information about the clients' current and past eating patterns,

Give a person a fish and you feed him for a day. Teach a person to fish and you feed him for a lifetime.

history of health problems, readiness to change, interest in wanting to make dietary changes or reasons for wanting to keep current eating patterns. Discuss concerns about changing dietary intake, feelings about specific changes, and past experiences with dietary change or attempts to make change. Inquire about strategies that helped in past experiences and those that did not.[2]

The dietetics practitioner should use open-ended questions that will assist in tailoring the intervention. Open-ended assessment questions include but are not limited to: How do you feel about your current diet? What problems have you had because of your diet? What would you like to change about your diet now? What would motivate you to maintain your current diet? Have you ever made changes in your diet? What helped? What situations make it hard for you to achieve your goal?[2]

Advise

When helping clients change their eating behaviors, the advice should be personalized to health concerns or clinical conditions and include reasons for change, personal preferences, and other benefits that modify dietary intake. Advice should be personalized and should validate what the patient is stating.

"Mr. Atkinson, as your dietitian, I am concerned that your diet is affecting your health. Are you aware that a major risk factor for heart disease is diet and genetics and your diet suggests risk? I would like to help you make some nutritional changes in your diet, such as decreasing the amount of saturated fat."

"Mrs. Jones, as your counselor, I need to advise you of the importance of following your diet for diabetes management. You expressed concern of complications from uncontrolled diabetes. That is important and I would be happy to assist you in reducing these risks with diet education on carbohydrate counting. What do you know about carbohydrate counting?"[2]

Assist

The type of assistance provided to help with dietary and behavior change is dependent on the patient's stage of change, as discussed in Chapter 4, and the intervention should be appropriate to the stage. The dietetics practitioner provides nutrition information and corrects misunderstandings, addresses and validates feelings about dietary changes, provides support, and expresses realistic optimism and motivational statements in regard to change. For example: "I know it's hard to adhere to your dietary goals during vacation." "It is difficult to make dietary changes when your job involves taking clients out to lunch and dinner."

Follow-up

Dietary and behavioral changes can be difficult. Therefore, follow-up visits are important. Evaluating and monitoring of progress is imperative as goals may need to be revised or new strategies implemented for success.[2]

NUTRITION CARE PROCESS

The Nutrition Care Process (NCP) consists of four steps: assessment, diagnoses, intervention, and monitoring and evaluation.

Nutrition Assessment

Nutrition assessment is the first step in the nutrition care process. Nutrition assessment is used throughout the NCP for obtaining, verifying, and interpreting data needed to make decisions about the nutrition-related problem[3] **(Figure 5-1)**.

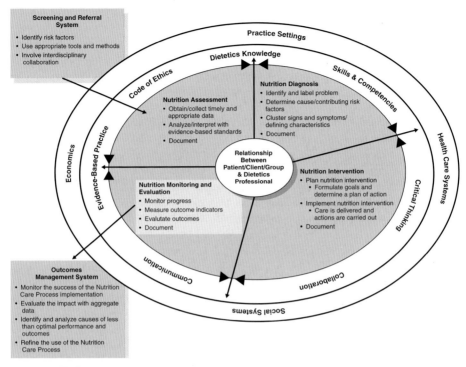

FIGURE **5-1** ADA Nutrition Care Process and Model. With permission from the American Dietetic Association.

The assessment process includes collecting biochemical data and results of medical tests and procedures; anthropometric measurements; physical examination findings; food and nutrition history; and client or patient history. The assessment assists in identifying a nutrition diagnosis, nutritional goals for change, the type of nutrition intervention designed to achieve the goals, and the evaluation of the outcomes.

The first step in nutrition assessment is to gather in advance data or information about the patient or client that may have an impact on treatment. In a hospital or clinical setting, the medical record is the source of data about the patient. Anthropometric measurements, biochemical data, and patient medical history should be noted. Many factors can have an impact on food and nutrient intake, such as role in family, occupation, socioeconomic status, educational level, cultural and religious beliefs, physical activity, functional status, cognitive abilities, and housing situation.

Information that is unavailable from the medical record may be obtained during the interview by using a self-administered questionnaire or by collecting anthropometric data and food and nutrition history. Dietetics practitioners are expected to understand their clients' physiological, psychological, social, cultural, and economical issues; that is, they should know what factors influence their clients' eating and lifestyle behaviors. Counselors must view their clients as individuals living and interacting in an environment that influences their motivation for and ability to change.

A second source of data is the provider's own professional records kept from previous counseling sessions or previous contact with the client. Since the purpose of nutrition counseling is to promote change, the dietitian should review all data before a follow-up session. Therefore, if changes need to be made or personal and lifestyle factors adjusted, they can be discussed with the client. Establishing good rapport with the client is an important step both in nutrition counseling and in developing a trusting relationship. For interviewing skills see Chapter 3.

The counselor may collect data on current eating patterns or habits; on physical, social, and cognitive environments; and on previous attempts to make dietary changes. (Behavioral assessment and cognitive assessment are discussed in Chapters 6 and 7.) The physical environment includes where meals are eaten (at home or in restaurants, and in which rooms of the home) and events that occur while eating (socializing, watching television, or reading). The social environment, which may or may not be supportive, includes family members, friends, social norms, and trends involved with eating behaviors (e.g., meeting friends for dinner, popular food items and beverages when tailgating). See Appendix A for a summary of questions to ask and not ask.

The cognitive or mental environment involves the client's thoughts and feelings about food and his or her self-image and self-confidence. It concerns what clients say to themselves about their food habits and life, since personal thoughts may or may not promote successful change. Positive thoughts, such as "I love a steak and baked potato," or "My favorite snacks are potato chips and beer" may support continued eating. There may be negative and self-defeating thoughts, or thoughts of failure, boredom, stress, and hunger. Examples include: "It's too difficult," "It's not worth it," "I can't do it," "I've been on diets before, always failed, and regained all of the weight I lost," or "I'm happy the way I am and don't want to change." These may also support continued eating. Since behavior is influenced by beliefs and attitudes, you need to explore these in relation to the medical condition, nutrition, food choices, and health. The client's educational level and any language barriers should also be noted.

The assessment may have several important functions, such as making both parties aware of the current food patterns, problems, knowledge, and misinformation, as well as obtaining the health history. The assessment also provides baseline information from which to determine the nutrition diagnosis and determine interventions that are realistic. Once all of the data for the assessment have been collected,

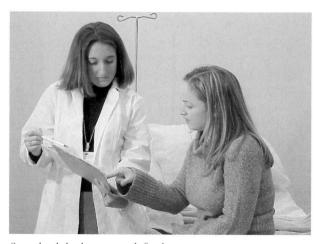

Counselors help clients set goals for change.

the counselor must integrate and assimilate what she or he has read, heard, and observed to distinguish relevant from irrelevant data, identify discrepancies and gaps in the data, and finally organize the data in a meaningful way and document the assessment.[3]

Nutrition Diagnosis

The second step, the nutrition diagnosis, is not the medical diagnosis. The nutrition diagnosis is what the registered dietitian is treating independently. For example, for a dialysis patient, the medical diagnosis is "renal failure," but the nutrition diagnosis may be "excessive intake of potassium (K^+)," "not ready for diet/lifestyle change." Appendix B lists the currently endorsed American Dietetic Association (ADA) lists of nutrition diagnoses. These diagnoses will evolve over time.

Besides selecting the most essential diagnoses to work on, the ADA recommends that the system of charting be reoriented to capture, in one to two sentences, the diagnostic focus based on the assessment. The recommendation is to document the diagnosis in a three-step process called the PES.

> **P**roblem—or diagnoses,
> **E**tiology—or the cause, and
> **S**igns and Symptoms or defining characteristics[4]

Mathieu and colleagues[4] studied the effects on implementation of switching from the traditional SOAP method of charting to the newly recommended approach. SOAP stands for Subjective, Objective, Assessment, and Planning. The new recommendation was to use the ADI template (assessment, diagnoses, and intervention) with the PES statements. The goal of the revised system is to reduce extraneous information, enabling the professional to focus on what is pertinent to the nutrition diagnosis or diagnoses. This new method of charting will evolve, and both methods are acceptable at this time. The Mathieu study showed that the new method of charting requires education, causes discomfort, and requires reinforcement similar to other changes. Another study, by Hakel-Smith and colleagues, reinforces the need for education to improve documentation.[5]

The problem or diagnosis is selected from the ADA's list of nutrition diagnoses (see Appendix B) or rarely, if necessary, a new diagnosis (Dx) is used and then shared with the ADA for potential use. The problem (P) is followed by the etiology (E) which includes the risk factors and the potential cause of the problem. The signs and symptoms (S) are included in the PES. **Table 5-1** shows the format for the PES statement.[3]

T A B L E **5-1** | **Example of the PES System**

Problem (P)	Etiology (E)	Signs and Symptoms (S)
Specific Nutrition Dx	Related to Etiology	As evidenced by Signs and Symptoms
Overweight	Related to excessive energy intake	As evidenced by significant fast food consumption and weight gain to 10 lbs in 3 months

Nutrition Intervention

The third step in the nutrition care process is intervention. It has two phases: goal setting, which includes selecting the nutrition intervention and implementation.

Goal Setting

The counseling relationship was described in the previous chapter. Counselors should clarify that the responsibility for change rests with the client, but that they are willing to assist in solving problems and helping with goals and new plans. It is recommended that nutrition interventions be based on the self-management approach. This involves clients in their own health care and has them take an active part in their treatment.

Before problems are explored and goals are set, it is advisable to discuss with the client, show approval for, and reinforce those current food choices that do not need changing, that is, what the individual is already doing right according to the diet assessment. Foods that should be limited or foods—or cooking practices that should be changed—may be discussed next, perhaps starting with the counselor's estimation of what is most important as well as what the client is willing to consider. Goals should be mutually negotiated based on the nutrition care plan, desired clinical outcomes, or, in the case of normal nutrition, the Dietary Guidelines for Americans[6] **(Box 5-1)**. The conditions and circumstances surrounding food behaviors need to be explored. This stage of counseling requires listening, questioning, accepting, clarifying, and helping clients find solutions to their problems and develop their own plan of action.

Box **5-1**

2005 Dietary Guidelines for Americans

Adequate Nutrients Within Calorie Needs

- Consume a variety of nutrient-dense foods and beverages within and among the basic food groups while choosing foods that limit the intake of saturated and *trans* fats, cholesterol, added sugars, salt, and alcohol.
- Meet recommended intakes within energy needs by adopting a balanced eating pattern, such as the U.S. Department of Agriculture (USDA) Food Guide or the Dietary Approaches to Stop Hypertension (DASH) Eating Plan.

Weight Management

- To maintain body weight in a healthy range, balance calories from foods and beverages with calories expended.
- To prevent gradual weight gain over time, make small decreases in food and beverage calories and increase physical activity.

Physical Activity

- Engage in regular physical activity and reduce sedentary activities to promote health, psychological well-being, and a healthy body weight.
  - To reduce the risk of chronic disease in adulthood: Engage in at least 30 minutes of moderate-intensity physical activity, above usual activity, at work or home on most days of the week.

- For most people, greater health benefits can be obtained by engaging in physical activity of more vigorous intensity or longer duration.
- To help manage body weight and prevent gradual, unhealthy body weight gain in adulthood: Engage in approximately 60 minutes of moderate- to vigorous-intensity activity on most days of the week while not exceeding caloric intake requirements.
- To sustain weight loss in adulthood: Participate in at least 60 to 90 minutes of daily moderate-intensity physical activity while not exceeding caloric intake requirements. Some people may need to consult with a healthcare provider before participating in this level of activity.

- Achieve physical fitness by including cardiovascular conditioning, stretching exercises for flexibility, and resistance exercises or calisthenics for muscle strength and endurance.

Food Groups to Encourage
- Consume a sufficient amount of fruits and vegetables while staying within energy needs. Two cups of fruit and $2\frac{1}{2}$ cups of vegetables per day are recommended for a reference 2,000-calorie intake, with higher or lower amounts depending on the calorie level.
- Choose a variety of fruits and vegetables each day. In particular, select from all five vegetable subgroups (dark green, orange, legumes, starchy vegetables, and other vegetables) several times a week.
- Consume 3 or more ounce-equivalents of whole-grain products per day, with the rest of the recommended grains coming from enriched or whole-grain products. In general, at least half the grains should come from whole grains.
- Consume 3 cups per day of fat-free or low-fat milk or equivalent milk products.

Fats
- Consume less than 10 percent of calories from saturated fatty acids and less than 300 mg/day of cholesterol, and keep *trans* fatty acid consumption as low as possible.
- Keep total fat intake between 20 and 35 percent of calories, with most fats coming from sources of polyunsaturated and monounsaturated fatty acids, such as fish, nuts, and vegetable oils.
- When selecting and preparing meat, poultry, dry beans, and milk or milk products, make choices that are lean, low-fat, or fat-free.
- Limit intake of fats and oils high in saturated and/or *trans* fatty acids, and choose products low in such fats and oils.

Carbohydrates
- Choose fiber-rich fruits, vegetables, and whole grains often.
- Choose and prepare foods and beverages with little added sugars or caloric sweeteners, such as amounts suggested by the USDA Food Guide and the DASH Eating Plan.
- Reduce the incidence of dental caries by practicing good oral hygiene and consuming sugar- and starch-containing foods and beverages less frequently.

Sodium and Potassium

- Consume less than 2,300 mg (approximately 1 teaspoon of salt) of sodium per day.
- Choose and prepare foods with little salt. At the same time, consume potassium-rich foods, such as fruits and vegetables.

Alcoholic Beverages

- Those who choose to drink alcoholic beverages should do so sensibly and in moderation—defined as the consumption of up to one drink per day for women and up to two drinks per day for men.
- Alcoholic beverages should not be consumed by some individuals, including those who cannot restrict their alcohol intake, women of childbearing age who may become pregnant, pregnant and lactating women, children and adolescents, individuals taking medications that can interact with alcohol, and those with specific medical conditions.
- Alcoholic beverages should be avoided by individuals engaging in activities that require attention, skill, or coordination, such as driving or operating machinery.

Food Safety

- To avoid microbial foodborne illness:
  - Clean hands, food contact surfaces, and fruits and vegetables. Meat and poultry should not be washed or rinsed.
  - Separate raw, cooked, and ready-to-eat foods while shopping, preparing, or storing foods.
  - Cook foods to a safe temperature to kill microorganisms.
  - Chill (refrigerate) perishable food promptly and defrost foods properly.
- Avoid raw (unpasteurized) milk or any products made from unpasteurized milk, raw or partially cooked eggs or foods containing raw eggs, raw or undercooked meat and poultry, unpasteurized juices, and raw sprouts.

Source: Dietary Guidelines for Americans, 2005. Available at: http://www.health.gov/dietaryguidelines/dga2005/recommendations.htm.

Note: These guidelines contain additional recommendations for specific populations. The full document is available online.

Counseling should not be directed solely at the client's knowledge, but also at feelings, attitudes, beliefs, and values, which have strong and powerful influences on dietary behaviors. Several reasonable and appropriate alternatives may be suggested by the counselor, leaving the final decision to the client on which alternative is preferred. Knowledge is a tool only if and when a person is ready to change and is motivated to change. You may ask any of the following questions:

> EXAMPLE: *"Which of these alternatives or changes do you think you could try?"*
> *"What would be the easiest?" "The hardest?"*
> *"Is this the right time to make changes?"*
> *"Do you think you can succeed?"*

"What foods could you substitute?"
"How will things be better or worse after you make the change?"
"How do you feel about making this change?"

The client weighs the pros and cons of the options.

Clients (not the counselor) at the preparation, action, and maintenance stages of change, as discussed in Chapter 4, should select one or two priorities or goals for change for the next week or so. Clients who are at the precontemplation and contemplation stages of change or who are enthusiastic about making total changes immediately are setting themselves up for frustration and possible failure, which may lead to abandoning the dietary changes altogether. The counselor should guard against this and use other interventions instead. Slow, steady changes that will persist over time are preferable.

The session with a client needing a meal pattern limited in sodium, for example, may uncover the following obstacles:

1. Uses salt in cooking and at the table.
2. Snacks include crackers and potato chips.
3. Uses some high-sodium spices and flavorings.
4. Likes bacon, ham, and salami.
5. Eats lunch in a restaurant.
6. Is the only one in the family on a limited sodium diet.
7. Grocery shopping is done by the wife, who does not read labels.

Goal Identification

The first step in goal setting and nutrition intervention is identification. Appendix C outlines the current nutrition intervention terminology, which includes many options for nutrition counseling. "Goal setting" would be the choice for the examples that follow.

Personal goals can spur clients to new achievements and changes because they give the person something to strive for as well as a standard against which to judge progress. Because clients are more committed to changes that they select, the counselor may inquire which one or two of the potential changes the person wants to address first by saying, "Which one or two changes do you think that you can work on this week?" When people play a significant role in selecting goals, they hold themselves responsible for progress. If goals are imposed by the counselor, people do not accept them or feel personally responsible for fulfilling them.

Goals selected by the client should be positively stated as concrete behaviors. Goals should be specific, measurable, reasonable, attainable, and timely. A goal should specify what the person will do or is trying to achieve. Following are examples of goals:

> E X A M P L E : *"I will eat fruit instead of baked desserts today."*
> *"I will purchase salt-free pretzels for a snack."*
> *"I will walk for 20 minutes on Monday, Wednesday, and Friday this week."*

Clear, attainable goals produce higher levels of performance than do general intentions to do the best one can, which may have little or no effect. An example of the latter is a statement such as "I'll look for low-sodium foods the next time I am at the grocery store." When goals are set unrealistically high, performance may prove disappointing. If the client selects problems numbered 1 and 2 from the earlier list, for example, these can be reinterpreted into goals for change as follows:

EXAMPLE: *"I will use low-sodium seasonings in cooking and pepper at the table."* *"I will eat fruits and low-sodium crackers for snacks 4 days this week."*

Note that the positive statement of using low-sodium seasonings is preferable to the negative goal of avoiding salt. It is easier to do something positive than to avoid doing something.

Setting specific goals can be motivating and result in positive outcomes. For example: "I will walk for 15 minutes everyday;" "I will lift weights for 30 minutes every Monday, Wednesday and Friday." Goals should be written down and updated when accomplished or until they are no longer a challenge and have become a new behavior.

To be realistic and reasonable, goals should be based on the person's past and current behavior. The first challenge should be only a small step away, not a major change, from the current behavior and should be matched with the client's perceived capabilities for achieving it. The counselor should guide people toward those goals that they believe can realistically be accomplished.

In goal setting a distinction must be made between short-term goals and distal or end goals. Short-term goals that are challenging but attainable with effort are likely to be more motivating and self-satisfying. Self-motivation can be increased by progressively achieving short-term goals, even though the long-range goals are difficult to realize. For example, people need to commit themselves to the goal of following the dietary changes or goal today, rather than a long-term goal of never eating high-fat foods again. When the distant future is the focus, it is easy to put off the goal and decide to start tomorrow.

Persistence that leads to eventual mastery of an activity is thus ensured through a progression of short-term goals, each with a high probability of

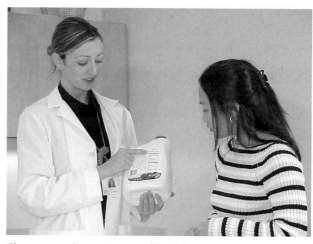

Clients may need an explanation of food labels.

success. When self-satisfaction is contingent upon attaining challenging goals, more effort is expended than if easy goals are adopted as sufficient.

Goal Importance and Acceptance

After identifying goals, the counselor assesses the goal importance by asking, for example: "On a scale of 1 to 10 with 10 being the highest, how important is that goal to you?" What the counselor thinks is important does not matter. Goals that are not perceived as important by the client are unlikely to be achieved.

Concerning nutrition diagnoses, if the diagnosis is "not ready for diet/lifestyle change," the goal of behavior change is unlikely. Instead the PES statement may be "not ready for diet/lifestyle change related to not seeing the importance of change" as evidenced by the indication of the importance of the goal on a numerical scale. Client intervention is difficult when the client does not see the need for change. In this example, the intervention might be "team meeting" to determine best approach with the client.

The strength of a person's goal commitment is affected by several factors. The practitioner needs to inquire about these:

"Do you think you can do it?"
"How important is it to you?"
"Is there someone else with whom you can share your plans?"

Goal Analysis and Overcoming Obstacles

It is important to discuss how the impact of physical, cultural, social, and cognitive environments will affect goals. You may ask: "What problems do you see in achieving this goal?" "What may interfere?" "How do you feel about this change?" It is advisable to tell the client to expect some problems, since some obstacles may come up that were not considered during the counseling session. If the client is aware of the possibility of problems, he or she may avoid abandoning the diet with the first lapse or obstacle. After all, basketball players do not make a basket every time they shoot the ball. But they keep on trying. Supplying a phone number or e-mail address for questions or a web site for resources may resolve unexpected problems. However, e-mail should be used cautiously, since there can be issues and potential problems related to the question asked, possible misinterpretations, legal and ethical implications, and economic reimbursement.[7]

Goal Implementation

In the final step in the intervention process, if obstacles are overcome, clients can discuss what specific steps they plan to take to maintain the goals. For example, the goal of using

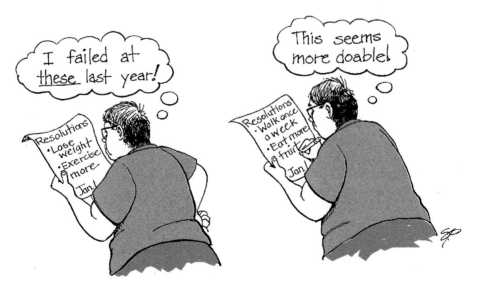

Goals should be specific, measurable, and short-term.

low-sodium seasonings may require identifying and purchasing them, acquiring new recipes for using them, and modifying favorite recipes to replace salt.

By selecting a level of performance, people create their own incentives to persist in their efforts until their efforts match the standards of the goals. Clients compare results against the goals continually so that they know when they are succeeding. The personal standards against which performance attainments are compared affect how much self-satisfaction or self-efficacy is derived for the goal. Feedback on progress is provided by mental comparison with the goal and self-evaluation. The counselor should also provide positive feedback.

The attainment of short-term goals builds motivation, competencies, interest, and self-perceptions of efficacy. Motivational effects do not derive from the goals themselves, but from accomplishing them. When individuals commit themselves to goals, perceived negative discrepancies between what they are doing and what they seek to achieve create self-dissatisfactions that can serve as incentives motivating enhanced effort.

Without standards against which to measure performance, people have little basis for judging how well they are doing nor do they have a basis for judging their capabilities. Short-term attainments increase self-perceptions of efficacy, and self-satisfaction sustains one's efforts. Attainments falling short of the goals lower perceived self-efficacy and the way one feels about oneself.

The nutrition intervention is determined based on the nutrition assessment, diagnosis, and the client's goals. The goals suggest the information, knowledge, and skills the client needs to make dietary changes. The counselor judges what information to provide, how much information can be absorbed at each session, at what educational or literacy level, and what handouts and media to use as supplements. The amount of information to provide and the best method of doing so must be individualized and matched to the client's stage of change and cultural influences.

The intervention may include nutrition education, for example, about the following topics and activities: reading food labels; adapting recipes; menu planning; restaurant or carry-out meals; principles of healthful eating; food safety; nutrients in selected foods; nutritional supplements; nutrition misinformation; fat, carbohydrate, sodium, or calorie counting; nutrient-drug interactions; managing appetite; and the relationship of nutrition to the health problem. In addition, the client needs to know about exercise, self-monitoring, and self-management. Problem-solving interventions for meal planning, food preparation, and food purchasing may be needed. Culturally sensitive interventions are important in meeting the needs, desires, and lifestyles of ethnic clients.

Obtain and document the client's commitment to specific action behaviors, at specific times. The counselor may suggest others with whom the client can discuss the goals, since a public commitment may make it more likely for goals to be accomplished. Practitioners frequently ask their clients to keep self-monitoring records of food intakes and environments, which they should bring to the next appointment as a way for them and the counselor to learn about factors affecting eating behaviors and as a demonstration of their commitment to change. Clients' personal records, observations, and analyses of their environment contribute to their personal awareness and understanding. (Chapter 6, Counseling for Behavior Modification, discusses this matter in more detail.)

By the end of the counseling session, the client should not only know what to do and how to do it, but also be committed to doing it. Clients should be asked to summarize their plans to check for understanding and commitment. The client has to perceive and accept the need for change to succeed. Motivation for change should be explored, as well as the dangers in continuing the current dietary patterns. Solely providing information about a dietary regimen is not usually enough to interest or enable people to improve their eating habits. Counseling involves much more than distributing printed diet materials to clients. Finally, the interventions should be documented.

Nutrition Monitoring and Evaluation

Monitoring and evaluation together comprise the fourth step in the nutrition care process. Monitoring is the follow-up step and evaluation is the comparison step, whether it is comparison to the last visit or comparison to a standard. The purpose of monitoring and evaluation is to ascertain progress and modify recommendations as needed to promote progress to goals. The determination of what the intervention should be as well as the evaluation mechanisms are individualized, but the ADA Evidence Analysis Library provides the framework for basing the nutrition care process on available evidence of best practice.[8] Appendix D provides the standardized terminology for documenting outcomes of care. These are the newest set of terms released in September 2007. As with the other terms, practitioner experience will evolve and refine the terminology.

An outcome is the measured result of the counseling process. Outcome data identify the benefits of medical nutrition therapy in patient and client care. In using these systems of quality control, nutrition counselors may wish to evaluate several things: (1) the success of the client in following the goals set and in implementing new eating behaviors; (2) the degree of success of the nutrition intervention, including its strengths and weaknesses; and (3) their own personal skills as counselors.

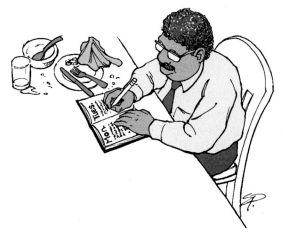

FOOD DIARY ENTRY:

Tues. dinner: skinless chicken breast, rice pilaf, green beans, 1 slice of bread with butter, and a bowl of vegetable soup.

Self-monitoring increases awareness.

The counselor should keep records of the client's issues and goals, the factors influencing them, and the intervention for future measurement of client change. Examples of outcomes are changes in weight, glycemic control, blood pressure, lipid and other laboratory values; patient acceptance and progress at self-management; improvements in knowledge, skills, and dietary changes; and lifestyle changes. These indicate the impact of the intervention and can be used to evaluate the effectiveness of the treatment. The counselor and client should engage in evaluation jointly.

Some measures of success are obvious, such as an overweight person who is now eating differently. Other outcome measures may be indicators of quality of care. The blood pressure and lipid levels of cardiovascular patients can be monitored, although they are more difficult to evaluate since they may depend on factors beyond dietary adherence. Despite the client's commitment to dietary change, results may not reflect adherence to the regimen. These outcomes can be used by the health care team working together to adjust the treatment to achieve or maintain treatment goals. Therefore, medical nutrition therapy is an ongoing process. Further information on evaluation is found in Chapter 12.

Frequent follow-up for reassessment, further intervention, coaching, and support is essential until the client is self-sufficient. Discussion at subsequent sessions should focus first on what went well, that is, the successful experiences and short-term goals reached—no matter how small. Such a positive focus helps clients feel that they can have some control over their eating, health, and life and builds a sense of personal mastery and coping ability. Self-monitoring records kept by the client should be examined jointly and discussed, and difficulties should be identified and resolved, as possible. Overlooking the records indicates to clients that they were not considered important. If progress is made, new short-term goals for change may be established jointly for the appropriate stage of change. Support and reinforcement to strengthen desirable habits along with gradual, planned changes should continue as long as necessary until the client is successful at self-management.

Enthusiasm for change may decline during the first week and even more during the second week, as obstacles develop. Therefore, frequent follow-up appointments should be scheduled if possible. Dietitians in acute care settings who do not have the opportunity for follow-up may need to refer patients to dietitians in outpatient settings or in private practice, since one session with a client is insufficient to promote long-term change in health practices.

DOCUMENTATION

The Joint Commission on Accreditation of Healthcare Organizations (JCAHO) sets standards that are required to address quality-of-care issues in the health care environment. Documentation is essential to quality patient care and reimbursement, and health care professionals need to meet the provisions in JCAHO standards. A summary of the medical nutrition therapy should be communicated to the medical team or other referral source in the medical record. The PES and interventions and the evaluation should be documented clearly and concisely in the permanent medical record. The format will be different in different institutions. All discharge instructions must be documented and provided to the organization or individual responsible for the patient's continuing care.

As the client returns for follow-up appointments, results of health outcomes and goals achieved should be noted. Changes in weight, meal intake, tolerance problems, results of new laboratory values, medications and their nutritional significance, and skills in self-management may be assessed. Follow-up reassessment with new goals and interventions should be recorded. Appropriate referrals should be included.

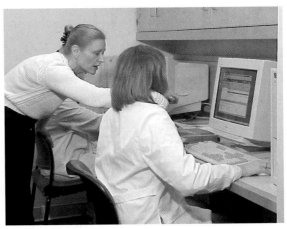

The professional documents in the medical record.

STUDIES ON STAGES OF CHANGE IN COUNSELING

Numerous studies are published annually on techniques and methods for effective counseling. A few such studies are summarized below. In the Diabetes Stages of Change (DSC) study,[9] investigators looked at a traditional family physician intervention as compared with a Pathways to Change (PTC) approach, which included a 12-month intervention with monthly mail or phone contact and intervention based on Transtheoretical Model (TTM) stage-matched interactions. For hemoglobin A_{1C} a significant change was only seen in those who reached the action stage of change. The PTC approach did better in moving the action stage of better self-care. The PTC group also did better in self-glucose monitoring, selecting low-fat foods, and stopping smoking. A study in rural Iowa[10] suggests that tools that measure stages of change can assist counselors in determining strategies to use in promoting a healthy diet. In a study of low-income, African-American mothers, stage of change tools were able to distinguish "decisional balance, processes of change and self-efficacy variables."[11] Women in the later stages of change saw more health benefits of healthier eating than women in earlier phases. The authors concluded that counseling should include practice skills to improve self-efficacy, as this related to stage of change.

EXPANDING ROLES FOR DIETETICS PRACTITIONERS

The concept of expanded roles first started 30-plus years ago and continues today as external opportunities change and entrepreneurial dietetics practitioners move out of "traditional" practice. Articles on key trends affecting the profession of dietetics provide an important source of ideas regarding new roles for dietetics practitioners.[12] Factors such as the increasing diversity of the population suggest that opportunities will expand for dietetics professionals with in-depth knowledge of cultures, foods, and languages.[13] The aging population suggests that geriatric specialists are needed. The busy lifestyles of today's families and consumer interest in nutrition are increasing the demand for personal chefs with nutrition expertise.

One particular new opportunity is for the health coach. Basically, a health coach gives "people the information they need to make informed decisions about how to lead health-ful lives."[14] Obviously, nutrition is a large part of that information. The health coach is pro-viding information and motivation rather than therapy. Those interested in the career may want to consider the Certified Health Education Specialist (CHES) credential.

Changes in technology are also creating new fields, such as the informatics specialist who will design decision-making clinical systems[15] and documentation systems. Computer programmers with nutrition expertise are needed to design interactive activi-ties for children. One such example is the MyPyramid for kids.[16]

Even traditional counseling roles are changing. Telephone-based counseling has been shown to reduce intake of dietary fat and improve fruit and vegetable intake.[17] This tech-nique may complement traditional counseling or may provide a way to broaden outreach.

All dietetics professionals need to be knowledgeable about the concepts, processes, and techniques of counseling, although they may apply them in different settings in professional practice. A comprehensive approach to counseling that considers lifestyle, environments, culture, and psychological and social factors is needed. Some dietitians, with added training, are expanding their roles to deal with long-term health behavior problems in addition to diet and are counseling to achieve patient adherence. Other chapters discuss the behavior modification approach to counseling and the importance of cognitions to change.

CASE STUDY

Connie, a registered dietitian, has worked at Sun Valley Hospital, a 200-bed community hospital for 3 years. Her immediate supervisor, Jill, the clinical manager, is preparing her performance evaluation. While preparing Connie's evaluation, Jill noted that more than 50% of the goals for Connie's performance had not been met. During the evaluation, Connie asked Jill why her merit increase was smaller than the year before. Jill indicated that since 50% of the goals were not met, she was receiving a merit increase based on partial achievement of her goals. Connie left the evaluation session angrily, stating "I don't think this is fair."

1. What could Jill have done to alter the evaluation process?
2. What is the role of Connie in the evaluation process?
3. What steps would you suggest to avoid a similar evaluation next year?

CASE STUDY

Len Howard is a 48-year-old male executive in a Fortune 500 company. In a recent physical exam, he was 5'11" tall and 175 pounds. His serum cholesterol was 290 (desirable: 200 mg/dL or less) with HDL of 50 (desirable: over 40 mg/dL) and LDL 220 (desirable: 100 mg/dL).

CASE STUDY 2

On the recommendation of his physician, he made an appointment with the dietitian in the corporate wellness program.

Mr. Howard's family history revealed that his father and older brother both died of heart disease. His wife is employed as an attorney, and they have a 15-year-old son.

Dietitian: "You mentioned that the doctor wants you to try modifying your diet before considering medication for your cholesterol level?"
Mr. Howard: "He said to reduce the fat and cholesterol in my diet."
Dietitian: "How much do you know about different foods and their effect on your cholesterol level?"
Mr. Howard: "I've heard of it, but don't know much about it."
Dietitian: "Let's talk about what you are eating now. Then we can identify what you are eating that is ok, and what, if any, changes you may be willing to make."

Mr. Howard' nutrition history revealed the following information:

Breakfast: Orange juice, 2 slices of toast with peanut butter, and black coffee
Mid-AM snack: Coffee and doughnut
Lunch: Beef sandwich or bacon cheeseburger, French fries, and cola
Mid-PM snack: Coffee
Dinner: Six- to 8-oz steak, baked potato with butter and sour cream, green vegetable, salad with blue cheese dressing, cookies, and wine
Evening snack: Beer and pretzels

1. What is Mr. Howard doing that is desirable and that you can encourage him to continue doing (foods reduced in cholesterol and saturated fatty acids)?
2. Using the goal-setting process described in the chapter, what are some possible short-term goals for change for him to consider with you?
3. How would you ask him to assess the importance of the choice of goals?
4. After he selects two goals, how would you discuss any obstacles he sees to reaching the goals?
5. Postulate some potential steps he could take to reach his goals. What key discussion points would you identify?
6. What type of follow-up would you recommend?
7. Develop written documentation for your session with this client, incorporating the nutrition care process model as applicable.

REVIEW AND DISCUSSION QUESTIONS

1. Explain the steps in the NCP.
2. What are the four steps in the patient-centered counseling model?
3. Explain the steps in the process of goal setting.

4. What should be included in the documentation of nutrition care and counseling?
5. Write a nutrition note using a PES statement and select an appropriate intervention term.
6. What are some of the newer roles that dietitians are assuming?

SUGGESTED ACTIVITIES

1. During the next week, make arrangements to observe a dietitian's counseling session. Afterward, discuss the philosophies of nutrition counseling.
2. Write both a paraphrase and an empathic comment to the following comments made by a counselee:
   A. "I feel uncomfortable discussing my eating habits with you. I don't know anything about nutrition."
   B. "People tend to think I'm fat and happy, but I don't believe they take me seriously."
   C. "I am at a point now where I don't believe I will ever lose the weight."
3. Form triads consisting of a counselor, counselee, and observer. Each person should take a turn in each of the roles for 7 minutes. The counselee should play the role of an obese client, and the counselor should use paraphrasing and empathizing along with open and closed questions to facilitate disclosure and problem solving. After each round, the observer should share reactions to the counselor's approach and encourage feedback from the counselee to the counselor. From the counselee's perspective, what did the counselor do that helped their interaction; what did he or she do that hindered it?
4. Write an open-ended question for each of the following statements:
   A. "I never have any fun at a family gathering anymore. Being on this diet has taken the fun out of my life."
   B. "Since I developed these health problems, it seems that all I do is think about my diet."
   C. "It seems easy every morning to promise myself that today I will stick to the goals we negotiated. By noon, however, I begin thinking that I'll never be able to comply with the diet for the rest of my life, so why bother?"
5. In groups of two, take turns discussing a lifestyle problem and restating it as a goal for change.
   A. Think of a lifestyle problem the counselee would like to change, such as eating too much; eating the wrong foods; needing to eat more fruits and vegetables, more fiber, or less fat; exercising too little; needing to budget better; drinking too much; smoking too much; or the like.
   B. Help the person discuss the problem and the conditions and circumstances surrounding it. Then have the counselee restate the problem as a positive goal for change, that is, "I will. . . ."
   C. Assess the importance of the goal on a scale of 1 to 10, with 10 being the highest importance. Revise the goal if necessary.
   D. Ask about and discuss the obstacles and barriers to accomplishing the goal, and try to have the person resolve these.

E. Have the person list the steps to achieving the goal. What will the person do, and when will it be done?

6. Visit one or more of the Internet sites that follow to determine what clients may find and how it may or may not help them change their food choices. Share your results with the class.

7. In groups of two, discuss the following client statements to determine what stage of change the person is in. Hint: look back at Chapter 4.

   A. "I have made some changes in my food choices within the past 6 months."
   B. "I am intending to change the foods I eat next month."
   C. "I intend to make some changes in the next 6 months."
   D. "I don't eat high-fat foods anymore."

8. Review the current key dietetics trends from the ADA and describe two or three future roles.

WEB SITES

Both professionals and clients may benefit from information on the Internet.

http://www.adaevidencelibrary.com/ American Dietetic Association evidence

http://www.americanheart.org/ American Heart Association

http://www.cancer.org/ American Cancer Society

http://www.cfsan.fda.gov/ U.S. Food and Drug Administration, Center for Food Safety and Applied Nutrition (site on food labeling, supplements, women's health, and more)

http://www.cholesterollowdown.org/ Cholesterol information

http://www.diabetes.org/ American Diabetes Association

http://www.dietary-supplements.info.nih.gov/ National Institutes of Health Office of Dietary Supplements

http://www.dole5aday.com/ Educates about fruits and vegetables

http://www.eatright.org/ American Dietetic Association

http://www.fightbac.org/ Partnership for food safety education

http://www.foodsafety.gov/ Government site on food safety

http://www.healthfinder.gov/ Consumer health information

http://www.mayohealth.org/ Mayo Clinic health information

http://www.merckhomeedition.com/ *Merck Manual of Medical Information,* Home Edition

http://www.nalusda.gov/fnic/ Food and Nutrition Information Center, U.S. Department of Agriculture; includes food guide pyramid, dietary supplements, and much more

http://www.nccam.nih.gov/health/supplements.htm/ National Center for Complementary and Alternative Medicine

http://www.nhlbi.nih.gov/ National Heart Lung Blood Institute information on cardiovascular diseases

http://www.nhlbisupport.com/bmi/ BMI calculator

http://www.nutrition.gov/ Nutrition-related material from various government agencies

http://www.shapeup.org/ Consumer weight control site

http://www.usda.gov/cnpp/ Center for Nutrition Policy Promotion, U.S. Department of Agriculture; includes dietary guidelines, interactive healthy eating index, and more

http://www.webmd.com/ Consumer health information

REFERENCES

1. American Dietetic Association. Nutrition Diagnosis and Intervention: Standardized Language for the Nutrition Care Process. Chicago: American Dietetic Association, 2007;191.
2. Rosal MC, Ebbeling CB, Lofgren I, et al. Facilitating dietary change: the patient-centered counseling model. J Am Diet Assoc 2001;101:332–338, 341.
3. Lacy K, Pritchett E. Nutrition Care Process and Model: ADA adopts road map to quality care and outcomes management. J Am Diet Assoc 2003;103:1061–1072.
4. Mathieu J, Foust M, Oullette P. Implementing nutrition diagnoses, Step two in the Nutrition Care Process and Model: Challenges and lessons learned in two health care facilities. J Am Diet Assoc 2005;105:1636–1640.
5. Hakel-Smith N, Newis N, Eskridge K. Orientation to nutrition care process standards improves nutrition care documentation by nutrition practitioners. J Am Diet Assoc 2005;105:1582–1589.
6. Dietary Guidelines for Americans, 2005. Available at: http://www.health.gov/dietaryguidelines/dga2005/recommendations.htm. Accessed March 17, 2007.
7. Rodriguez JC. Legal, ethical, and professional issues to consider when communicating via the Internet: a suggested response model and policy. J Am Diet Assoc 1999;99:1428–1432.
8. Evidence analyses nutrition topics. American Dietetic Association. Available at: http://www.adaevidencelibrary.com. Accessed March 17, 2007.
9. Jones H, Edwards L, Valles M, et al. Changes in diabetes self-care behaviors make a difference in glycemic control: the Diabetes Stage of Change (DSC) study. Diabetes Care 2003;26:732–737.
10. Nothwehr F, Snetselaar L, Yang J. Stages of change for healthy eating and use of behavioral strategies. J Am Diet Assoc 2006;106:1035–1041.
11. Henry H, Reimer K, Smith C, et al. Associations of decisional balance, processes of change, and self-efficacy with stages of change for increased fruit and vegetable intake among low-income, African-American mothers. J Am Diet Assoc 2006;106:841–849.
12. Jarratt J, Mahaffie JB. Key trends affecting the dietetics profession and the American Dietetic Association. J Am Diet Assoc 2002;102:1821–1839.
13. Harris-Davis E, Haughton B. Model for multicultural nutrition counseling competencies. J Am Diet Assoc 2000;100:1178–1185.
14. Lipscomb R. Health coaching: a new opportunity for dietetics professionals. J Am Diet Assoc 2006;106:801–803.
15. Charney P. Computer technology and the nutrition support professional: make it work for you! Nutr Clin Pract 2007;22: 421–427.
16. Peregrin T. Making MyPyramid for kids a successful tool in nutrition education. J Am Diet Assoc 2006;106:656–658.
17. Van Worner JJ, Boucher JL, Pronk NP. Telephone-based counseling improves dietary fat, fruit and vegetable consumption: a best-evidence synthesis. J Am Diet Assoc 2006;106:1434–1444.

Counseling for Behavior Modification

CHAPTER 6

OBJECTIVES

- Define and distinguish learning styles of classical conditioning, operant or instrumental conditioning, and observational learning or modeling.
- Apply learning styles to behavior change and specifically in clinical situations such as obesity, diabetes mellitus, and cardiovascular disease, and in human resource management.
- Analyze eating behaviors according to the "ABC" framework.
- Apply behavior modification to case study examples.

> *"Treat a man as he is and he will become who he is;*
> *treat a man as he can and should be and he will*
> *become as he can and should be."*
>
> —GOETHE

Lose weight! Quit smoking! Control your blood sugar! This advice is easily uttered but requires a process to implement and maintain. This process is referred to as behavior modification. Changing behaviors is one of the most difficult tasks for people because human behavior is quite complex. Complex behaviors usually are based on a combination of inherited and acquired characteristics. The inherited characteristics cannot be changed, just as it is impossible to alter any genetic attribute. However, the acquired characteristics, those shaped by a person's environment and experience, can be altered. Behaviors that are learned or acquired can be changed or modified, but this usually requires the right approach at the appropriate time.

This chapter reviews the principles of learning and the process of behavior modification that have evolved from research. Included are classical conditioning, operant or instrumental conditioning based on positive reinforcement or rewards, and observational learning or modeling after others. The role of cognition—the individual's mental perceptions of events, and their effect on behavior—a newer area of research, is covered in more detail in Chapter 7.

Consequences drive behavior. Most undesirable behavior is acquired and maintained by the same principles as optimal behavior, and in some cases the unhealthy behaviors will naturally change.[1] However, the role of a counselor in behavior change is warranted in some situations to highlight for the patient the cost–benefit trade-off or reveal how the "pros" outweigh the "cons" of change. In behavior modification, the therapist attempts to alter previously learned behavior or to encourage the development of new behavior.[2] For example, it is often difficult to influence patients who may not see the health danger in their current habits. Food preferences and eating behaviors have deep roots within the individual and may be highly resistant to change. In addition, behaviors may define individuals in terms of what they think and feel and how they react to certain situations.[3] Reluctance to make changes may occur when a good rationale and a stepwise process to change are not identified. Counseling for behavior change can help reduce the resistance to change.

Simply furnishing information about what to eat often is insufficient to promote alterations in eating behaviors or adherence to medical nutrition therapy. In these instances, it may help to differentiate between diet instruction and behavior modification. Contrary to traditional diet instructions, nutrition counseling for behavior modification steers the client into assuming responsibility for change.[4] The transfer of decision-making power from the professional to the client reduces the risk of relapse and failure. Over time, even individuals in the best-designed, short-term intervention can relapse after the formal program ends. If the responsibility for decisions is transferred to clients, they are much more likely to modify eating choices. As difficult as this seems, it is even more challenging to effectively implement this approach in acute care nutrition intervention settings. Along with information on nutrition, behavior modification principles may be used because they offer the dietetics professional an additional dimension to counseling—that of combining the sciences of psychology and physiology with the art of therapy.[4]

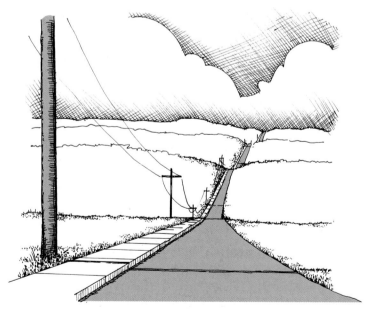

Behavior modification principles are applied in the treatment of various nutrition problems. One of the earliest and the most frequently used applications was in the treatment of

The road to long-term behavioral change is not easy.

obesity. Therapy for inappropriate eating behaviors related to diabetes mellitus and cardiovascular diseases and other chronic diseases are other potential uses of behavior modification.

In prevention, behavior modification can be applied in wellness and disease risk reduction. If unhealthy eating behaviors are modified in favor of healthy alternatives, the incidence of nutrition-related diseases could decrease.

In human resource management, supervisors may be interested in altering the behavior of subordinates and encouraging the development of new behaviors. More effective interaction between peers and superiors may also be a goal. Although the term *behavior modification* in the context of human resource management may sound manipulative, an honest and understanding supervisor may use the principles by sharing with employees the goals of the process. Modeling is a technique that is used frequently in employee training programs. Likewise people in leadership positions may use techniques to help employees assess situations and make adjustments, or behavior changes, as needed to obtain the desired results.[5]

CLASSICAL CONDITIONING

The methods of behavior modification are based on principles of learning that have been discovered mostly in the experimental laboratory. Perhaps the best-known animals in the history of psychology were the dogs housed in the laboratory of Ivan Pavlov, the Russian physiologist, who was conducting research on digestive processes.[6] Serendipitously, Pavlov noted that his laboratory animals salivated not only when food was presented, but also when the laboratory assistant who regularly fed them came into the room; at times, they even salivated at the sound of the laboratory door opening. Pavlov spent the rest of his life investigating a type of learning based on association, now known as classical conditioning.

Pavlov realized immediately that the response of salivation to laboratory assistants and noisy doors was not a part of the physiological makeup of the dog. The dogs were salivating when events occurred that had regularly and repeatedly come before the presentation of their food. An association was apparently formed between some event and the future appearance of food.

Pavlov noted that certain environmental events or stimuli would reliably trigger or elicit a particular behavioral response. For example, food in a dog's mouth would reliably produce saliva. The triggering event (food in the mouth) became known as the *unconditioned stimulus* (US), whereas the response that was triggered (salivation) was called the *unconditioned response* (UR). This relationship was built into the organism and hence unconditioned.

Conditioning occurs when a neutral stimulus—one that originally does not trigger a particular response (e.g., salivation)—eventually comes to produce that response. This occurs by pairing the originally neutral stimulus with the unconditioned stimulus. When conditioning has occurred, the *conditioned stimulus* (CS), which was originally neutral, produces the same response as the US, or one that is very similar. In the example, the CS was the presence of the laboratory assistant. Pavlov showed that bells, tones, lights, and many other stimuli could serve as the CS and could come to elicit the response of salivation, which is labeled a *conditioned response* (CR) because it is triggered by or produced by a CS.[6]

Many types of responses have been found to react to classical conditioning principles. Not only reflexive responses, such as salivation and eye blink, but complex emotional responses can be classically conditioned. The heart pounds and beads of perspiration appear on the forehead as one hears the siren of an ambulance approaching a neighbor's home. The same phenomenon may occur when the teacher passes out examination questions. Try to construct a scenario to account for this response in terms of classical conditioning principles, or think of situations in dietetics in which classical conditioning might play a part in human behavior or emotional responses.

OPERANT CONDITIONING

At about the same time that Pavlov was delineating the principles of classical conditioning, a young American scientist, Edward Thorndike, was pursuing the investigation of learning principles from another perspective. Thorndike used many types of animals in his research and designed and constructed "puzzle boxes" for cats. A hungry cat was placed inside the box with food located outside. To have access to the food, the cat had to solve the puzzle of how to escape from the box. Thorndike observed that the cats made trial-and-error responses until escape was achieved and the food consumed. Gradually, the time required to complete the puzzle decreased. Furthermore, the behavior that achieved success in solving the puzzle became dominant, and unsuccessful behaviors were eliminated.[7]

Thorndike proposed an explanation for this phenomenon based on a principle he called the Law of Effect. This law stated that behaviors could be changed by their consequences. Responses that were followed by satisfying consequences would be strengthened. Behaviors not followed by satisfying consequences, or behaviors followed by annoying consequences, would be weakened and less likely to occur in the future. Thorndike's Law of Effect led to much research in principles of learning and formed the foundation for the study of operant or instrumental conditioning, which is learning based on reinforcement or reward.

The focal point of research on the Law of Effect is the relationship between responses, or behaviors, and the consequences of those behaviors. Four types of response–consequence outcomes have been characterized.[7] First, responses or behaviors may produce positive outcomes, a consequence known as *positive reinforcement*. An example of reinforcement would be the praise and attention an overweight person may receive after losing a noticeable amount of weight. Second, responses may produce negative outcomes; this consequence is known as *punishment*. Punishment decreases the future likelihood of a response. Examples of punishment include the receipt of a traffic ticket for an improper left turn, or the inability to fit into a favorite outfit after gaining weight. Third, responses may result in the removal of adverse stimuli that are already present. This consequence is known as *negative reinforcement* or escape and is similar to positive reinforcement in that it increases the future likelihood or probability of a response. Examples of negative reinforcement include escaping devastating cold by going into a heated building, escaping a boring television show by changing channels, or eliminating or reducing hypoglycemic agents in type 2 diabetes by losing weight and following a sound meal plan. Finally, responses may prevent an unpleasant event from occurring. Examples include avoiding the cold by staying indoors, or engaging in regular physical activity to prevent weight gain. The avoidance of adverse events increases the likelihood of the response, as does positive reinforcement.

Behaviors that are neither positively nor negatively reinforced should typically decrease in strength.

Later behaviorists continued where Thorndike concluded. B.F. Skinner is best known for championing a set of methods and terms to explain behavior on the basis of the principles of operant conditioning. Skinner developed a situation in which behavior could be observed in discrete units and subsequently recorded. This situation was an operant chamber, which has been dubbed a "Skinner box." The lever presses of rats and key pecks of pigeons have been the most fre-

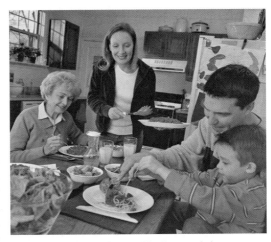

Parents and caregivers shape children's eating habits.
Source: United States Department of Agriculture.

quently studied responses. Skinner's enthusiasm for the behavioristic approach was not limited to lower animals, however, as he proposed wide application for the principles that were established. In recent years, the behavioristic approach has become an increasingly important practical technique in many settings, such as classrooms, mental health interventions, prisons, offices, and self-management situations.[1,8]

MODELING

In addition to classical and operant conditioning as modes of behavior change, a third form of learning is known as observational learning, or modeling. Learning by modeling involves the observation of some behavior or pattern of behaving, which is followed by the performance of either the same or a similar behavior. Albert Bandura is associated with this method of learning by modeling.[9] In behavior modification for weight reduction, for example, a person could "eat like a thin person" to model after the appropriate food choices, portion sizes, and duration of meals of someone who demonstrates the skill.

The effectiveness of learning by modeling appears to be directly related to certain characteristics of the model. The two characteristics found to be most relevant are the observer's similarity to the model and the status of the model. The more similar the characteristics of the model are to those of the observer, the higher is the probability that learning by modeling will occur. Movie and television stars and other well-known persons capitalize on modeling by producing books and videotapes of their fitness and nutrition programs. Many people model after the behavior of a person with "status," even though equally effective or superior programs could be developed by relatively unknown but professionally trained nutritionists and exercise physiologists.

Shaping behavior begins at an early age. Parents and caregivers of children serve as role models in forming good eating habits and healthy behaviors. Long-term food choices of children can stem from the dietary patterns of parental figures. Nutrition counseling may be geared toward parents for their benefit and for the health of the children.[10,11]

To take advantage of modeling, dietetics professionals may try sharing success stories of people who have made permanent dietary modifications for the benefit of their health. In group therapy, clients who have succeeded in changing eating practices may serve as models for others. Keep in mind that the client often views the counselor as a model, and, to this end, dietetics professionals should be following the healthy nutrition recommendations given to others.

Behavior modeling is used in employee training programs to teach basic supervisory techniques, selling skills, and a variety of other verbal skills through observation of films and videotapes. New employees may be assigned to work with current employees who serve as models of desirable behaviors. Managers should make sure that their own behaviors exemplify what they expect of subordinates.[12] If the supervisor adds an extra 10 minutes to the allowed time for a coffee break, for example, employees may model after the example set.

A great deal of human learning and behavior undoubtedly is a result of modeling, even though traditionally emphasis has been placed on the stimulus–response (or behavior–consequence) approach to explaining changes in behavior, or the acquisition and extinction of responses.[6,7] These three approaches—conditioning, operant conditioning, and modeling—form the basis of behavior modification. The behavioristic position is that many behaviors are learned or alterable through use of these three learning principles.

Note, however, that individuals might be more or less resistant to behavior change depending on where they are on the continuum of Stages of Change (see Chapter 4 for in-depth discussion of the Stages of Change model). One barrier to effective communication is that a counseling approach may be implemented erroneously in a particular stage, but may be effective in a different stage. Consequently, counseling for behavior change may employ various approaches to counseling at particular stages.[4,8]

CHANGING EATING BEHAVIORS

As the principles that govern behavior and behavior change became more clearly defined, it became increasingly apparent that nutritionists and behavioral scientists should work together to provide methods of using these principles in applied settings where changes in dietary habits are the primary goal. The National Heart, Lung, and Blood Institute (NHLBI) has been one of the leaders in encouraging this type of collaboration.[13] The most common application has been the behavioral management of obesity, but cooperative programs have led to application in such diverse areas of concern as cardiovascular diseases, eating disorders, and diabetes mellitus.

Dietary behaviors should be studied in terms of the client's total environment, which includes physical, social, cultural, psychological, physiological, and environmental factors compounded by all conditions and events that precede and follow eating. Behavioral scientists have referred to this as the "ABC" framework, derived from analysis of the **A**ntecedents (stimuli or cues), the **B**ehavior (response itself or eating), and the **C**onsequences (reinforcement or reward) of the behavior.[14]

$$A \rightarrow B \rightarrow C$$

For an example of the ABC framework, consider the following: a man at home alone notices a package of cookies left on the kitchen counter; this may be considered the antecedent or cue. Next the man eats some or all cookies in the kitchen; this is considered the behavior. After eating the cookies the man may experience the consequence, that of satisfaction from the taste of the cookies, with reduced feelings of hunger or frustration to reinforce the behavior. The dietetics professional and the client must find ways to decrease unhealthy eating behaviors and increase new desirable ones.

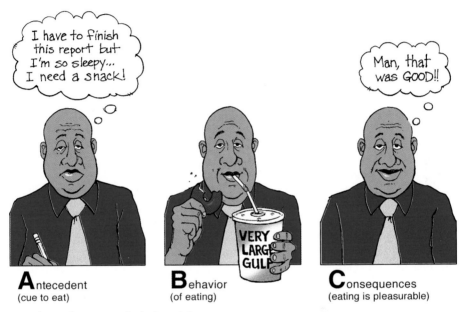

Antecedent
(cue to eat)

Behavior
(of eating)

Consequences
(eating is pleasurable)

Counselors need to examine the As, Bs, and Cs.

Antecedents

Behavior modification techniques work by regulating the antecedents, the behavior of eating itself, and the consequences or rewards. Analysis of antecedents of behavior seeks to control or limit the stimuli or cues to eating. For example, a cue may be seeing or smelling food, watching television, arriving home from work or school, attending a social event, or noticing the presence of extra food on the table at mealtime. Behavior may be influenced by both internal and external factors. There may be internal cues, such as physiological feelings of hunger or psychological feelings of loneliness or boredom. Various external variables may cue eating, such as noting the time of day or passing an ice cream shop in the street. Both internal and external factors may be mediated by cognitive factors, such as not caring about current weight levels or not wishing to dull one's appetite for the next meal.[15]

Once the antecedents are identified, the mediating variable theory calls for identifying the variable most strongly associated with the behavior.[16] The premise is that if one alters the mediating variable, one would expect to influence the behavior associated with that variable. Conversely, if behavior is only weakly associated with a variable, changes to the mediating variable are not expected to manifest in successful behavior change.

SELF-ASSESSMENT

1. What are your cues for eating?
2. What are strong mediating variables to your eating behaviors?
3. The introductory paragraph included the example of a man eating cookies in the kitchen. How could the cues in this situation be modified?

The behavior-modifying strategy involves decreasing the exposures to situations in which food is used as a reward or as a focal point of an activity. A list of suggestions for changing behavior that have been recommended by various authors for persons desiring to lose weight is found in **Box 6-1**.[15,17,18] To modify antecedents, the dietetics professional may suggest removing negative cues (not buying inappropriate foods); introducing new, more positive cues (exercising instead of eating); restricting behavior to one set of cues (eating only at designated times); cognitive restructuring, discussed in Chapter 7; and role-playing new responses to old antecedents (telling a friend you would rather go to a movie than out for pizza). Breaking response chains and preplanning behavior are other strategies.[19]

Preplanning meals and snacks and having only appropriate foods in the house are preferable to expecting self-control when hungry. Preplanning social occasions and exercise are helpful. Small portions of favorite foods may need to be included in the diet to avoid feelings of total deprivation and potential abandonment of dietary changes. Doing the right thing is enhanced by stimulus control. The goal of preplanning to control antecedents is to decrease the number of times the person is exposed to tempting situations so that the client's behavior is tested as seldom as possible.[20]

In some instances, responses occur in chains in which each response produces the stimulus for the next response. An example of a chain is watching television, going to the kitchen at commercial breaks, getting a snack, eating the snack, and feeling satisfied or less bored (reinforcer). The components of the chain should be identified, and then a break in the chain should be planned, such as doing stretching exercises or laundry at commercials.

Behavior

After identifying antecedents, the dietetics professional and client can explore the eating behavior itself by investigating the speed of eating, the reasons for eating, the presence of others, and activities carried on during meals or snacks, such as watching television. The chain of eating too rapidly, for example, can be broken by introducing delays in eating, such as resting the utensils after a bite of food or pausing for conversation. Also, eating behaviors can be modified by encouraging the person to focus on eating as a single event in which he or she concentrates on the act of eating and enjoying the flavors of the foods.

Consequences

Consequences of eating are described as reinforcements or rewards. Because behavior may be maintained by its consequences, efforts are made to arrange consequences that

BOX **6-1**

Techniques for Behavior Modification [4, 17, 24, 30]

I. Provide Incentives to Aid Patients In Maintaining Commitment

    A. Determine ways to focus attention on successful experiences. A positive comment by the counselor is helpful, and you can always find something positive to say.

    B. Encourage people to tell others about dietary goals. This public commitment often will aid in maintaining a course of action.

    C. Have the person anticipate problems that might come up and consider possible solutions before a problem arises. Having a plan ready will make focusing on the goal easier.

    D. Concentrate on allowed foods and portions rather than the disallowed. Be positive.

    E. Keep reminding the person that dietary change is a gradual process. Dietary habits were not developed in a brief period of time and probably will not be significantly changed in a short time. Set realistic goals for immediate and long-term change. Encourage successive approximations to the desired behavior.

II. Learn Eating Habits (and Exercise Habits) by Record Keeping

A person cannot change a habit until he or she knows what it is. Self-monitoring with accurate records of the foods consumed is necessary for behavioral control of eating. Information to consider recording would be:

    A. What food was eaten

    B. Quantity of each food

    C. What the person was doing just before eating (to help identify cues)

    D. Place of eating (cue providing)

    E. With whom eating occurs, or alone (cue providing)

    F. How the person felt (cue providing)

    G. Time of eating (cue providing)

This record-keeping exercise can identify the person's patterns of food intake and those cues that are associated with food consumption as well as the emotional outcome of eating. The person will become more aware of the environmental stimuli that are associated with eating behavior.

III. Control the Stimuli (Cues) and Restructure the Environment

    A. Physical environment

        1. Based on the records kept, have the person identify physical stimuli in the environment that are associated with, and therefore are cues to, inappropriate eating behaviors. Different stimuli become associated with the act of eating and can become signals for appropriate or inappropriate food consumption.

        2. Ask the person to identify physical stimuli that could remind him or her to eat properly. Examples of these would be charts or graphs, cartoons, signs, and the like. The presence of appropriate foods in the home is probably the best cue to appropriate eating, supplemented by the elimination of inappropriate foods.

3. Have the person specify a special place where food should be consumed, such as at the dining table, and not in front of the television set or kitchen sink.
4. Make those foods that are acceptable in the nutrition plan as attractive as possible. Use good dishes, crystal, and so forth to make dining a pleasant event.
5. Set up shopping trips based on the following suggestions:
   a. Shop for food only after eating.
   b. Use a shopping list.
   c. Avoid ready-to-eat foods.
   d. Do not carry more money than needed for shopping list.
6. Set up specific plans and activities:
   a. Substitute exercise for snacking.
   b. Eat meals and snacks at scheduled times.
   c. Do not accept food offered by others.
   d. Store food out of sight.
   e. Remove food from inappropriate storage areas in the house.
   f. Use smaller dishes.
   g. Avoid being the food server.
   h. Leave the table immediately after eating.
   i. Discard leftovers.
7. Regarding special events and holidays:
   a. Drink fewer alcoholic beverages.
   b. Plan eating before parties.
   c. Eat a low-calorie snack before parties.
   d. Practice polite ways to decline food.
   e. Do not get discouraged by occasional setbacks.
B. Social environment
   1. Have the person identify the types of social situations that contribute to poor eating habits. Examples of stimuli in the social environment that might contribute to difficulty for the person would be negative statements from family members or friends, and social situations in which there are expectations for eating inappropriate or disallowed foods.
   2. Have the person identify the kinds of social interactions that would support good eating habits and following the nutrition plan. Role-playing, in which the person practices how he or she will ask others to help change his or her eating habits, can be useful.
C. Cognitive or mental environment
   1. Have the person identify the thoughts and feelings that are likely to make attempts to change eating habits unsuccessful.
   2. After the person has identified possible negative thoughts that could lead to discouragement, help him or her develop some positive thoughts that can be used to counteract the negative ones.
   3. Avoid setting unreasonable goals.

IV. Change Actual Eating Behavior
   A. Slow down.
      1. Take one small bite at a time.
      2. Put the fork down between mouthfuls.
      3. Chew thoroughly before swallowing.
      4. Take a break during the meal. Stop eating completely for a short period.
   B. Leave some food on the plate.
   C. Make eating of inappropriate foods as difficult as possible.
   D. Control snacks.
      1. Save allowable foods from meals for snacks.
      2. Establish behaviors incompatible with eating.
      3. Prepare snacks the way one prepares meals—on a plate.
      4. Keep on hand a quantity of low-calorie foods such as raw vegetables; have them ready to eat and easy to get.
   E. Instruct the person that when eating, he or she should not be performing any other act. The cues associated with eating should be restricted to that act, so the person should not eat while reading, sewing, watching television, and so on.
   F. Have the person continue self-monitoring.
 V. Change Exercise Behavior
   A. Routine activity
      1. Increase routine activity.
      2. Increase use of stairs.
      3. Keep records of distance walked daily.
   B. Exercise
      1. Begin a supervised exercise program under a specialist's direction.
      2. Keep records of daily exercise.
      3. Increase exercise gradually.
VI. Set Up a Reward-and-Reinforcement System
   A. Have family and friends provide this help in the form of praise and material rewards.
   B. Clearly define behaviors to be reinforced.
   C. Use self-monitoring records as a basis for rewards.
   D. Plan specific rewards for specific behaviors. Use written contracts.
   E. Gradually make rewards more difficult to earn.
   F. Use creative reinforcers, such as dropping quarters in a bank, putting money away for each goal reached and earmarked for something desirable. Take money back as a punishment if the goal is not reached.

will maintain desirable behaviors. The consequences of eating may be positive, negative, or neutral. In general, positive consequences are more effective in promoting change than negative or punishing consequences. Reinforcers may be earned over a long period of time, or they may be short term. For example, a long-term reinforcer may be fitting into smaller clothes size after a weight loss program. A short-term reinforcer may be avoiding purchasing "empty calories" from the snack machine, setting the money that would have been spent on the snack aside, and then purchasing a book at the end of the week with the money saved. Alternatives to eating may be included, such as walking or exercising, calling a friend, gardening, or working on a hobby.

If the client's current eating habits are pleasurable and if food is considered its own reward, then new and different rewards must be established. Eating is a powerfully motivated behavior, the occurrence of which is necessary to maintain life, a positive reinforcement. The dietetics professional needs to identify new reinforcers with clients and introduce healthier food choices. Acquired taste can be developed for a broader selection of foods and can steer choices to healthier selections. In some cases, a client may be aware of foods prepared only one way, which were not pleasing to eat. If a new preparation method is described, the client may be receptive to trying the food. For example, a client may dislike asparagus because he or she knows it only as the long skinny vegetable that is boiled and covered with Hollandaise sauce. If the client is told that asparagus can be grilled for a delicious flavor, he or she may be open-minded enough to try it again and perhaps develop a taste for this low-fat vegetable. Changes in eating patterns that are pleasurable are self-reinforcing. If new patterns are a chore and are disliked, they will fail to provide self-reinforcement.

The counselor can work with the client to establish reinforcers. Asking, "What do you like to do with your leisure time?" may identify activity reinforcers. Reinforcers may be walking; attending movies, plays, or sporting events; taking a bath; gardening; knitting; playing cards; or reading. Social reinforcers may be found by asking, "Whom do you like to be with?" Reinforcers may include visiting family or friends or phoning. Other questions are, "What do you find enjoyable?" and "What do you like to buy when you have extra money?" (other than unhealthy foods, of course).[4] **Box 6-2** summarizes the identification of reinforcers.

A very important point here is to recognize that the counselor is also part of the reinforcement. Rather than focusing on failures, the counselor should emphasize what the person has done right with verbal reward and praise. Remind clients to reward themselves cognitively by telling themselves they are making progress and have done something right. For the obese, the ability to fit into smaller-sized clothes hanging in the closet and the weight loss itself are reinforcing. New reinforcers need to be established and introduced for weight maintenance, such as engaging in enjoyable activities, joining

---

BOX 6-2

Identifying Reinforcers

1. Make a list of leisure-time activities and hobbies that you enjoy.
2. Make a list of people you like to be with.
3. Make a list of things you would like to purchase with small amounts of extra money.
4. What do you find relaxing?
5. What do you do for fun?
6. What are your favorite possessions?

SELF-ASSESSMENT

1. What rewards do you get from eating?
2. What rewards do you think others receive from eating?
3. Identify one or two reinforcers that may help you change an eating behavior.

a gym for physical activity, engaging in social events not centered on eating, or walking laps around shopping malls. The reinforcement provided by significant others and self-monitoring are discussed later in this chapter.

After one or two eating changes or goals are identified, a schedule of reinforcement needs to be discussed and established. The schedule specifies which behaviors, if any, will be reinforced and how frequently reinforcement will be provided. Continual reinforcement is the simplest method, but this may lose its effectiveness if the reinforcer is used excessively. An alternative is intermittent reinforcement, such as reinforcement three times a day, or once a day. Eventually, the time may be lengthened between reinforcements. The schedule should be appropriate to the behavior one is trying to strengthen, convenient for the person to apply, and applied immediately for the greatest effect. Never reinforcing a behavior leads to its extinction.[21]

In some cases, contracts may be desirable. Contracts are clear statements of target behaviors of the individual; they specify the type of reinforcers to be used, the person who will deliver the reinforcers, and the frequency of reinforcement. They are signed and dated by the counselor and the client. Contracts ensure that all parties agree on the goals and procedures and provide a measurement of how close the client is to reaching the goals. The signatures help to ensure that the contract will be followed, since signing is a commitment and may provide added motivation to change.[4] **Figure 6-1** is an example of a contract.

An alternative to a formal contract is encouraging the client to write out a list of behaviors to change and a few strategies to implement the change. Also, a simple list of pros and cons of modifying food choices can become a key eye-opener to some.

Completion of behavioral assessment, including a consideration of the Stage of Change, is needed before counseling begins. Examination of the ABC framework (antecedents, behaviors, and consequences) by the nutrition counselor and the client assists both parties in understanding current eating behaviors and allows discussion of what can be changed. Maintaining new behaviors when under pressure or stress is especially difficult. The counselor may consider assessing client self-confidence and ability to cope with stress or anxiety. This evaluation may help identify clients who will need additional support at particularly stressful times.

The role of the counselor is to provide an integrated plan for the total nutrition program of each client. The nutrition counselor serves as a guide or facilitator of change rather than a director or controller of change by suggesting behavioral techniques appropriate to the situation. The counselor should assist the client in assessing the triggers to eating problems and should suggest possible goals, strategies, and techniques to deal with them.[17] Ultimately, the client must determine which suggestions seem manageable at that time and must be willing to implement them. It is also a good idea to ask the client to give an example of the specific behavior change rather than the concept by stating, for example, "the

Patient/Client Name _____

Date _____

Goals:

Example: Increase physical activity 3 times a week.

1.

2.

Strategy to Modify Goal:

Time Frame:

Example: Get up a half-hour earlier than usual for a brisk walk in the neighborhood Tuesdays, Thursdays, and Saturdays.

Use the stairs instead of the elevator, especially if only one floor.

1.

2.

_____   _____
Patient/Client Signature   Dietitian's Signature

FIGURE **6-1**   Example of a Behavioral Contract for Change.

next time I am out of milk I will buy low-fat milk instead of whole milk." This is a concrete action plan compared with merely stating "I'll try to follow a low-fat diet."

Goal setting is one of the critical steps of behavior modification. Goals must be set realistically yet high enough to provide significant change. Cullen and colleagues[22] suggest using a multiple-step goal-setting process. The four-step process encompasses (1) recognizing the need for change, (2) establishing a goal, (3) monitoring goal-related activity, and (4) rewarding yourself for goal attainment. These components can be easily adapted to nutrition interventions.

Since clients are not routinely in daily contact with the counselor, they must be ready to assume personal responsibility for sound dietary changes and eventually become independent. They must learn to analyze and solve their own eating behavior problems. Have the client start with small, easy changes, which are most likely to be successful, and progress incrementally to more difficult ones in later sessions. To be self-reinforcing, the eating changes should be pleasurable ones. If clients enjoy potato chips, ice cream, pizza, and beer, they have to find substitutes they enjoy, such as baked chips, fresh grapes, unbuttered popcorn, and calorie-free beverages or light beer. It may be sufficient to start by reducing the quantity of favorite foods consumed. However, some people may elect to avoid a food item entirely to reduce the temptation of having more. Needless to say, strategies must be highly individualized, and what is appropriate for one client may be inappropriate for another.

Nutrition therapists have the opportunity to share the experiences of others. By having counseled patients and clients on various issues and using customized approaches, counselors learn to assist patients at every point of change. The process of counseling can be compared to making bread. Every baker knows that particular ingredients, kneading, and rising time are essential to making a loaf of bread, but he or she

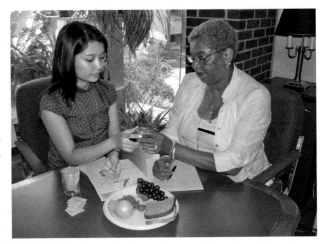

The goal of counseling is self-management.

also introduces artistic expression and ingredient variation to make a unique loaf of bread that meets the distinct tastes of loyal customers. When preparing a new recipe, it is often helpful to see pictures of the finished product; however the baker or chef must sometimes adjust the recipe for cooking at different altitudes or varying ingredients. Similarly as counselors, we need to be cognizant of the right things to convey at the right time and able to customize along the way.

The client should be told to expect problems and some inappropriate eating episodes, especially when under physical or emotional stress. Expecting immediate, total control over change is unrealistic and may lead to diminished self-esteem in clients who have problems following diets, with eventual abandonment of the dietary changes. Learning any new skill requires practice over a period of time. Repetition of the same new behaviors gradually becomes reinforcing and habitual. Support and forgiveness should be provided during any lapses. Enthusiasm for change may be expected to drop rapidly after the initial period, especially if frustration and disappointments arise. Weekly appointments with the counselor may be needed and are desirable in the beginning, tapering to bimonthly and monthly.

SELF-MONITORING

Self-monitoring, or keeping records of eating behaviors to be controlled, was intended originally as a means of supplying the counselor and client with data for analysis. Clients record what, where, when, and how much they eat; the circumstances (e.g., eating while watching television or while feeling bored); and the persons present **(Table 6-1)**. The exercise of keeping records has additional value of its own; it increases client awareness and understanding of current eating behaviors and the influences on them and leads to such realizations as, "I'm eating too much during evening hours while I watch television." Data provide a basis for setting goals for change ("I'll eat a low calorie snack instead") and finding ways to reinforce new behaviors ("I'll tell myself how well I'm doing"). Keeping records serves as a measure of the person's commitment to change. In addition, by having

T A B L E **6-1** | **Self-Monitoring Food Record**

Time	Food/ Amount/ Prep Method	Room/ Place	Others Present	How You Felt Before Eating	Activities at Same Time
Example: 9:30 PM	8 cookies, 10 oz milk	Family room	Husband	Bored, tired	Watching TV

to write down the foods and beverages consumed, the client may think twice about actually consuming an item rather than eating it out of habit or while distracted. Weight loss graphs for the obese and records of physical exercise, blood sugar, and blood pressure are other self-monitoring techniques. However, knowledge of the relation between muscle mass and weight and the concepts of weight plateaus are essential to avoid misinterpretation regarding total health.

SELF-MANAGEMENT

In most behavior modification programs for weight control, the client and counselor are together only for a brief duration at specified intervals. Consequently, the counselor cannot be continually in control of dispensing rewards and punishments or withholding them for appropriate and inappropriate behavior, which is the basis of behavior modification. Therefore, self-regulation or self-management techniques are taught to clients so that they can regulate and control their own behavior. In this way, progress may be achieved in the interval between meetings of the client and counselor.

Research has shown the importance of developing behavioral self-management techniques. Skinner explained that self-management or "self-control" occurs when the individual manipulates the variables on which the behavior rests.[23] Self-management programs have been designed to help persons become aware of and modify antecedents of eating and to self-administer rewarding consequences for eating differently. As self-management programs have evolved, more emphasis has been placed on cognitive change. People have been helped to modify thoughts and beliefs that interfered with adherence to specific dietary regimens and to make use of self-reinforcing thoughts when appropriate behaviors occur. Becoming aware of one's inner state can assist in achieving the desired self-management. For example, referring to a diet has connotations of an ephemeral event, whereas adapting a lifestyle change leads to a more permanent behavior modification.

SOCIAL SUPPORT

Clients' social environments consist of people they are in contact with daily. It is important to include the person's family and significant others when planning lifestyle and dietary changes. The food and nutrition professional should include family members in counseling for change whenever possible, since the changes in food plans at home may affect them as well. Cultural and social factors may be contributing factors to obesity. If the family system supports an obese lifestyle with high-calorie foods and little physical activity, change will be difficult for the client unless the whole family participates in the challenge.[3,4,24] The involvement and support of spouse and family play an important role in weight loss.[25]

Ideally, family and friends are supportive of the client's efforts to change eating behaviors. The counselor may need to discuss with clients the important role of support in achieving permanent change. The professional may suggest that clients request help from family or friends by seeking their agreement not to eat inappropriate foods in front of them or not to purchase or prepare the unhealthy foods. In addition, clients might ask their spouses, families, and friends to offer positive reinforcement for their efforts. Role-playing some of these situations with clients may be helpful.

When family members are present at the counseling session, they should be asked to

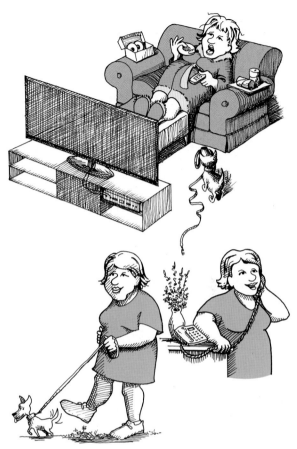

The counselor can assist the client in identifying new behaviors. (Top) Old behavior. (Bottom) New behaviors.

discuss ways in which they can contribute to the client's lifestyle change. Reinforcing proper behavior by the use of praise is an example. Controlling antecedents by having proper foods available is of great assistance. Family and friends should avoid acting the role of judge. "You shouldn't eat that," "It's bad for you," and "I told you so" are not helpful remarks. Jealous and envious reactions may also be expected. "You've lost enough weight," "Just this once won't hurt your diet," and "Your skin is getting to look awful" are remarks that the client may need to tolerate or confront.

APPLICATIONS

Obesity

The most common application of behavioral principles and methods to the treatment of nutritional problems has been in the management of obesity. Although there has been much success using behavior modification in weight loss regimens, weight regain is common and is a result of the failure to impose weight maintenance behaviors.[26] Research into the characteristics among people who successfully maintain weight loss reveals that weight regain is due in part to not fully implementing behavior change.[27]

Opinions differ regarding the efficacy of behavior modification techniques developed for use in treating overweight clients. Brownell reports that behavior therapy is an essential part of any weight reduction program.[28] Obesity is a complex state and is not treated easily. The obese may be overweight for a variety of reasons, only one of which may be related to inappropriate eating behaviors.[29] This does not mean, however, that it is futile to attempt to control one's weight.

The American Dietetic Association's position on weight management states that a successful approach "requires a life-long commitment to healthful lifestyle behaviors emphasizing sustainable and enjoyable eating practices and daily physical activity."[24] The American College of Sports Medicine, in a position statement, stressed that lifelong weight control requires commitment, an understanding of your eating habits, and a willingness to change them.[30] Realistic goal setting, combined with a reduction of caloric intake plus a sound exercise program is recommended. Tailoring practical applications to a client's lifestyle achieves the greatest success.

However, long-term weight maintenance remains a difficult task. Clearly, improved methods to facilitate a higher level and longer duration of success are needed. According to research by Hill and Wing, from the National Weight Control Registry, four common behaviors among dieters who have been successful in weight maintenance are (1) eating a low-fat, high-carbohydrate breakfast, (2) eating breakfast almost every day, (3) self-monitoring (weighing, food journals), and (4) engaging in high levels of physical activity (approximately 1 hour a day).[31]

Motivation and readiness must be present for behavior change. This is particularly true of eating behaviors and physical activity. Several factors are relevant to the prediction of success in weight control, one of which is motivation to reduce weight. After the Stages of Change model is applied to assess the readiness to change behavior, realistic and individual goal setting is critical.[32]

Explaining realistic weight loss achievements is essential. Clients should consider weight loss successful with an initial reduction of about 10% of their body weight over a 6- to 12-month period.[33,34] To expect more than that initially would be a setup for disappointment; however, weight goals can be reevaluated after successful weight loss. Requiring a fee for treatment is another approach; a deposit-refund system may also be used.[4] In the latter system, patients are asked to deposit money, which is later returned if the patient attends meetings faithfully, or achieves a previously determined weight loss, or both. This system appears to be effective in reducing the dropout rate.

An added benefit of significant weight reduction based on cognitive-behavioral treatment in a long-term therapeutic setting has been the reduction in psychosomatic symptoms, anxiety, and depression in treated clients. More adaptive behavioral alternatives in longer goal-oriented programs seem effective in promoting continued weight loss.[35] Research results, therefore, emphasize the fact that there is no quick-fix in weight reduction and that the outlook must be long term.[36]

Diabetes Mellitus

Behavior modification methods have proved to be a useful component in the management of diabetes mellitus. Historically, patient adherence to appropriate dietary regimens to control glucose has been challenging. Behavioral interventions such as cueing, self-monitoring, and reinforcement for appropriate behavior can be successfully implemented to improve glycemic control and reduce risks of complications in patients with diabetes.[34] As previously noted, though, the problem of control of obesity from the standpoint of any particular treatment is complex.

Behavioral management techniques may be used to reduce the burden of diabetes complications.[37] Proactive management by care providers and patients is warranted and has demonstrated positive outcomes.[38–40] Implementation of Internet technology to increase therapist and social support is on the rise as care providers continue to seek better ways to achieve optimal behaviors.[41]

The National Diabetes Education Program (NDEP) supports the work of the other organizations in diabetes management and sets forth initiatives for comprehensive care. These initiatives and additional resources can be viewed on its web site at http://ndep.nih.gov.

Behavioral interventions, when used in the management of diabetes mellitus, should be geared to the developmental stage of the individual in treatment.[39] An understanding of life-span changes (i.e., preadolescence, adolescence, and adulthood) in relation to life role, peer conformity pressure, eating disorders, and hormonal changes needs to be taken into account. A strategy that is effective for an adolescent with diabetes struggling with peer conformity pressures may differ markedly from one that will be of assistance to a pregnant woman with diabetes. There is a definite need to individualize interventions directed toward behavior change.[42]

Cardiovascular Diseases

In the Multiple Risk Factor Intervention Trial (MRFIT), behavioral scientists and nutritionists worked cooperatively with the aim of changing behaviors related to diet and smoking on a long-term basis to reduce the risk of cardiovascular disease. A self-evaluation system for monitoring food intake was developed so that the counselor could estimate the subject's progress in making appropriate dietary changes. A scoring system was used to classify foods according to their fat and cholesterol content as well as their predicted effect on blood cholesterol. Subjects could use the system and select alternative food choices to meet appropriate eating goals. The self-monitoring records were used as a method of measuring compliance and also served to reinforce change and provide positive feedback for appropriate behavior.[43]

More recently, a randomized trial to reduce hypertension was conducted in four clinics to compare the effects of behavioral interventions on blood pressure.[44] The PREMIER trial randomized adults with hypertension to receive one of three interventions. One group of volunteers received "advice only," which consisted of the established recommendations for reducing blood pressure in two 30-minute sessions. A second group received "established recommendations," which included lifestyle recommendations for physical activity. The third group received the "established plus DASH," which included the established recommendations plus the DASH dietary pattern, emphasizing fruits vegetables and low-fat dairy. Participants in both the "established recommendations" group and the "established plus DASH" group received more intensive counseling than those in the "advice only" group. These two groups kept food diaries for total calories and sodium, plus physical activity logs, and received support for behavior change, problem solving, and reinforcement. Over an 18-month period, the adults in the "established recommendations" group and the "established plus DASH" group showed improved blood pressure, weight status, and dietary intake patterns when compared with the "advice only" group. The "established plus DASH" group had the best nutrient intake profile for dietary cholesterol, calcium, magnesium, folate, and fiber when compared with the other two groups. The PREMIER trial showed that lifestyle interventions can be effective in reducing blood pressure and decreasing the risk of cardiovascular disease in adults.[44,45]

Studies of healthy populations, of those at increased risk, and of patients with cardiovascular disease have shown that risk-related behavior can be altered and, in some cases, the incidence of cardiovascular disease can be reduced.[46,47] Since it is generally recognized that cardiovascular disease may result from self-selected behaviors such as smoking, inappropriate eating behaviors, and the pursuit of stress-prone lifestyles, it is encouraging that the initiation of the behavior is by choice and that modification of these self-defeating behaviors is possible. Because the risk factors are behavioral in nature, it is particularly appropriate to attempt to alter them using psychological methods based on behavior modification. The degree of difficulty with such behavior modification partially depends on how long the undesirable behavior has been in place.

Human Resource Management

The behavior of employees is of major concern to supervisors interested in productivity and good human relations. Blanchard and colleagues provide examples of behavioral modification strategies.[5] Setting observable, measurable goals and noting the discrepancy between actual and desired performance promotes new behaviors. Supervisors need to convert ambiguous affective goal statements into a format that is useful for producing improved performance. In this way, employees are encouraged to periodically assess their own performance and adjust behavior as needed for improved results. Rather than attempting to catch subordinates doing things wrong or inefficiently, managers are encouraged to positively reinforce when employees are doing something right or approximately right and then gradually move them toward the desired behavior. Positive reinforcers include:

- Praise
- Positive feedback
- Recognition (employee of the week, month)
- Added responsibility
- Compliments
- Special assignments
- Social events
- Knowledge of results
- Thank-you letter
- Salary increase
- Bonus
- Promotion

Praise is used immediately to reinforce proper behavior. Eventually, some employees begin to praise themselves for the proper behavior, which provides additional reinforcement. A gentle reprimand may also be used, concentrating on the improper behavior, not on the person.

An important aspect of job satisfaction and performance is the employee's sense of personal control; therefore, it is imperative that supervisors refrain from using behavior modification in ways that are seen as manipulative and degrading to employees. Intrinsic motivation should be encouraged to emphasize the importance of a self-reinforcing loop.[5]

There are numerous applications and major advantages of behavior therapy. Programs integrating behavioral approaches appear to hold the most promise for effecting lasting changes. In particular, comprehensive programs that consider psychological, cultural, environmental, and behavioral factors are more apt to be successful.

Eating patterns are not altered easily, but behavior modification therapy offers promising techniques that may be helpful to both the client and the counselor. Analysis of the ABCs— the antecedents of eating, the eating behavior itself, and the consequences of eating—by the counselor and client leads to understanding of the problems, the setting of goals, and the development of strategies for change. Efforts should be made to arrange consequences that reinforce and maintain desirable changes, with an ultimate goal being independent client self-management. Behavior modification may be used in conjunction with other counseling and education strategies.

CASE STUDY 1

Gail is a 23-year-old single woman who has landed her first professional job as a lawyer in a large New York City law firm. She is 5′4″ and weighs 105 pounds. She lives alone in a small apartment and spends most of her time at work or out with friends. Typically, she consumes three cups of black coffee in the morning at work before 9:00 AM. Gail usually works through lunch and may eat a light yogurt or a banana while doing other things. After work she meets with clients or friends for dinner, where she will pick at a tossed salad but rarely finishes the meal. She accompanies the meal with several martinis and a half-pack of cigarettes. On the advice of a friend, Gail has chosen voluntarily to see a dietetics professional for nutrition advice.

1. What are they key factors to consider in your evaluation of Gail's nutritional status?
2. What are the health risk factors for Gail?
3. What tool(s) or intervention(s) for behavioral change could be implemented in Gail's lifestyle?
4. Develop written documentation for your session with this client, incorporating the Nutrition Care Process (NCP) model as applicable.

CASE STUDY 2

Steve is a 45-year-old banker at a small local bank. He has recently been found to have high cholesterol. He is 6′1″ tall and weighs 255 pounds. His wife Susan is employed full-time in the same bank and is also overweight. They have no children.

The dietetics professional discovers that Steve enjoys eating and looks forward to his meals. He skips breakfast, but has coffee with cream and sugar and one or two doughnuts or rolls at his desk at work. He usually eats at a local restaurant for lunch. One of his most

(continued)

CASE STUDY 2

(continued from previous page)

common meals at lunch is a cheeseburger with French fries, a large cola, and an ice cream sandwich for dessert. If time permits, he may have an afternoon snack of another large cola and some cookies. He looks forward to arriving home after work and relaxes with one or two glasses of wine. A typical dinner includes fried chicken, baked potato with sour cream, corn, a roll and butter, and apple pie for dessert. Steve and Susan watch television in the evening and snack on popcorn and potato chips with cola or beer.

1. Identify Steve's antecedents or cues to eating.
2. Identify the relevant information upon which to plan your education activities for Steve.
3. Eating is enjoyable and a reward for Steve. What could the dietetics professional do to help Steve identify new rewards?
4. Describe your recommended nutrition interventions.
5. Develop written documentation for your session with this client, incorporating the NCP model as applicable.

REVIEW AND DISCUSSION QUESTIONS

1. Describe the similarities and differences in learning styles of classical conditioning, operant conditioning, and modeling. Are there situations or cases in which you would prefer using one style over another?
2. Give two examples of a chain of events using the ABC framework.
3. Describe two methods of self-control discussed in the chapter, and discuss how each aids in successful behavior modification.
4. List one important behavior modification strategy for each of the applications discussed: obesity, diabetes, cardiovascular disease, and human resource management.

SUGGESTED ACTIVITIES

1. Complete a food diary for 3 days. Identify your cues for eating. Identify your reinforcers. Set one goal for change with identified reinforcers.
2. Record and identify your own ABCs related to an activity other than eating, such as studying, exercising, smoking, and the like. How can these behaviors be made to occur more or less often by rearranging the antecedents, consequences, or both?
3. Role-play and record a counseling session. How often did you reinforce positive behaviors?
4. Arrange to watch an adult interact with a child or children for half an hour. Tally the number of times the adult attends to desirable behaviors, which reinforces them, versus the number of times desirable behaviors are ignored, which may lead to their extinction. Note whether the adult responds to undesirable behaviors, which reinforces them.

5. Identify your own reinforcers by making a list of leisure-time activities that you enjoy, people you like to be with, and things you would purchase with extra money. Select an appropriate reinforcer for yourself for the next time you have a book to read or a paper to write. Identify a time schedule for dispensing the reinforcer.

6. Select an undesirable behavior of your own that you would like to diminish. Record the situations in which the stimulus or the behavior occurs for 3 days. Identify the controlling stimulus conditions just before the behavior and the reinforcement.

7. Identify three situations in which modeling occurs.

8. In a social situation with friends, tally the number of times in a half-hour that you dispense social approval (smiles, nods, appreciative words) compared with disapproval (frowns, disparaging words).

9. List 10 phrases of social approval that you are comfortable using with others.

10. Discuss your personal experiences at work and compare them with those of others. Does your supervisor praise or punish? What are the consequences of the supervisor's actions on your behavior and that of other employees?

WEB SITES

http://www.diabetes.org   American Diabetes Association

http://www.nationaleatingdisorders.org   National Eating Disorders Association

http://ndep.nih.gov   National Diabetes Education Program

http://www.nhlbi.nih.gov   National Heart, Lung, and Blood Institute

http://www.nwcr.ws/   National Weight Control Registry

http://www.renfrew.org   Renfrew Center for eating disorders

REFERENCES

1. Peltier B. The Psychology of Executive Coaching: Theory and Application. New York: Brunner-Routledge, 2000.

2. Sundel M, Sundel SS. Behavior Change in the Human Services: Behavioral and Cognitive Principles and Applications. 5th Ed. Thousand Oaks, CA: Sage, 2005.

3. Brownell KD. The central role of lifestyle change in long-term weight management. Clin Cornerstone 1999;2:43–51.

4. Helm KK, Klawitter BK. Nutrition Therapy: Advanced Counseling Skills. 3rd Ed. Baltimore: Lippincott Williams & Wilkins, 2007.

5. Blanchard KH, Miller M. The Secret: What Great Leaders Know—And Do. San Francisco: Berrett-Koehler, 2004.

6. Nairne JS. Psychology: The Adaptive Mind. 4th Ed. Belmont, CA: Thomson/Wadsworth, 2006.

7. Rathus SA. Psychology: Concepts and Connections. 9th Ed. Belmont, CA: Thomson/Wadsworth, 2005.

8. Miller WR, Rollnick S. Motivational Interviewing: Preparing People for Change. 2nd Ed. New York: Guilford Press, 2002.

9. Bandura A. Self-efficacy: The Exercise of Control. New York: WH Freeman, 1997.

10. Haire-Joshu D, Brownson RC, Nanncy MS, et al. Improving dietary behavior in African Americans: the parents as teachers high 5, low fat program. Prev Med 2003;36:684–691.

11. Nicklas TA, Baranowski T, Baranowski JC, et al. Family and child-care provider influences on preschool children's fruit, juice, and vegetable consumption. Nutr Rev 2001;59:224–235.
12. Pearce CL, Manz CC. The new silver bullets of leadership: The importance of self- and shared leadership in knowledge work. Organizational Dynamics 2005;34:130–140.
13. National Heart Lung and Blood Institute. Mission Statement. Available at: http://www.nhlbi.nih,gov/about/org/mission.htm. Accessed December 27, 2006.
14. Mahoney MJ, Caggiula AW. Applying behavioral methods to nutritional counseling. J Am Diet Assoc 1978;72:372–377.
15. Stone NJ, Saxon D. Approach to treatment of the patient with metabolic syndrome: lifestyle therapy. Am J Cardiol 2005;96(4A):15E–21E.
16. Baranowski T. Advances in basic behavioral research will make the most important contributions to effective dietary change programs at this time. J Am Diet Assoc 2006;106:808–811.
17. Foreyt JP. Need for lifestyle intervention: how to begin. Am J Cardiol 2005;96(4A):11E–14E.
18. Nothwehr F, Snetselaar L, Wu H. Weight management strategies reported by rural men and women in Iowa. J Nutr Educ Behav 2006;38:249–253.
19. Baranowski T, et al. Are current health behavioral change models helpful in guiding prevention of weight gain efforts? Obes Res 2003;11(Suppl):23S–43S.
20. Wing RR. Behavioral weight control. In: Wadden TA, Stunkard AJ, eds. Handbook of Obesity Treatment. New York: Guilford, 2001.
21. Sadock BJ, Sadock VA, Kaplan HI, eds. Kaplan & Sadock's Comprehensive Textbook of Psychiatry. 8th Ed. Philadelphia: Lippincott Williams & Wilkins, 2004.
22. Cullen KW, Baranowski T, Smith SP. Using goal setting as a strategy for dietary behavior change. J Am Diet Assoc 2001;101:562–566.
23. Skinner BF. Science and Human Behavior. New York: Macmillan, 1953.
24. American Dietetic Association. Position of the American Dietetic Association: weight management. J Am Diet Assoc 2002;102:1145–1155.
25. Poston WS 2nd, Foreyt JP. Successful management of the obese patient. Am Fam Physician 2000;61:3615–3622.
26. Latner JD, Stankard AJ, Wilson GT, et al. Effective long-term treatment of obesity: a continuing care model. Int J Obes Relat Metab Disord 2000;24:893–898.
27. McGuire MT, Wing RR, Klem ML, et al. What predicts weight regain in a group of successful weight losers? J Consult Clin Psychol 1999;67:177–185.
28. Brownell KD. Diet, exercise and behavioural intervention: the nonpharmacological approach. Eur J Clin Invest 1998;28(Suppl 2):19–21; discussion 22.
29. Hill JO, Catenacci V, Wyatt HR. Obesity: overview of an epidemic. Psychiatr Clin North Am 2005;28:1–23.
30. Jakicic JM, Clark K, Coleman E, et al. American College of Sports Medicine position stand. Appropriate intervention strategies for weight loss and prevention of weight regain for adults. Med Sci Sports Exer 2001;33:2145–2156.
31. National Weight Control Registry. Available at: http://www.nwcr.ws/default.htm. Accessed December 27, 2006.
32. Nothwehr Snetselaar J, Yang J, et al. Stage of change for healthful eating and use of behavioral strategies. J Am Diet Assoc 2006;106:1035–1041.
33. U.S. Department of Health and Human Services. Identification, Evaluation, and Treatment of Overweight and Obesity in Adults. Available at: http://www.nhlbi.nih.gov/guidelines/obesity/prctgd_c.pdf. Accessed December 27, 2006.
34. Wing RR, Goldstein MG, Acton KJ, et al. Behavioral science research in diabetes: lifestyle changes related to obesity, eating behavior, and physical activity. Diabetes Care 2001;24:117–123.
35. Fabricatore AN, Wadden TA. Psychological aspects of obesity. Clin Dermatol 2004;22:332–337.
36. Jeffery RW, Drewnowski A, Epstein LH, et al. Long-term maintenance of weight loss: current status. Health Psychol 2000;19(Suppl):5–16.

37. Clark CM Jr, Fradkin JE, Hiss RG, et al. The National Diabetes Education Program, changing the way diabetes is treated: comprehensive diabetes care. Diabetes Care 2001;24:617–618.

38. Mayer-Davis EJ, D'Antonio A, Martin M, et al. Pilot study of strategies for effective weight management in type 2 diabetes: Pounds Off with Empowerment (POWER). Fam Community Health 2001;24:27–35.

39. Clark CM Jr, Snyder JW, Meek RL, et al. A systematic approach to risk stratification and intervention within a managed care environment improves diabetes outcomes and patient satisfaction. Diabetes Care 2001;24:1079–1086.

40. Ridgeway NA, Harvill DR, Harvill LM, et al. Improved control of type 2 diabetes mellitus: a practical education/behavior modification program in a primary care clinic. South Med J 1999;92:667–672.

41. Jackson CL, Bolen S, Braneati FL, et al. A systematic review of interactive computer-assisted technology in diabetes care. Interactive information technology in diabetes care. J Gen Intern Med 2006;21:105–110.

42. Glasgow RE, Fisher EB, Anderson BJ, et al. Behavioral science in diabetes. Contributions and opportunities. Diabetes Care 1999;22:832–843.

43. Remmell PS, Gorder DD, Hall Y, et al. Assessing dietary adherence in the Multiple Risk Factor Intervention Trial (MRFIT). I. Use of a dietary monitoring tool. J Am Diet Assoc 1980;76:351–356.

44. Elmer PJ, Obarzanek E, Vollmer WM, et al. Effects of comprehensive lifestyle modification on diet, weight, physical fitness, and blood pressure control: 18-month results of a randomized trial. Ann Intern Med 2006;144:485–495.

45. Svetkey LP, Erlinger TP, Vollmer WM, et al. Effect of lifestyle modifications on blood pressure by race, sex, hypertension status, and age. J Hum Hypertens 2005;19:21–31.

46. Klieman L, Hyde S, Berra K. Cardiovascular disease risk reduction in older adults. J Cardiovasc Nurs 2006;21(Suppl 1):S27–39.

47. Linden W, Moseley JV. The efficacy of behavioral treatments for hypertension. Appl Psychophysiol Biofeedback 2006;31:51–63.

Counseling for Cognitive Change

OBJECTIVES

- Identify the types of cognitions a person may have and their effect on behavioral change.
- Discuss the types of cognitive distortions and the effects they have on people's behaviors.
- Explain the three phases of cognitive restructuring.
- Discuss self-efficacy's role in the initiation and maintenance of health behavior changes and in a person's choice of activities.
- List the advantages and disadvantages of the four sources of efficacy information.
- Explain how people appraise information cognitively.
- Define relapse prevention and the difference between a lapse and relapse.
- Explain high-risk situations and the cognitive-behavioral model of the relapse process.
- List determinants and predictors of lapse and relapse and how to assess them.
- Identify treatment strategies to prevent lapses and relapse.

"If you think you can't, you're right."

—HENRY FORD

Behavior modification focuses on the influence of external environmental factors on an individual's behaviors and places little weight on cognitive processes. A person's eating choices are linked to cues in the external environment and shaped by the immediate consequences (positive reinforcement) without requiring conscious thought. Another psychological approach, which can be classified as internal rather than external, is exploring the relationship between cognitive processes and the problem in question, such as the need for changes in health behaviors.

Cognitions may be defined as one's thoughts or perceptions at a particular moment in time. Thinking patterns can profoundly influence people's behavior and feelings.[1] Many emotions we feel are preceded and caused by a thought.[2] When strategies for dealing with a client's cognitions are incorporated into behavioral programs, the term "cognitive-behavioral therapy" is used. Cognitive-behavioral therapy techniques are established treatments for eating disorders and other conditions. For bulimia nervosa, cognitive-behavioral therapy is the most effective treatment to date.[3]

The major aim is to produce changes in the cognitive process that maintains a behavior that needs to be changed. Combining several approaches to treatment holds the promise of better results. Weight control programs, for example, may include treatment components of assessing readiness to change, stimulus control, self-monitoring, cognitive restructuring, self-efficacy, outcome evaluations, realistic goal setting, physical activity, stress management, relapse prevention, contracting, body image, social support, and dietary change.[4–9]

As part of the American Dietetic Association's required knowledge of counseling theories and methods, this chapter explores three interrelated areas—cognitions and cognitive restructuring, self-efficacy, and relapse prevention.[10] Negative thoughts, such as "It's not worth the effort," inhibit behavioral change, affect people's feelings, and may decrease self-efficacy or people's beliefs about their ability to perform specific behaviors ("I can't do it"). This can lead to lapses or relapse in the behavior change process ("I'll eat whatever I want."). Individuals with positive cognitions, such as "Losing weight is worth the effort," and perceived self-efficacy ("I can do it") tend to call upon their coping skills and regulate their behavior better.

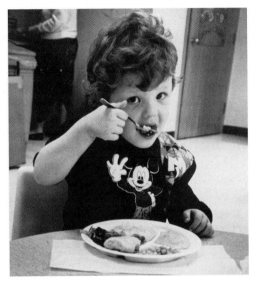

"This tastes good" is a positive cognition.
Source: United States Department of Agriculture.

COGNITIONS

Cognitions are thoughts that occur in one's stream of consciousness. Beck refers to them as "automatic thoughts," since they run through the mind automatically.[11] Meichenbaum calls them ongoing "internal dialogue," and others refer to them as "self-talk."[12] The conversation you have within your head continues all day, and a portion of it is negative. Since our thoughts are seldom noticed, we are barely aware of them even though they can create powerful feelings.[2] They are usually believed to be true and are not analyzed logically. An example of a neutral internal dialogue is: "Shall I cook supper or eat out? I guess I'll cook in. I wonder what's in the freezer that won't take too long to cook. I'll check as soon as I get home."

While people do not engage in self-talk all of the time, on many occasions they do. Times when individuals are more likely to engage in self-talk include when they are integrating new thoughts and actions, such as making lifestyle and dietary changes or performing a new job; making choices and judgments, as in novel situations; and anticipating or experiencing intense emotions.[12] According to Albert Bandura, cognitive processes play a major role in the acquisition and retention of new behavior patterns.[13] See **Box 7-1** for examples of self-talk.

Box 7-1

Examples of Self-Talk

"I'm going to get a college degree so I'll have a successful career."

"I need to get up earlier tomorrow so I'll arrive on time."

"It's the holidays so I'm going to eat whatever I want."

"My New Year's resolution is to get more exercise."

"I'd be in better health if I lost some weight, but it's hard to do."

"I look fat."

"I hate to exercise because it makes me sweat."

"I have no will power."

Cognitive therapy is based on the hypothesis that people's feelings and behaviors are influenced not by events, but by their perception of events or situations.[11] The perception is often expressed in internal dialogue that affects and influences subsequent feelings, behaviors, and even physiological responses. For example, someone who has already lost 5 pounds on a new eating plan (situation) may be thinking that dieting is difficult and not worth the effort (thoughts), and feeling deprived and hungry (feelings). Successfully losing the weight is not as influential as the perception that it is difficult and not worth the effort, resulting in feelings of deprivation and hunger. As a result, the individual may decide to abandon plans for further weight loss even though successful.

Cognitive Distortions

Since negative thoughts inhibit behavioral change, it is necessary for individuals to first become aware of distortions in their thought patterns. Faulty thinking almost always contains gross distortions, often has little to do with actual reality, and may be self-defeating and destructive. Burns and others identify 10 common cognitive distortions.[1,11]

1. **All-or-Nothing Thinking.** This refers to the tendency to evaluate oneself, one's experiences, people, and things in as either black or white, good or bad, and is the basis of perfectionism. One is either perfect or a failure. For example: "I ate this piece

---

SELF-ASSESSMENT

What is the result of each of the following cognitions?

1. "I don't feel like studying tonight."
2. "I might as well do my homework now and get it over with."
3. "I don't have time to exercise today."
4. "I'll feel better if I take a break and walk for 20 minutes."

Your understanding of cognitive restructuring will improve if you start applying it to yourself when you identify negative and dysfunctional thoughts.

of pie, and I shouldn't have. I'm a weak person and a failure." Or "I am too fat." Those with eating disorders are likely to have "all-or-none" cognitions.[3]

2. **Overgeneralization.** If one isolated negative event happens, one concludes that it will extend to other broad situations or events. For example: "I ate too much at the restaurant. It's no use. I will never be able to lose weight." Or "I tried to lose weight once before and was unsuccessful, so I might as well not bother again."

3. **Mental Filter.** In spite of positive experiences, a single negative detail in a situation is dwelt upon, causing the whole situation to be perceived as negative. For example: "If I can't eat whatever I want at the party, the party won't be any fun."

4. **Discounting the Positive.** Some individuals transform neutral and even positive experiences into one's that don't count. For example: "I am following the diet now, but I probably won't be able to do it tomorrow."

5. **Jumping to Conclusions.** People assume the worst even though there are no facts to support it. There are two types: (A) Mind Reading—People assume they know how others are feeling, and that others are looking down on them. For example: "People don't want to be my friend because I am so fat." (B) Fortune-Teller Error—A person predicts that things will turn out badly and assumes that this is a fact. For example: "I don't think I can follow the diet." A positive prediction is: "I'll feel less lonely if I eat this bag of cookies." This is not entirely true, and later the person may feel guilty and have less self-respect. These negative feelings may lead to more binge eating.

6. **Magnification and Minimization.** One tends to magnify the negative, called "catastrophizing," and minimize the positive. For example: "Everyone will hear I goofed up. I'm ruined" (enlarging a situation). Or, "I lost weight this week, but

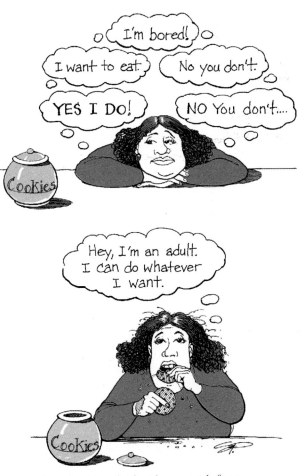

The counselor needs to have the client keep a record of cognitions.

such a small amount that it doesn't amount to anything" (minimizing it). The anorexic client, for example, overinterprets small increases in weight and has distorted beliefs about shape, body weight, and eating.[3,14]

7. **Emotional Reasoning.** Negative feelings are taken as evidence of the truth even if there is evidence to the contrary. For example: "I feel inadequate. Therefore, I must be inadequate." Or "I'm so tired that I need a hot fudge sundae for energy."

8. **Should Statements.** Individuals try to motivate themselves with "should," "must," and "shouldn't" statements. For example: "I should eat fruit," and "I shouldn't eat cake." When behavior falls short of one's personal standards, guilt results. To assert their independence when others tell people what they "should" or "shouldn't" do, some individuals feel rebellious and do just the opposite.

9. **Labeling and Mislabeling.** Instead of describing an error, individuals attach a label to themselves no matter the evidence. Instead of thinking that a lapse occurred on the diet, for example, the person thinks, "I'm a pig," "I'm an idiot," or "I'm a failure."

10. **Personalization.** One sees oneself as the cause of some negative external event when this is not true. For example: "What happened was my fault because I am inadequate."

Cognitive distortions are thinking traps that have been learned. These negative thoughts create feelings that may lead to a negative self-image or sense of worthlessness. In addition, they can become a self-fulfilling prophecy. Because they have been learned, they can be changed or relearned with practice. Since some people have had these thoughts for years, however, change may require extended effort and counseling.

Cognitive Restructuring

Cognitive restructuring techniques refer to a variety of approaches involved with modifying the client's thinking and the assumptions and attitudes underlying these cognitions. While much self-talk is harmless, the focus is on the false thoughts, inferences, and premises. Thus the counselor attempts to become familiar with the client's thought content, feelings, and behaviors in various situations or events. The dietitian needs to help the client identify specific misconceptions and distortions and to test their validity and reasonableness.[12,15] Changing the thoughts to positive ones can modify one's feelings and behaviors.

The client's internal dialogue is viewed as a learned response that may be positive and supportive, negative and upsetting, or neutral. Positive cognitions support behaviors, as for example, "These dietary changes are not so bad." Negative cognitions, such as, "This dietary regimen looks difficult to follow" inhibit people's ability to change behaviors. Thoughts can be self-critical, such as "I'm fat," or self-indulgent, such as "I deserve a treat." In eating disorders such as anorexia nervosa and bulimia nervosa, dysfunctional thoughts and beliefs about "fattening" foods, fear of weight gain, body image distortion, and feelings of low self-worth, require identification, challenging, and restructuring.[3,14] In managing subordinates, an employee may be thinking, "I like my job," or "This job is boring."

Because cognitions are learned responses, the counselor may view the client's cognitions as behaviors that can be modified or changed. Many people cannot improve their eating habits until they change their thoughts about food, eating, and drinking. Overeating and drinking can be an individual's way of coping with stress, depression, and other emotions. The approach is to help the client get rid of unproductive, debilitating thoughts or beliefs and adopt more positive, constructive ones.

Phases of Cognitive Behavior Modification

Cognitive modification consists of three phases, not necessarily in progression. They include recognizing the problem, exploring it, and making changes. The major aim is to produce changes in the cognitive processes that maintain a behavior that needs to be changed.

Recognizing the Problem

The first step involves helping the client recognize and understand the nature of the problem.[7] A basic principle is that people cannot change a behavior without increasing their awareness, raising their consciousness, or noticing a pattern in how they think, feel, and behave, and the impact of their behavior in various situations or events. The client's recognition is a necessary first step, although not a sufficient condition to bring about change.

Rarely does a client recognize that thinking processes are a source of the eating problems. This is true in eating disorders and other eating changes. Homework is necessary. The counselor should enlist clients in a collaborative, investigative effort to understand. Clients need to self-monitor by keeping a written log of self-observations to heighten the awareness of the relationship between self-defeating thoughts, feelings, and eating choices in various situations as a source of material to discuss in counseling sessions. Avoiding the terms "maladaptive" and "dysfunctional" thoughts with clients is advisable.

Burns suggests self-monitoring records with three columns, including first the false thought or self-criticism, then the type of cognitive distortion or thinking error it represents, and finally a self-defense response or the substitution of a more objective, coping, self-enhancing thought.[1] See **Table 7-1** for an example.

People have a mixture of healthy and self-critical thoughts and beliefs and need to identify positive thoughts and modify self-defeating ones.[16] Self-monitoring aims to promote self-efficacy, increase awareness of the effect of thoughts on food intake in various situations, and monitor progress.[17] The counselor should reinforce any positive and coping thoughts, and should help clients recognize and restructure the negative ones. This can increase the client's desire to change.

In addition to written records, the counselor can discuss with clients the range of eating situations, past and present, during which they have false thoughts, such as hopeless thoughts about previous attempts to lose weight or follow specific dietary changes.

TABLE **7-1** | Assessing and Altering False Thoughts

Daily record of _____ Date: _____		
False Thought or Belief	**Type of Distortion**	**Self-Defense, Coping Thought**
"I shouldn't have eaten those cookies. I'm a failure."	All-or-none thinking	"Eating 3 cookies does not make me a failure. I can improve."
"I ate the pie. I'm a pig."	Mislabeling	"Pigs are animals and I am human. I don't have to be perfect."
"I don't have time to eat right or exercise."	Fortune-teller error	"I have just as much time as anyone else. I can make time."

Using the Socratic method, the professional should ask questions so clients verbalize their thoughts and feelings concerning food, eating, and the dietary goal or change during the counseling session by asking, "How do you feel about . . .?" and "What do you think about . . .?" to determine what individuals are thinking to themselves about the eating behavior to be changed, about their ability and desire to change it, and at follow-up appointments, about their progress.

> EXAMPLE: "How do you feel about eating more fruits and vegetables?"
> "How do you feel about cutting down on the amount of fried foods you eat?"
> "What do you think about your ability to make these changes starting tomorrow?"
> "On a scale of 1 to 10 with 10 being the highest, how important is this to you?"

In group counseling, cognitions can be discussed as, for example, the negative self-talk of obese people. Clients need to realize the false, self-defeating, and self-fulfilling aspects of their self-statements. These beliefs have a strong influence on self-esteem and behavior.

Exploring the Problem

During the second phase, the counselor helps the client to explore and consolidate the cognitive problem found in self-monitoring records. As the client reports negative, self-defeating, and self-fulfilling prophecy aspects of thoughts, the counselor can ask how these affect actual behavior and how they can be modified into more positive, coping thoughts.

> EXAMPLE: "What happens when you are thinking you are bored and want to eat something?"
> "What happens when you think you are too tired after working all day to do any cooking?"
> "What happens when you think the food isn't as good tasting or satisfying as before?"
> Note that the counselor does not provide answers or solutions to the problem and must resist this temptation.

The client needs to interrupt the automatic nature of negative self-talk and appraise the situation. The negative cognitions are viewed as hypotheses worthy of testing rather than as facts. The client can be encouraged to ask the following questions:[1]

- What good does it do to focus on negative thoughts? Is there another way to look at the situation or a different explanation?
- What is the worst that could happen versus the likeliest? What if it happens?
- What is the factual evidence supporting or challenging this negative thought? Is it really true?
- How helpful or hurtful is this to my goals?
- Do I benefit from thinking this way?
- What can I say about myself in self-defense?
- Am I exaggerating a negative situation?
- Is it as bad as it seems? What is more realistic?

While the counselor may be tempted to give advice, it is not helpful. Rather than providing answers, asking clients questions about their thoughts promotes self-discovery, thus helping people learn to solve their own problems. Clients need to recognize that negative

T A B L E **7-2** | **Log of Cognitions**

Date	Time	Place	Food Eaten	Thoughts About Eating Before/During Eating	Thoughts About Eating After Eating
1/10	2:15 PM	Home	6 cookies, cola	"I feel hungry and tired. The cookies taste great."	"I'm not hungry any more. I feel better."

thoughts sabotage lifestyle change and decrease motivation. An example of a client log of cognitions is found in **Table 7-2**.

Making Changes

In the third phase, actual change takes place. The counselor helps clients to modify their internal dialogue or self-statements to produce new, more adaptive thoughts and behaviors. Clients are encouraged to control negative self-destructive statements, to talk back with positive self-statements as a coping strategy, and to reinforce themselves for having coped. An obese woman who is eating differently, for example, can tell herself how well she is doing and to keep it up. The "power of positive thinking" greatly enhances motivation and results.

Cognitive rehearsal with visual imagery permits attention to the important details of a future, desired behavior. A client may rehearse, for example, his or her food order at a restaurant or the amount of food and beverages to consume at a party. If individuals think about or imagine themselves overcoming barriers and performing adequately, actual performance is likely to improve.

Motivation is partly influenced by cognitions. People form beliefs about what they can do, set goals for themselves, and plan actions to achieve the results they value. The ability to represent future consequences or outcomes in positive thoughts provides a source of motivation.[13] For example, positive thoughts that one will feel better, look better, or be in better health may contribute to motivation.

Other Counseling Techniques

Besides these techniques, it may be necessary to teach the person other coping skills. Examples are problem-solving skills, mental rehearsal, and "thought stopping."

Problem-solving approaches help to teach a client to stand back and systematically analyze a problem situation. A problem solving method called "STOP" requires the individual to (1) **S**pecify the problem behavior in detail; (2) **T**hink of all possible options or solutions and the advantages and disadvantages of each; (3) **O**pt for the best solution; and (4) **P**ut the solution into practice.[18]

Another technique is "thought-stopping." Clients are trained to self-instruct themselves by saying "STOP!!" whenever they are having false thoughts or negative self-talk and to focus on a positive thought instead. In addition, some of the same behavioral techniques for modifying overt behaviors discussed in Chapter 6, such as identifying cues to thoughts, modeling, and using self-rewards for reinforcement can be used.[2,4]

SELF-EFFICACY

Given a choice, would you be more likely to take on a task if you believed you might be unsuccessful or would you select a task where you were confident of success? The concept of self-efficacy is a useful part of social cognitive theory in predicting and promoting behavior change.

Self-efficacy (SE) is a situation-specific judgment or confidence in one's ability to perform specific behaviors or tasks, such as eating differently, exercising more, or coping in high-risk situations without relapsing.[19] These perceptions about performing a behavior and overcoming barriers, not necessarily one's true capabilities, influence whether people consider changing, whether they mobilize the perseverance and motivation to succeed, their ability to recover from setbacks, and how well they maintain changes they achieve.[20] A client on a weight reduction or diabetic regimen, for example, may have a strong degree of SE when eating at home, but a weaker degree when eating in a restaurant, thus affecting motivation and performance. There are many things people do not pursue because they think they are not capable and harbor self-doubts about their abilities.

Does will power have anything to do with behavior change? Albert Bandura does not believe that appropriate behavior, such as healthful eating, is achieved by a feat of will power. He recognized that learning and behavior change are influenced not only by external cues and rewards that are discussed in Chapter 6, but also by the interaction of demands on one's coping capabilities. In his view, successful therapies work by increasing an individual's confidence in his or her ability to engage in or practice a specific behavior.[13] This, in turn, allows individuals to exercise greater control over their own behavior, motivation, and environment.

SELF-ASSESSMENT

On a scale of 1 to 5, with 5 the highest, rate your level of confidence (self-efficacy) in your ability to do the following:

1. Exercise 3 times a week.
2. Give a 45-minute speech.
3. Make healthful food choices.
4. Lift 10-pound weights.
5. Ski downhill.
6. Control your weight.
7. Give a dinner party for 20 people.
8. Meet new people at a party.

What effect does a high or low rating have on your choice of activities?

Bandura distinguishes between "efficacy" expectancies ("Can I do it?") and "outcome" expectations ("What will happen if I do it?").[21,22] An "outcome" expectancy is a person's estimate or belief that a given change will or will not lead to an outcome the person values. For example, the behavior of reducing dietary sodium will lead to an outcome of lower blood pressure and better health; following a dietary regimen will lead to an outcome of weight loss and better physical appearance; reducing dietary fat will lead to a lower cholesterol level in the blood and prevent heart disease; or successfully completing a project for one's superior will lead to a salary increase or promotion. Besides cost and benefit outcomes, people weight the outcomes of social approval or disapproval, pleasurable or aversive expectations, and personal standards against which one evaluates oneself.[20]

An SE expectation is the belief that one is or is not capable or performing the change in behavior required to lead to the desired outcome. It affects how much effort a person gives, what level of performance is attained, and whether or not healthful behavior changes are maintained.[23] A male client may or may not believe, for example, that he can reduce his dietary sodium intake continuously to attain the outcome of lower blood pressure. Among staff, an employee may believe that performing work optimally will lead to the desired "outcome" of a promotion but may or may not believe that he or she is capable (SE) of optimum performance on a continuous basis.

SE and outcomes are differentiated because people may believe that certain actions can produce the outcome, but they may have serious doubts about whether or not they can cope with the necessary changes and overcome barriers to reach the outcome. These evaluations may apply to performing a desired behavior as well as abstaining from a problem one.[24]

Choice of Behaviors and Activities

Efficacy expectations are a major determinant of people's choice of activities.[13] The client involved in a change of behavior, such as eating or exercise, must make decisions about whether or not to attempt different food choices, how long to continue, how much effort to make, and in the face of difficulties or aversive experiences, whether or not to persist. Bandura believes that these decisions are partly governed by judgments of SE. People tend to avoid situations that they believe exceed their coping capabilities, but are willing to undertake activities they judge themselves capable of executing.[13] The stronger the perceived SE, or sense of personal mastery, the more persistent are the efforts, even in the presence of obstacles. When difficulties arise, those with lower perceptions of SE make less effort or may give up entirely.[20]

A person's SE is generally a good predictor of how that individual is likely to behave on specific tasks.[13] SE affects whether or not people consider changing a health habit, whether they mobilize the motivation and perseverance to succeed, whether they are able to recover from setbacks and relapses, and how well they maintain the changes they have made.[20]

The evidence is overwhelming that there is a close association between SE and nutrition and health behavior change, and that SE is a powerful predictor of change. An important goal of diabetes care and education is enhancing SE of patients to self-manage their diabetes.[25] In exploring self-care in diabetes, SE was a strong predictor of self-care and enhanced metabolic control.[26] In people with type 1 diabetes, SE was a predictor of self-care practices and HbA_{1c} and metabolic control.[27]

In an obesity study, higher SE with respect to eating behavior predicted greater weight loss among subjects. Less weight reduction was associated with poor SE and the beliefs that obesity was not under behavioral control, but had a physical origin.[28] A weight loss intervention program found that when SE improved, there were greater improvements in eating behaviors.[29] In a study of postpartum women, higher exercise SE was associated with more frequent exercise, and food intake SE was associated with reductions in food intake.[30] A study of bulimic women found that those high in perfectionism who believed they were overweight and who had low SE reported the highest number of weeks of binge eating.[31] According to Bandura: "Unless people believe they can master and adhere to health-promoting habits, they are unlikely to devote the effort necessary to succeed."[21]

In addition, perceived SE and personal goals enhance performance.[20] Motivation to perform a task can improve in part through one's self-evaluation of performance as compared with the adopted goal or standard. A person with strong SE increases effort and persistence in achieving subgoals and that results in higher performance. For this client, the counselor needs to break down tasks into easily mastered steps that are within the person's capabilities while requiring some degree of effort.

People commonly have a higher sense of confidence about one type of activity than another. For example, a woman may feel confident in increasing daily walks, but doubt that she can sustain the effort to reduce her fat intake in the face of family food preferences. A male employee may feel confident in his ability to perform one aspect of his job, such as using a computer, but not another, such as giving a 30-minute oral presentation.

Dimensions of Efficacy Expectations

The practitioner needs to assess clients' thoughts about their abilities to make changes in eating and exercise behaviors or employees' thoughts about work behaviors. Different dimensions of thoughts may be examined, such as level of difficulty of the task, strength of SE to succeed at the task, and generalization to other situations. When tasks have different levels of difficulty, efficacy expectations may limit some people to the simple tasks, while others may feel comfortable with the moderately difficult or difficult ones. SE differs also in strength or confidence for regulating eating behaviors. Weak self-beliefs are easily extinguished by disconfirming experiences, whereas those with strong efficacy expectations will persevere in their coping efforts even through difficulties. Perceived efficacy may or may not be generalized to other activities or behaviors requiring similar skills.[22]

Measuring SE

A two-step approach to measuring SE is suggested. First, given a group of tasks of varying levels of difficulty, ask clients which dietary goals or changes they can undertake. It is preferable to start off with the simpler ones in order to guarantee success as that will increase SE. Then one can work up slowly to more difficult ones.

Second, for each designated task in the behavior change, ask clients to rate the strength of their confidence of success in making a specific change on a 5-point scale, with 5 being very confident to 1 being not at all confident. If not confident, a different task or goal should be found. Self-appraisals are reasonably accurate, because people successfully execute tasks within their perceived capabilities but shun those that exceed their perceived coping abilities.

Efficacy varies with the situation or event. Efficacy expectations and performance should be assessed periodically during the dietary change process, because the stronger the perceived efficacy, the more likely people are to persist in their efforts until they succeed. In the Transtheoretical Model (TTM) or Stages of Change, discussed in Chapter 4, SE scores have generally been found to increase in the later stages. They are low in the precontemplation and contemplation stages, where people with little confidence in their ability to change can be stuck.[24,32] SE was significantly higher for those in the later stages of change, such as action and maintenance.

Sources of Efficacy Information

When planning interventions with clients, it is important to consider the four major sources of efficacy information. Clients' beliefs about efficacy are based on (1) actual performance accomplishments, (2) vicarious experiences (modeling) by observing the performance of others, (3) verbal persuasion, and (4) physiological and emotional states.[13,22] All four have been used in food and exercise interventions.[30]

Actual Performance

The most influential and effective way to increase SE is actual performance accomplishments. The counselor needs to divide changes into many small steps, let the client select the ones to try first, and be sure the person has the confidence to succeed. Setting goals and self-rewards may be beneficial. One should structure goals that bring success and avoid situations in which people are likely to fail. The increase in efficacy is based on the experience of successfully performing the behavior in question.[22] "Nothing succeeds like success" reinforces this idea. Personal successes raise mastery expectations while failures lower them, especially early in the course of a change. Repeated success in overcoming obstacles through perseverance strengthens SE. People also perfect their coping skills and lessen their vulnerability to stress. Success begets success; failure begets failure.

Modeling

A second source of efficacy information comes from modeling followed by guided performance. Clients can learn how to handle situations by observing a model demonstrating the appropriate behavior, such as ordering healthful food from a restaurant menu or saying "no thank you" to dessert offerings. The vicarious experience of seeing another perform can generate expectations that if another can do it, "so can I."

To enhance SE, the model should be perceived as similar to oneself or possessing competencies to which one aspires. Clients should then be given an opportunity to perform the modeled behavior successfully. In educational classes where recipes are prepared, for example, clients can participate. Negative role models are a problem in group counseling and should be avoided. Employees also learn by observing and modeling after other employees who, it is hoped, are following proper procedures. Stronger efficacy expectations, however, are produced by personal performance accomplishments than by only observing a model.

Verbal Persuasion

A third approach, verbal persuasion, is widely used by counselors in attempts to influence behavior, but is among the least effective approaches. Telling people what to do, that they possess the ability to do it, and informing them of the benefits, is not as effective, however, especially if the individual has had a previous disconfirming experience, such as a failure to follow dietary changes or perform a task at work. The impact of verbal persuasion, the encouragement of the counselor, or support from others, may vary greatly depending on the perceived credibility of the persuaders, their prestige, trustworthiness, and other factors. "If you try, I know you can be successful in making dietary changes and exercising more often" may not persuade the client to mobilize efforts to change.[13,22]

Physiological and Emotional States

Finally, people partly judge their capabilities from physiological states and emotions. Situations in which an individual has to cope with lifestyle changes may produce anxiety, stress, hunger, fatigue, and tension. Whether or not the person can perform in the face of negative signals varies with the individual. Individuals who diet and regain the weight, for example, may have lowered self-esteem. Those susceptible to anxiety may become self-preoccupied with their perceived inadequacies in the face of difficulties rather than with the task at hand. Stress-reducing exercises and discussion of correct interpretation of body signals may be of help when these problems arise.[13,22]

In summary, an effective intervention program should increase SE as well as increase the value of the outcome.[30] The dietitian may help clients use one or more of the four sources of efficacy information to raise or strengthen self-perceptions. Personal mastery of a dietary change or accomplishment of a goal is the most compelling. Small "wins" build confidence for additional changes. Good role models, such as former clients, may be enlisted to explain how they overcame difficulties by determined effort. Persuasive information is given by informing people that they are capable. The meaning of physiological information, such as anxiety, hunger, and stress, should be explained to make sure that the individual does not misread body signals and abandon efforts.

With employees, personal accomplishments give better efficacy information than telling people that they are capable of performing a job. Modeling after the performance of others, such as seeing that hard work leads to a promotion, is another source of efficacy information. Behaviors, whether good or bad, may be adopted from seeing what others are doing.

Cognitive Appraisal of Efficacy Information

Many factors affect successful performance. The extent to which success raises SE depends in part on the amount of effort expended. Laborious effort suggests less SE than success achieved through minimal effort. One's performance suggests higher SE if attained through continuous progress rather than through discouraging reversals and plateaus.

In addition, various factors enter into personal appraisals. People with high SE set higher goals with a firmer commitment, attribute failure to lack of effort, and may increase effort and persistence in achieving a goal. If people are not fully convinced of their personal efficacy, they abandon the skills they have learned when they fail to get quick results or when they experience obstacles to success. Those with low SE may attribute it to low ability. Those with negative self-beliefs do not discard them readily.[20] Even when actual performance attainments are beyond their previous expectations, they may discount their importance through faulty thoughts and evaluation or credit their achievements to factors other than to their own capabilities.

Perceived SE and personal goals enhance performance. The counselor can guide individuals to increased SE by guiding them through small, easily managed steps or goals requiring only a small effort, gradually lead them to do more difficult ones. Attainment of subgoals indicates personal mastery that can enhance SE and motivation through one's self-evaluation of performance as compared with the goal. Distant future goals are not as effective, as they are too far removed to have an effect.[13] For example, attaining the subgoal of following the dietary change today is an immediate commitment rather than a future goal of never eating desserts again. With employees, a goal of improving performance today is better than a more distant goal of improving during the month.[22,33]

Thus, in their daily lives, people approach, explore, and try to deal with situations within their self-perceived capabilities, but avoid situations they perceive as exceeding their ability. People weigh and integrate various sources of information about their capabilities, regulating their choices of behaviors, how much effort they put forth, and how long they will persist in the face of difficulties.[13,22] Efficacy expectations are presumed to influence the level of performance by enhancing intensity and persistence of effort. Thus the dietitian needs to discuss with clients and employees their judgments of their capabilities to perform a variety of tasks and the strength of the belief.

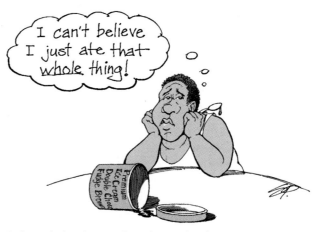

Unless one's thoughts are redirected positively, a lapse can turn into a full-blown relapse.

RELAPSE PREVENTION

"I ate the whole thing!"

The problem of giving in to temptation is a challenge for clients engaging in diet and other health behavior changes. Most people making lifestyle changes experience temporary setbacks. When they don't know how to recover, they may give up all efforts to change.

Relapse prevention (RP) refers to a group of cognitive and behavioral strategies for helping people who are changing a behavior. The self-management program is designed to help individuals anticipate and cope in high-risk situations.[34–36]

A central component of RP is a distinction between a "lapse" and a "relapse."[24,35] A lapse, such as one overeating episode at a restaurant, is a slight error, or one instance of return to a previously discontinued food behavior. It is a slip, not a total failure. A lapse may provide a learning experience if one examines the immediate precipitating circumstances and ways to correct them in the future. A relapse is a complex process and may be defined as the individual's response to a series of lapses, a loss of control, and a return to previous eating behaviors. The major goal is to notice the possibility of a lapse or relapse and find techniques for preventing it or managing it when it occurs. The dietitian works with the client to anticipate and prevent lapses that may occur during high-risk situations, and to help the individual recover from minor slips before they become a full relapse or total breakdown in self-control.

Negative cognitions and low SE ratings are of concern to counselors because they are predictive of relapse. Individuals with positive cognitions and perceived SE tend to call upon their coping skills and regulate their behavior better. Albert Bandura does not believe that appropriate behavior, such as eating what one should, is achieved by a feat of willpower. When people do not behave optimally even though they know what they should do, thoughts or cognitions may be mediating the relationship between what one knows and what one does.[13,21]

RP includes both behavioral and cognitive components.[34] In this view, behaviors may be seen as overlearned, maladaptive habits that can be analyzed and modified. The eating behavior of individuals with anorexia nervosa, bulimia, and obesity, for example, may be viewed as overlearned, maladaptive habit patterns with maladaptive coping mechanisms.[37] These maladaptive behaviors are generally followed by some sort of immediate gratification, such as feelings of pleasure or the reduction of anxiety, tension, boredom, or loneliness. When eating takes place during or prior to stressful or unpleasant situations, it represents a maladaptive coping mechanism.

A Relapse Model

The model of relapse is based on the response to high-risk situations.[34] An individual's control continues until the person encounters high-risk situations, defined as "those that challenge the individual's ability to cope."[37] See **Figure 7-1** for a simplified model.

High-Risk Situations

High-risk situations for a person on a restricted diet are of several types. Common tempting situations are emotional distress, negative emotions, moods, feelings, cravings, social situations, and negative physiological states.[35]

Negative emotional moods and feelings, such as depression, anxiety, stress, frustration, anger, boredom, loneliness, and feelings of deprivation prior to or at the time of the lapse are related to relapse. Uncontrolled eating is a common response when a person is alone. The emotional reactions increase the chance that a slip will occur and become a relapse.

Positive emotional states in which one desires to increase feelings of pleasure or celebrate an event are also a problem. A study of dieters found that negative emotional states

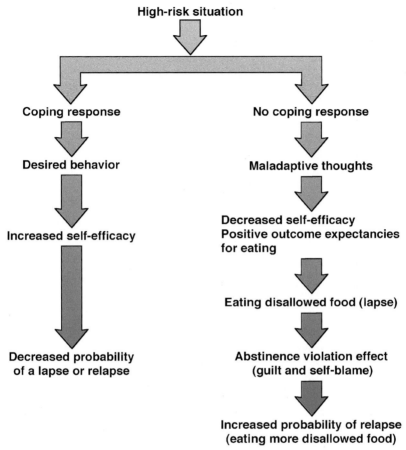

FIGURE **7-1**   Cognitive-Behavioral Model of the Relapse Process. (Modified from Marlatt GA, Gordon JR, Eds. Relapse Prevention. New York: Guilford Press, 1985.)

occurring when the individual was alone and positive emotional states involving other people, such as at social gatherings, were both difficult high-risk situations to handle, suggesting that emphasis on managing these situations should be incorporated into nutrition counseling programs.[38]

Besides individual factors, situational or environmental factors also play a role in relapse. These include social support and environmental cues. The support of family, friends, or self-help groups is associated with better success in several studies, while the opposite situation, interpersonal conflicts, such as disagreements or hassles, in relationships with family, friends, or an employer, signals the possibility of relapse.[39,40] In addition, events in the environment may provoke a relapse. Eating cues in the environment, for example, may include holidays, restaurants, and social gatherings where overeating is socially acceptable. Social pressures from others occur when individuals tempt or coax ("Eat it. Just this once won't hurt you.") and when a person sees others consuming foods not on his or her dietary regimen. ("Everyone else is eating it. Why shouldn't I?")

Box **7-2**

Examples of High-Risk Situations

Physiological feelings of hunger, fatigue, food cravings, tension
Attending social affairs, parties, eating in restaurants
Holidays
Low self-efficacy or inadequate motivation
Stress
Negative self-talk
Lack of social support from family, friends, or coworkers
Interpersonal conflicts
Positive emotional states (i.e., fun and celebration of an event)
Negative emotional states or moods (i.e., depression; anxiety; frustration; anger; boredom; loneliness; feeling deprived, upset, sad, or worried)

Finally, negative physiological factors may contribute to relapse. Urges and cravings for foods, feeling of hunger, fatigue, or headache, changes in metabolic rate during weight loss, and metabolic tendencies toward weight regain when lapsing from a diet may increase the likelihood of relapse. **Box 7-2** summarizes examples of high-risk situations.

Researchers studying problem situations that create obstacles to dietary adherence in adults with diabetes identified 12 such situations: negative emotions and stress, which tempted people to overeat; food, food cues, or cravings, which made it difficult to resist temptation; eating in restaurants; feeling deprived; time pressures; feeling tempted to give up; lack of time for advance planning of what and when to eat; competing priorities; social events; lack of family support; inability to refuse inappropriate food offered; and lack of support of friends. An individual's ability to cope in these high-risk situations should be assessed so that problem-solving strategies can be a part of counseling.[41]

In adolescents with diabetes mellitus, 10 obstacles were found, including being tempted to stop trying; negative emotional eating; seeing forbidden foods; peer interpersonal conflict; competing priorities; eating at school; social events and holidays; food cravings; snacking when home alone or bored; and social pressures to eat. The counselor can assist clients in dealing with these situations.[42] Among postpartum women, barriers to reducing food intake included emotional and physical stress, social situations including food, lack of time, and eating snacks and convenience foods with a high energy density.[30]

High-risk situations for failure to exercise were identified. They include bad weather, lack of time or inconvenient time of day, negative emotions, safety concerns, child care, money, fatigue, and being alone.[43]

SELF-ASSESSMENT

Using the examples of high-risk situations in Box 7-2, identify those that are high-risk situations for your own eating.

Identification and Assessment of High-Risk Situations

Assessment of high-risk situations may be viewed as a two-stage process.[44] In the first stage, an attempt is made to identify specific situations that may pose a problem for a client in terms of lapse or relapse. The use of self-monitoring records is helpful in identifying these situations as well as in raising the individual's level of awareness of food choices made. Self-monitoring is an intervention in itself and may reduce some of the behaviors.

Eating may be an automatic response that cannot be dealt with until there is a conscious awareness that one is eating without any conscious decision to do so. SE ratings can be assessed by giving the client a series of descriptions of specific situations and asking him or her to rate how difficult it would be to cope. The counselor may ask the client to identify the difficulty on a 5-point scale, with 5 being the most difficulty. Autobiographical statements about the history and development of the dietary problem and descriptions of past relapses are other techniques that may be used.[44] People who coped successfully may have relied on behavioral avoidance of events or on cognitive strategies, such as thinking positively about goals for change or the negative consequences of a slip.

Responses to High-Risk Situations or Coping Versus Failure to Cope

There are two possibilities when a person is in a high-risk situation—a coping response or lack of a coping response (see Figure 7-1). If the individual copes, SE is increased and there is less probability of a lapse or relapse. For example, the client thinks: "I'm not hungry so I won't eat," "I'll take a walk instead of eating," or "I'll phone my friend instead of eating."

After identifying high-risk situations, the second stage is an assessment of the client's coping skills or capacity to respond involving both thoughts and actions. One can evaluate these in simulated situations with role-playing or in written form. The individual can role-play responses to high-risk situations with the counselor or fellow group members. Videotapes of these sessions may be helpful if they are available.

Abstinence from less preferable foods is frequently viewed

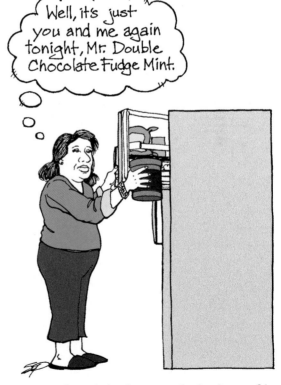

An individual faces a high-risk situation related to the time of day (arriving home from work) and the cognition.

by individuals from an all-or-nothing perspective. Marlatt postulates a cognitive "abstinence violation effect" (AVE) when a person violates the commitment to change food choices and consumes a food that he or she should not eat.[36]

Possible responses to giving in to temptation are[45]:

- One feels guilty, has lowered self-esteem, and blames oneself for the loss of control or indulgence in food. ("I shouldn't have eaten it, but I did. I'm guilty.")
- An obese individual may continue to eat to relieve the guilt ("I ate one cookie and I blew it. I might as well eat the whole bag.")
- A person may alter his or her cognition from being a restrainer to an indulger. ("I never could follow the diet anyway.")
- The person may rationalize. ("I deserve a break today. I owe myself this food.")
- The person may change his or her commitment to save face. ("I changed my mind about following this dietary regimen and decided to eat whatever I want.")

Lapses affect both people's thoughts and their feelings. If there is no coping response and the person feels unable to exert control, he or she experiences a decrease in self-efficacy, sometimes coupled with a sense of helplessness and passive giving in to the situation. ("It's no use. I can't stop myself.") In this all-or-nothing perspective, a single lapse leads to giving up. If the person has positive outcome expectancies of immediate gratification from eating ("It will taste delicious. I will feel better if I eat this.") and ignores the negative health consequences, the probability of lapse or relapse is enhanced. The individual experiences a conflict of motives between a desire to maintain control and the temptation to give in.[45,46] The person consumes less desirable foods and a slip or lapse has occurred. There can be a problem in reestablishing control.

It is important to educate clients about the relapse process since it is unlikely that people will recognize the range of situations that may trigger eating.[35] When the individual's unique high-risk situations (thoughts, feelings, people, situations) are identified, the dietitian can teach the person to look for cues, such as an upcoming party, vacation, or stressful time at work. The client can take preventive action and make advance decisions about how to cope. The goal of treatment is to help the client learn to anticipate and prevent the occurrence of lapses and relapse or help the individual recover from a lapse before it escalates into a full-blown relapse or total breakdown in control.[44] When high-risk situations, temptations, and urges occur, relapse prevention techniques are designed to enhance SE in coping.

Lapses are inevitable. The counselor needs to advise clients to expect this possibility and prepare them to handle it. Failure to do so deprives the client of the opportunity for developing skills to cope with a lapse or relapse or minimize damage if one occurs. Using the term "lapse" avoids the value judgment associated with a term like "cheating" on the diet. Everyone will, on occasion, overeat or eat tempting foods. Marlatt and Gordon use the metaphor of a fire drill: a person practices to escape a fire even though fires are rare.[36]

Each mistake is viewed as an opportunity for new learning, not a personal failure. The goal is to teach the individual involved in a behavior change program how to identify situations with a high risk for lapse and relapse, to use problem-solving and coping strategies when confronted with these situations, and to deal with the negative thoughts that accompany a lapse.

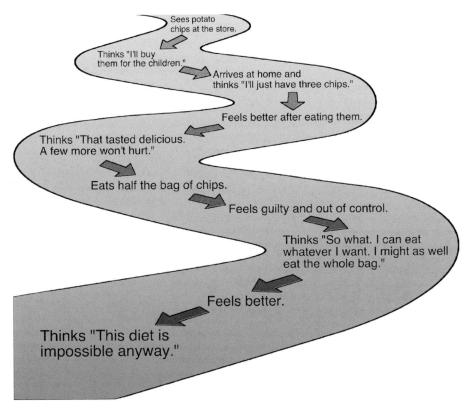

FIGURE 7-2 In Failing to Cope, One's Thoughts Affect Eating.

The reward of instant gratification may far outweigh negative health effects in a distant future. Thus, a single lapse, or series of lapses, may snowball into a full-blown relapse from which it is more difficult to recover. **Figure 7-2** is an example of failing to cope at the grocery store and at home in the presence of the external cue of potato chips. The loss of control and dysfunctional self-talk result in binge eating and relapse.

Cognitive restructuring may be used also to counter the cognitive and affective components of the abstinence violation effect. Instead of seeing the first lapse as a sign of failure characterized by conflict, guilt, and personal attribution, the client is taught to view it as a single event or small mistake rather than a total disaster, and to recognize that it is possible to resume the lifestyle change right away and learn from mistakes.

Clients initiate dietary changes with varying degrees of motivation and commitment. In addition, some who appear to be highly motivated initially may discover that long-term change is more difficult than first imagined. Initial response to treatment may predict later lack of success if much backsliding occurs early on. Low levels of SE are predictive of relapse.[35] Patients on weight reduction diets who lose some weight, for example, and those who struggle but adhere to their dietary regimens, may be able to cope with temporary setbacks. The construct of motivation may differ among people from collectivistic cultures where people interact in the group.[47]

Coping skills include cognitive responses, such as positive self-talk ("I can do it."), behavioral responses, such as calling a friend instead of eating less preferable foods, and beliefs about SE, or judgments concerning whether or not one can respond effectively in a situation. In one study, abstinence-violation effects were more strongly associated with lapses than with temptations.[48]

Other Treatment Strategies

Food habits or eating behaviors are assumed to be shaped by prior learning experiences. Changing these habits involves the active participation and responsibility of the client, who eventually becomes the agent of change. In a self-management program, the individual acquires new skills and cognitive strategies so that behaviors are under the regulation of higher mental processes and responsible decision making.

Coping skill training implies the actual acquisition of a new behavior through overt practice and rehearsal. One does not acquire a new skill, such as playing tennis, by verbal instruction alone. Actual practice of coping skills is essential.[44] Both cognitive and action coping strategies may be needed—"Practice makes perfect," as an old saying goes. Baseball players do not hit a home run every time they are at bat. In fact they may not even get a hit. If they strike out once, they just try again the next time.

Modeling, behavioral rehearsal, use of positive self-talk, direct instruction, and coaching and feedback from the counselor are useful. Role reversal with the client teaching the practitioner how to cope with a high-risk situation and handle a lapse will give the client more convincing arguments than any counselor could provide. Increasing SE through successful performance and modeling of positive self-statements are recommended, such as "I can handle it."[44]

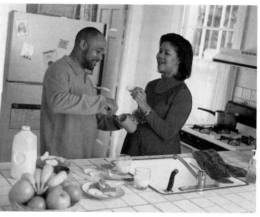

When you are hungry or upset, the availability of high-calorie foods presents a high-risk situation.
Source: United States Department of Agriculture.

Covert modeling—mental rehearsal through imagined scenarios in which the client engages in coping responses when temptations are present and feels good about it—may be used to cope with reactions to a slip or lapse.[44] Another strategy is called "urge surfing." When confronted with an urge to binge, clients are asked to imagine their urge is an ocean wave building to a crest. The challenge is to ride the wave and remain in balance without being "wiped out."[49] One continues until the urge to eat has passed.

As an antidote to stress, relaxation training; positive self-talk; meditation; exercise instead of eating; visualization of relaxing, pleasant scenes or of carrying out coping behaviors when tempted; and stress management procedures may be needed.[37] In visualization, clients are asked to close their eyes and think of a stressful or tempting situation in which they might find themselves. The counselor can help them create a mental image of the situation by asking questions that create a visual picture of the situation and the accompanying emotions. If imagining a party, for example, the counselor may ask: "What do the surroundings look like?" "What are you doing?" "What are other people doing?" "Where are the foods and beverages?" "What will you choose?" "Who can you turn to for support?" "What will you say?" "How do you feel?"

Patients with eating disorders can make written plans for lapses and relapses, identifying early warning signs of a slip and strategies to stay on track. These can be carried on reminder index cards for referral.[14]

Adopting a problem-solving orientation to stressful situations or modeling problem solving by thinking out loud with clients is helpful. The counselor and client can review the events and emotions in past lapses and relapses since patterns may repeat themselves. When lapses are discussed, it is preferable to discuss how the individual might have succeeded in preference to focusing on the failures.

MODELS AND THEORIES OF CHANGE

In the TTM, or Stages of Change, recycling to a previous stage is expected as people go through the five stages of precontemplation, contemplation, preparation, action, and maintenance. RP strategies are important, especially in the action and maintenance stages of change. Patients with eating disorders and other nutritional problems can be expected to progress through all five stages with frequent backsliding.

People in the action stage will encounter high-risk situations, stresses, and temptations that tax coping efforts.[24] They may slip or lapse in one situation and resist in another. The majority are not successful at the first attempt at change. Relapse commences with recycling to an earlier stage and can be viewed as a learning opportunity. In a study of obese women, poor coping or problem-solving skills and low SE had an important effect on weight maintenance behaviors and relapse.[50]

Chronic problems may require long-term treatment even in the maintenance stage of change. Just as Rome was not built in a day, neither is successful dietary change established in a short period of time. It may not be sufficient to teach new ways of eating and turn people loose and unaccountable on a maintenance program.

Clients need to learn strategies to cope with the normal urge to lapse into old habits. Self-monitoring and self-management skills are needed. They should be more successful when they keep in contact with a counselor, at least by phone, for a year or more. The model of life-long treatment is used by several groups, such as Alcoholics Anonymous, Overeaters Anonymous, and the lifetime membership offered in Weight Watchers.

One would hope that our models and theories of health behavior change would explain and predict change and better direct interventions. Social cognitive theories, the Health Behavior Model, the TTM, and other theories have limited success in explaining dietary change. Food practices are the result of a number of interacting variables.

Baronowski suggests that interventions do not change behaviors directly, but can be designed to change mediating variables. The change in strongly related mediating variables (psychosocial, behavioral, environmental, and biological) can result in behavioral change.[51] Changes in family food practices, for example, may be a strongly related mediating variable resulting in change.

Brug suggests that nutrition and physical activity are complex collections of specific behaviors, each with its own specific determinants related to abilities, opportunities, and motivation. Thus behavior change is not merely a case of convincing clients that the pros of change outweigh the cons.[52]

Resnicow and Vaughan offer the Chaos Theory and Dynamic Systems Theory as competing views of health behavior change. They argue that behavioral change is not linear, but instead is a chaotic system that occurs in quantum leaps from a surge in inspiration or motivation, sudden insights, mini-epiphanies, an "aha!" event, and tipping points that may be random and impossible to predict. They suggest that motivation "arrives" rather than being planned. While they recognize that factors such as knowledge, attitude, belief, and efficacy exert some influence on health behavior change, these factors interact in a complex system altered by many variables. They conclude that behavior change includes both chaotic and rational, linear processes. Periodic exposure in counseling models, such as motivational interviewing, allows clients to explore life both with and without behavioral change.[53]

While all theories and models are valuable, additional scientific research is needed as a basis for planning more effective interventions. This research would contribute to solving the rising epidemic of obesity and to health behavior change.[54]

In summary, the counselor may use a number of counseling approaches with clients. This chapter describes the use of cognitive restructuring of negative and dysfunctional thoughts, and outlines methods that increase the client's SE or self-confidence to change a behavior.

Counselors should give clients a summary or overview of the relapse process. Clients with an increased level of awareness in high-risk situations are better prepared to utilize their coping skills and take remedial action to avoid a lapse or relapse. People need to see themselves as capable agents of control rather than as helpless victims in situations beyond their control.

CASE STUDY 1

Carol Jones is a 50-year-old woman recently diagnosed with type 2 diabetes mellitus. Her maternal grandmother had diabetes. Mrs. Jones was an overweight child and is an overweight adult at 5'4" and 180 pounds. She is married and works part-time at a retail clothing store at a local mall.

Dr. Smith referred her for counseling to lose weight. The dietitian, Joan Stivers, notes in her assessment that Mrs. Jones seems to have a problem with low self-image and negative cognitions. Her diagnosis is overweight related to cognitive distortions. As a result, her current priority is cognitive restructuring.

1. Complete the professional's response to each of the client's statements. Do not give advice. Instead seek further information with a paraphrase of the thought or the feeling or a summary of what she said.

CASE STUDY 1

Professional: "The doctor referred you because losing weight will help to improve your blood sugar levels."

   a. Mrs. Jones: "I've always been heavy. I don't think I can lose weight."

     Professional: _____.

   b. Mrs. Jones: "My husband likes me the way I am. He does not think I am overweight."

     Professional: _____.

   c. Mrs. Jones: "I lost 10 pounds once before. But it was just a fluke. I couldn't do it again."

     Professional: _____.

   d. Mrs. Jones: "When I go out to eat at a restaurant, I won't get my money's worth if I don't eat the food they serve."

     Professional: _____.

   e. Mrs. Jones: "When the holidays come, my friends bring me candy and other goodies. So my husband and I eat them. We can't waste food."

     Professional: _____.

2. What nutrition diagnosis would you make?
3. What nutrition intervention(s) would you make?
4. Develop written documentation for your session with this client, incorporating the Nutrition Care Process (NCP) model as applicable.

CASE STUDY 2

Betty has been off and on diets to control her weight for the past 10 years and always regained the weight. She is 45 years old and employed full-time as a librarian. Currently, she is 5'5" and weights 185 pounds. She is married to Stan, who is 25 pounds overweight, and they have one son who is 15 years old. Before her son was born, she weighed 150 pounds.

Betty has sought the advice of Joan Stivers, a registered dietitian in private practice, in order to lose weight. She expresses confidence that she can lose weight with the dietitian's help. The dietitian is concerned with Betty's "yo-yo" dieting and has decided to counsel her on lifestyle modification, emphasizing relapse prevention so that she can maintain any weight she loses.

1. What Stage of Change is Betty in?
2. How would you help her in preventing lapses and relapse as she loses weight with lifestyle modification?
3. Develop written documentation for your session with this client, incorporating the NCP model as applicable.

REVIEW AND DISCUSSION QUESTIONS

1. What is cognitive-behavioral therapy?
2. What effect do negative cognitions have on behavioral change?
3. What types of cognitive distortions do people have?
4. Explain the three phases of cognitive restructuring.
5. Describe examples of coping skills the counselor may teach to the client?
6. What is the relationship between an outcome expectancy and an efficacy expectancy?
7. How do self-perceptions of efficacy affect a person's choice of activities?
8. Explain an individual's four sources of efficacy information. How does each affect behavior?
9. What is the difference between a lapse and a relapse?
10. Explain the relapse model.
11. What are examples of high-risk situations?
12. What strategies can help to prevent relapse?

SUGGESTED ACTIVITIES

1. Keep a log of what you eat during one day noting your thoughts about food before eating, during eating, and after eating. Are the thoughts positive or negative? What percent are positive? Negative? This will increase your awareness.
2. Identify you own high-risk situations for eating and how you respond. What happens if you cope with the situation? What happens if you are unable to cope with the situation? How do you feel?
3. For each of the following client cognitions, forecast how the client will behave. Then develop a more positive, coping thought.
   A. "I've never been able to stick to any low calorie diet for more than a week."
   B. "The food doesn't taste any good without salt."
   C. "There are chocolate chip cookies in the cupboard, and I sure could use a few after the day I've had. I deserve a treat."
   D. "Here is a commercial break on my television show. Guess I'll check the refrigerator."
   E. "That leftover pie looks good, but I don't need it."
   F. "I've blown my whole diet eating that apple pie with ice cream. What's the use?"
   G. "I don't have time to prepare all of that special food today."
4. For 2 days, keep a tally of the number of times people use the terms "should," "shouldn't," "must," "have to," or "ought to" in statements about themselves. Or keep a tally of the number of times you use these terms.
5. For 2 or more days, consume a modified diet (low fat, low calorie, restricted sodium, high fiber, etc.). Keep a log of your thoughts. Identify any high-risk situations.
6. Each evening for 2 days, make a written list of all of your successes or things you accomplished. Give yourself a verbal pat on the back with a positive cognition.

WEB SITES

http://www.anred.com/relpr.html   Relapse prevention in anorexia nervosa and eating disorders

http://www.beckinstitute.org   Beck Institute for Cognitive Therapy and Research

http://www.cognitivetherapynyc.com   American Institute for Cognitive Therapy

http://www.cttoday.org   Cognitive therapy today blog

http://www.des.emory.edu/mfp/BanEncy.html   Information on self-efficacy

http://www.des.emory.edu/mfp/bandurabio.html   Biographical sketch of Albert Bandura

http://www.mirror-mirror.org/relprev.htm   Relapse prevention, eating disorders

http://www.nacbt.org/whatiscbt.htm   National Association of Cognitive-Behavioral Therapists

http://nationalpsychologist.com/articles/art_v9n5_3.htm   Article on relapse prevention from the *National Psychologist*

http://patienteducation.stanford.edu/research/sediabetes.html   Stanford Patient Education Research Center, Diabetes Self-Efficacy Scale

http://www.umbc.edu/psyc/habits/TTM-O.html   Self-efficacy scales for weight management, eating, and exercise and some available for public use

http://www.uri.edu/research/cprc/Measures/Exercise04.htm   Cancer Prevention Research Center, Exercise Self-Efficacy Scale

REFERENCES

1. Burns DD. The Feeling Good Handbook. New York: Plume, 1999.
2. McKay M, Fanning P, Davis M. Thoughts & Feelings: Taking Control of Your Moods and Your Life: A Workbook of Cognitive Behavioral Techniques. Oakland, CA: New Harbinger Publications, 1997.
3. Position of the American Dietetic Association. Nutrition intervention in the treatment of anorexia nervosa, bulimia nervosa, and eating disorders not otherwise specified. J Am Diet Assoc 2006;106:2073–2082.
4. Cooper Z, Fairburn CG, Hawker DM. Cognitive-Behavioral Treatment of Obesity: A Clinician's Guide. New York: Guilford Press, 2003.
5. Teixeira PJ, Going SB, Houtkooper LB, et al. Pretreatment predictors of attrition and successful weight management in women. Int J Obes Relat Metab Disord 2004;28:1124–1133.
6. Costain L, Croker H. Helping individuals to help themselves. Proc Nutr Soc 2005;64:89–96.
7. Wisotsky W, Swencionis C. Cognitive-behavioral approaches in the management of obesity. Adolesc Med 2003;14:37–48.
8. Greenwald A. Current nutritional treatments of obesity. Adv Psychosom Med 2006;27:24–41.
9. Foreyt JP. The role of lifestyle modification in dysmetabolic syndrome management. Nestle Nutr Workshop Ser Clin Perform Programme 2006;11:197–205.
10. Commission on Accreditation for Dietetics Education. 2002 Eligibility Requirements and Accreditation Standards. Chicago: American Dietetic Association, 2006.
11. Beck JS. Cognitive Therapy: Basics and Beyond. New York: Guilford Press, 1995.

12. Meichenbaum D. Cognitive-behavior modification. In: Kanfer FH, Goldstein AP, eds. Helping People Change. 3rd Ed. New York: Pergamon Press, 1986.

13. Bandura A. Exercise of personal and collective efficacy in changing societies. In Bandura A, ed. Self-Efficacy in Changing Societies. New York: Cambridge University Press, 1995.

14. Peterson CB, Mitchell J E. Cognitive-behavioral therapy for eating disorders. In: Mitchell JE, ed. The Outpatient Treatment of Eating Disorders: A Guide for Therapists, Dietitians, and Physicians. Minneapolis: University of Minnesota Press, 2001.

15. Fabricatore AN. Behavior therapy and cognitive-behavioral therapy of obesity: is there a difference? J Am Diet Assoc 2007;107:92–99.

16. Wright JH, Basco, MR, Thase ME. Learning Cognitive-Behavior Therapy: An Illustrated Guide. Washington, DC: American Psychiatric Publishing, 2006.

17. Mossavar-Rahmani Y, Henry H, Rodabough R, et al. Additional self-monitoring tools in the dietary modification component of the Women's Health Initiative. J Am Diet Assoc 2004;104: 76–85.

18. Glasgow RE, Tooberi DJ, Mitchell DL, et al. Nutrition education and social learning interventions for type II diabetes. Diabetes Care 1989;12:150–152.

19. Prochaska JO, Redding CA, Evers KE. The transtheoretical model and stages of change. In: Glanz K, Rimer BK, Lewis FM, eds. Health Behavior and Health Education: Theory, Research, and Practice. 3rd Ed. San Francisco: Jossey-Bass, 2002.

20. Bandura A. Health promotion by social cognitive means. Health Educ Behav 2004;31:143–164.

21. Bandura A. Social Foundations of Thought and Action: A Social Cognitive Theory. Englewood Cliffs, NJ: Prentice-Hall, 1986.

22. Bandura A. Self-Efficacy: The Exercise of Control. New York: WH Freeman, 1997.

23. Baranowski T, Perry CL, Parcel GS. How individuals, environments, and health behavior interact: social cognitive theory. In: Glanz K, Rimer BK, Lewis FM, eds. Health Behavior and Health Education: Theory, Research, and Practice. 3rd Ed. San Francisco: Jossey-Bass, 2002.

24. DiClemente CC. Addiction and Change: How Addictions Develop and Addicted People Recover. New York: Guilford Press, 2003.

25. Anderson RM, Funnell MM, Fitzgerald JT, et al. The diabetes empowerment scale: a measure of psychosocial self-efficacy. Diabetes Care 2000;23:739–743.

26. Sigurdardottir AK. Self-care in diabetes: model of factors affecting self-care. J Clin Nurs 2005; 14:301–314.

27. Johnston-Brooks CH, Lewis MA, Garg S. Self-efficacy impacts self-care and HbA_{1c} in young adults with type I diabetes. Psychosom Med 2002;64:43–51.

28. Wamsteker EW, Geenen R, Iestra J, et al. Obesity-related beliefs predict weight loss after an 8-week low-calorie diet. J Am Diet Assoc 2005;105:441–444.

29. Roach JB, Yadrick MK, Johnson JT, et al. Using self-efficacy to predict weight loss among young adults. J Am Diet Assoc 2003;103:1357–1359.

30. Hinton PS, Olson CM. Postpartum exercise and food intake: the importance of behavior-specific self-efficacy. J Am Diet Assoc 2001;101:1430–1437.

31. Bardone-Cone AM, Abramson LY, Vohs KD, et al. Predicting bulimic symptoms: an interactive model of self-efficacy, perfectionism, and perceived weight status. Behav Res Ther 2006; 44:27–42.

32. Henry H, Reimer K, Smith C, et al. Associations of decisional balance processes of change and self-efficacy with stages of change for increased fruit and vegetable intake among low-income, African-American mothers. J Am Diet Assoc 2006;106:841–849.

33. Bandura A, Locke EA. Negative self-efficacy and goal effects revisited. J Appl Psychol 2003;88: 87–99.

34. Marlatt GA, Witkiewitz K. Relapse prevention for alcohol and drug problems. In: Marlatt GA, Donovan DM, eds. Relapse Prevention: Maintenance Strategies in the Treatment of Addictive Behaviors. 2nd Ed. New York: Guilford Press, 2005.

35. Donovan DM. Assessment of addictive behaviors for relapse prevention. In: Donovan DM, Marlatt GA, eds. Assessment of Addictive Behaviors. 2nd Ed. New York: Guilford Press, 2005.

36. Marlatt GA. Relapse prevention: theoretical rationale and overview of the model. In: Marlatt GA, Gordon JR, eds. Relapse Prevention. New York: Guilford Press, 1985.

37. Collins RL. Relapse prevention for eating disorders and obesity. In: Marlatt GA, Donovan DM, eds. Relapse Prevention: Maintenance Strategies in the Treatment of Addictive Behaviors. 2nd Ed. New York: Guilford Press, 2005.

38. Sternberg B. Relapse in weight control: definitions, processes, and prevention strategies. In: Marlatt GA, Gordon JR, eds. Relapse Prevention. New York: Guilford Press, 1985.

39. McCann BS, Retzlaff BM, Dowdy AA, et al. Promoting adherence to low-fat, low-cholesterol diets: review and recommendations. J Am Diet Assoc 1990;90:408.

40. DeWolfe JA, Shannon BM. Factors affecting fat consumption of university students: testing a model to predict eating behavior. J Canadian Diet Assoc 1993;54:132.

41. Schlundt DG, Rea MR, Kline SS, et al. Situational obstacles to dietary adherence for adults with diabetes. J Am Diet Assoc 1994;94:874–876, 879.

42. Schlundt DG, Pichert JW, Rea MR, et al. Situational obstacles to adherence for adolescents with diabetes. Diabetes Educator 1994;20:207–211.

43. Stetson BA, Beacham AO, Frommelt SJ, et al. Exercise slips in high-risk situations and activity patterns in long-term exercisers: an application of the relapse prevention model. Ann Behav Med. 2005;30:25–35.

44. Marlatt GA. Situational determinants of relapse and skill-training interventions. In: Marlatt GA, Gordon JR, eds. Relapse Prevention. New York: Guilford Press, 1985.

45. Marlatt, GA Cognitive factors in the relapse process. In: Marlatt GA, Gordon JR, eds. Relapse Prevention. New York: Guilford Press, 1985.

46. Marlatt GA. Cognitive assessment and intervention procedures in relapse prevention. In: Marlatt GA, Gordon JR, eds. Relapse Prevention. New York: Guilford Press, 1985.

47. Blume AW, Morera OF, DeLaCruz BG. Assessment of addictive behaviors in ethnic-minority cultures. In: Donovan DM, Marlatt GA, eds. Assessment of Addictive Behaviors. 2nd Ed. New York: Guilford Press, 2005.

48. Carels RA, Douglass OM, Cacciapaglia HM, et al. An ecological momentary assessment of relapse crises in dieting. J Consult Clin Psychol 2004;72:341–348.

49. Marlatt GA, Baer JS, Quigley LA. Self-efficacy and addictive behavior. In: Bandura A, ed. Self-Efficacy in Changing Societies. New York: Cambridge University Press, 1995.

50. Byrne SM. Psychological aspects of weight maintenance and relapse in obesity. J Psychosom Res 2002;53:l029–1036.

51. Baranowski T. Advances in basic behavioral research will make the most important contributions to effective dietary change programs at this time. J Am Diet Assoc 2006; 106:808–811.

52. Brug J. Order is needed to promote linear or quantum changes in nutrition and physical activity behaviors: a reaction to 'A chaotic view of behavior change' by Resnicow and Vaughan. Int J Behav Nutr Phys Act 2006;3:29.

53. Resnicow K, Vaughan R. A chaotic view of behavior change: a quantum leap for health promotion. Int J Behav Nutr Phys Act 2006;3:25.

54. Baranowski T. Crisis and chaos in behavioral nutrition and physical activity. Int J Behav Nutr Phys Act 2006;3:27.

Cross-Cultural and Life-Span Counseling

OBJECTIVES

- Discuss the challenges of diversity.
- Describe the management of diverse employees.
- Identify the stages of cultural competence in nutrition counseling.
- List the barriers that may appear in counseling culturally diverse clients and identify strategies to handle them.
- Explore resources to learn about different cultures.
- Identify potential barriers in cross-cultural communication.
- Describe the nutritional issues that one should be aware of when counseling at different ages in the life span.
- Explain the strategies for working with individuals throughout the life span and for those with limited literacy.

In the United States, the population is 12.9% African American, 12.4% Hispanic or Latino, and 4.2% Asian.[1] The Hispanic population has increased by more than 50% since 1990.[2]

The issue of diversity is not new. After all, the United States has an increasingly heterogeneous population and has been called a "nation of immigrants." The government health objectives for the nation published in *Healthy People 2010* reflect the health needs of a diverse population.[3] Because dietetics professionals encounter diverse clients every day, they must make an effort to learn about customs and cultures different from their own so they can develop efficient methods and strategies for serving all of their clients.

What is diversity? According to Arthur, diversity consists of the many ways in which individuals are unique or different while at the same time being similar in other ways.[4] The United States is home to individuals and families of varied cultural and ethnic backgrounds, who speak many different languages. Its population encompasses people of different races, religions, genders, sexual orientations, body sizes, physical abilities, health status, educational levels, ages, work experiences, lifestyles, values, marital status, socioeconomic status, and the like. It is important to value and understand all types of diversity.

This chapter begins by examining the dietetics professional's role in communicating with culturally diverse clients and workplace employees. Next, it explores the challenges that dietitians encounter while counseling individuals and families at various stages in the life span. Lastly, this chapter provides information on communicating with those of limited literacy.

WORKPLACE DIVERSITY

Although there has always been diversity in the workforce, federal legislation mandating equal employment opportunities, affirmative action, and access for people with disabilities spurred changes in the 1960s and beyond. In addition, the annual influx of new immigrants, most recently people of Hispanic descent, has contributed to cultural diversity. In earlier years, most immigrants came from Europe and Canada.[4] More recently, immigrants have come from Asia, Mexico, Latin America, and Central America. For example, in 2002, 52% of U.S. immigrants were from Latin America, 25% were from Asia, and only 14% were from Europe.[5] By 2010 it is estimated that almost half the nation's new workers will be people traditionally classified as "minorities."[6]

Challenges of Diversity

Many immigrants who choose to make the United States their home face issues of assimilation. Generally, the first generation of immigrants has the most difficulty adapting to American culture. Many of them experience problems in speaking and interpreting the English language. Literacy can often be the biggest problem for non-native learners or clients who must now read or write in English, rather than in their native language. Thus, health care professionals may experience difficulty in communicating with their workers.

Food service departments employ a large proportion of immigrant populations and ethnic groups. As this pool of available employees continues to become more culturally diverse, dietetics professionals face numerous challenges. First, health care professionals and managers are faced with the challenge of integrating this diverse population into the workforce. Second, dietetics professionals are faced with the challenge of developing strategies and training programs that allow all workers to communicate with one another and with their clients. As many different types of immigrant populations are employed within the industry, a non-English language barrier might also exist between managers, staff, and clients who often speak different languages. This language barrier may translate into a literacy problem because non–English-speaking people may have difficulties reading and writing in a language different than their native language. Third, food service professionals are faced with the challenge of cultural assimilation. Many new immigrants intent on making the United States their home encounter difficulties adapting to American culture because of the language barrier or resistance to changing their cultural customs. Therefore, bilingual kitchens and cultural assimilation are a modern challenge faced by all health care employers and employees.

Another area of diversity in the workplace involves age. As more people attend and graduate from college, an influx of skilled, young professionals enters the workforce.[7] Younger workers in their 20s and 30s may seem to have more opportunities for advancement than older workers because they are thought to be knowledgeable about the latest theories and innovations within their field. Moreover, the aging worker may appear to have a greater interest in balancing work and career with family responsibilities and outside interests. Older workers may be seeking jobs that are more fulfilling and may be willing to seek other employment if job satisfaction falls or fails to satisfy. Therefore, their values, priorities, and goals may differ from those of younger workers.

Benefits of Diversity

There are many benefits to a diverse organization. First, organizations that are composed of diverse employees are better able to develop and implement a variety of ideas, policies, and programs.[4,8] By hiring people from a multitude of backgrounds, who possess different viewpoints, experiences, and ideologies, an organization can better meet the needs and demands of the population at large. Second, a diverse staff can be essential for companies that serve diverse consumers or customer groups. Studies have shown that customers better identify with service providers whose gender and ethnic background is similar to their own. This finding may be attributed to imbedded norms that enable the customer to better understand and relate to the service provider. An organization composed of diverse employees is also good for business because it enables the company to better understand a certain segment of the market that it is targeting for a product or service. If the organization reflects the community it serves, there is an increased chance that it will provide the goods and services that are needed or wanted.

Management professionals need to be committed to developing and supporting diverse groups and teams so they can effectively create a culturally diverse workforce.[9] In an effort to create a culturally diverse organization, managers must consider diversity in job interviews, supervision of employees, staff development programs, and in the creation of a harassment-free work environment. For example, in recruitment practices managers should advertise job descriptions in places where minority groups might see them.[10] All members of the organization, including those of the dominant culture, must not only accept diversity, but also make a commitment to it and value it.

Managing Diversity

The goal of an effective organization and operative workplace is to foster an environment in which all employees maximize their potential by contributing a variety of talents and abilities.[8] To do so, managers must harness cultural differences and create a productive environment where people feel their skill set is being efficiently utilized and valued.[11] As such, all employees must be viewed as assets who work together toward achieving the universal goals and objectives of the organization, while prospering individually.

Although it is necessary to treat everyone within the organization with respect, some members of the organization may have difficulty developing cultural sensitivity and may inadvertently treat employees differently. Moreover, when dealing with colleagues or clients who are different from them, some people may have a tendency to make assumptions or generalizations about the behaviors of these individuals.[10] For example, in some professional environments there is a tendency to label workers by their race, ethnicity, or sexual orientation.[4] Specifically, people might still refer to a colleague as being the black supervisor, white waiter, Mexican cook, Japanese hostess, gay dishwasher, or Puerto Rican manager. In order to rectify this ethnic labeling, people must be made aware of their biases, examine their own prejudices and work to overcome them. It is important not just to accept diversity, but also to value it and demonstrate acceptance of it through words and actions.

In diversity-driven environments, individuality is nurtured. Thus, differences in ideas and experiences can lead to more creative solutions to problems and better decisions.[4] Collaboration, consensus, and shared power, whereby professional authority is shared and determined by one's knowledge and skill set, make everyone feel more equal.[12] In these types of work environments, the employees are more productive and the company is more competitive in achieving it objectives.

The permanent change in how employees work together may take time; however, it is the responsibility of professionals to establish a workplace where cultural acceptance is the norm. The following are some questions to consider when evaluating workplace diversity:

- Are all employees viewed as assets?
- Are there lower expectations of any employees because of their ethnicity?
- Is there an overall atmosphere of acceptance and encouragement for all workers?
- Do diverse workers have levels of responsibility comparable to the dominant group?
- Are managers' expectations lower for certain ethnic groups or individuals?
- Are certain ethnic groups overrepresented or underrepresented in some departments or areas?
- Are hiring and promotion opportunities open to all? What percent of management positions are filled by women and minorities? Are minorities or women regarded as "token" employees or are they respected? Are they resented?
- Are everyone's ideas, proposals, and suggestions taken seriously?
- Do all groups participate in the normal socialization and networking during work hours?
- Are English-speaking employees impatient with those who speak English slowly or poorly?
- Are different cultural mannerisms and body language accepted or misunderstood and ridiculed?
- Are all people treated with patience, tolerance, and understanding?

HEALTH DISPARITIES IN DIVERSE POPULATION GROUPS

Among various ethnic, cultural, and life-span populations, there are particular health concerns, unmet needs, and barriers to meeting health and nutrition issues. In response to this the U.S. Department of Health and Human Services' Office of Disease Prevention and Health Promotion established national health objectives published in *Healthy People 2000*.[13] This document provided a framework to serve as a basis for developing community plans to improve the health of our nation and has been evaluated and updated in the subsequently published *Healthy People 2010*.

The two overall goals of *Healthy People 2010* are (1) to increase quality and years of life and (2) to eliminate health disparities. Both goals are aimed at improving health and wellness throughout the life span as well as for all population groups.

Two of the 10 leading health indicators that track and measure the health of our nation are physical activity and overweight/obesity.[3] Nutrition and overweight is one of the 28 focus areas with a set goal to "promote health and reduce chronic disease associated with diet and weight." Seventeen measurable objectives have set targets to attain this goal. These objectives are tracked, monitored, and measured over time to determine if the target has been met **(Box 8-1)**. Unfortunately, none of the objectives to achieve healthy weight and reduce the incidence of overweight and obesity are currently being met. In fact, data show that the percentages of people in the United States who are overweight and obese are increasing.

Therefore, the objective of achieving a healthy weight is moving away from the target number set, rather than moving toward the goal. For example, the target for the percentage of Americans who are at a healthy weight is 60% of the nation's population. At present, the number of individuals who are at their healthy weight is only 42%. Moreover, the data for different ethnic groups show that only 34% of blacks or African Americans are at a healthy weight and only 30% of Mexican Americans are considered to be a healthy weight.

Regarding the objective for individuals to consume the age-recommended calcium intake, only 46% of the overall nation is meeting this objective. Evaluating the data according to age, sex, and ethnicity identifies those groups that are more vulnerable to the problem of poor calcium intake. The population group with the lowest intake is females aged 9 to 19 years, with only 19% of this group achieving adequate intakes. Among ethnic and

---

Box **8-1**

Actions Fundamental to Achieving the Nutrition Objectives of *Healthy People 2010*

- Improving accessibility of nutrition information, nutrition education, nutrition counseling and related services, and healthful foods in a variety of settings and for all population groups.
- Focusing on preventing chronic disease associated with diet and weight, beginning in youth.
- Strengthening the link between nutrition and physical activity in health promotion.
- Maintaining a strong national program for basic and applied nutrition research to provide a sound science base for dietary recommendations and effective interventions.
- Maintaining a strong national nutrition monitoring program to provide accurate, reliable, timely, and comparable data to assess status and progress and to be responsive to unmet data needs and emerging issues.
- Strengthening state and community data systems to be responsive to the data users at these levels.
- Building and sustaining broad-based initiatives and commitment to these objectives by public and private sector partners at the national, state, and local levels.

Reproduced from the U.S. Department of Health and Human Services, *Healthy People 2010*. Available at: http://www.healthypeople.gov/document/.

racial groups, blacks or African Americans have the lowest intake, with only 30% meeting the recommended calcium intake levels. Examining individuals living above and below the poverty level shows that only 39% of those living below the poverty level have adequate calcium intake compared with 48% of those above it.[3]

The trends are similar for other objectives relating to nutrition and overweight. As a nation, we are falling short and, in many cases, moving backward in achieving these objectives. In addition, the data clearly indicate disparities between different ethnic populations, age groups, and males and females. These data are extremely helpful in planning community programs and counseling individuals of different ages and cultural or ethnic groups. Dietetics professionals need to determine which groups are the most vulnerable and create nutrition messages targeted to those groups. Although all groups may benefit from nutrition education, it is best to focus on particular populations that are most at risk, based on available consumption data. For example, when promoting calcium consumption, a target group could be females, aged 9 to 19 years, or low-income individuals. If a nutrition program is designed for Mexican Americans, data would suggest making education to help them achieve a healthy weight a priority. Food guide pyramids for various ethnic and cultural groups as well as those for children and older adults are available as resources in planning programs and counseling individuals from many different populations.

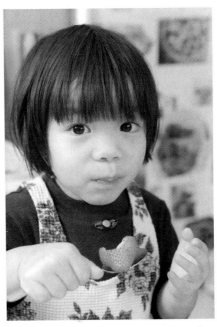

The professional counseling ethnic groups needs to be knowledgeable about their food practices.
Source: United States Department of Agriculture.

CULTURE AND ACCULTURATION

What is culture? Culture is broadly defined as "the values, beliefs, attitudes, and practices accepted by a community of individuals."[14] It is a "framework that guides and bounds life's practices."[15] Culture is integral to a person and enables a person to identify with a particular group of people or a population. As a deeply ingrained concept, cultural practices evolve gradually and affect and guide the activities and daily behavior of specific groups.

Culture influences many aspects of a person's identity; it shapes the foods served, ways holidays are celebrated, values, beliefs, spirituality, child-rearing practices, and expected family roles. Cultural roots influence attitudes and have a profound influence on behaviors.[15] Values differ related to cooperation versus competition, activity versus passivity, youth versus age, importance of family versus friends, and independence versus interdependence. For example, American culture encourages competitiveness. In contrast, in Asian cultures competition is seen as self-serving; these cultures instead encourage cooperation and teamwork.

Culture is learned, not inherited. It is passed from generation to generation in the home by a process called *enculturation*. Yet, within each culture there exist different customs, practices, ideologies, and viewpoints. Many countries throughout the world have populations that comprise one major group as well as many subgroups that differ from one another in various ways. For example, the Latino population is a major ethnic group in the Americas; yet within the Latino community are many subgroups, including Mexican Americans, Puerto Ricans, Cubans, and Central and South Americans. Within these subgroups are subcultures, and among these subcultures there are probably many similarities, but also distinct cultural differences.[16]

The process by which people from one cultural group modify their traditional behaviors, attitudes, and viewpoints as a result of contact with a new, dominant culture is termed *acculturation*.[17] Unlike the process of assimilation, in which members of a minority group adopt the practices and belief system of the dominant group, acculturation implies that both the traditional ethnic culture and the new, dominant culture play an important role in the process of cultural identity. As a result of this process, people may move toward the dominant culture, integrate the two cultures, reject the new culture while reaffirming their own traditional culture, or become alienated from both cultures.

As a nutrition practitioner it is important for various reasons to understand the concept of acculturation.[17] First, dietetics practitioners must understand acculturation so that they gain a better comprehension of the factors that hamper or enhance particular food choices. Second, practitioners must not assume that all dietary acculturation is healthy or unhealthy. For example, an Asian who acculturates to the dominant American culture by eating fast food would be viewed as making unhealthy food choices, yet an Asian who maintains the minority group's traditional diet rich in whole grains and rice would be seen as healthy. Third, dietetics professionals must identify whether acculturation to the American culture is influencing chronic disease factors, and if so, how.[16,17] For example, the United States is currently experiencing increasing obesity rates among both children and adults. In light of this trend, professionals must ensure that acculturation to the dominant culture does not cause members of minority groups to become obese.

To ensure that the diets of immigrants and minority groups are healthy, dietetics professionals should assess the degree of acculturation to American eating practices. In making this assessment, the practitioner should consult and listen carefully to the client, because he or she is the best source of information about the types of foods consumed.[18] Based on this assessment, the practitioner may determine that those who are more acculturated need more help in selecting healthy American foods. Similarly, those who are less acculturated may need help modifying their culture's traditional recipes, if they are unhealthy.

CULTURAL COMPETENCE IN COUNSELING

Dietetics professionals communicate with diverse clients, patients, and population groups. Consequently, it is essential that they not only learn how to manage diversity, but also understand the importance of cultural competence.

Three Principles of Cultural Understanding

As the United States becomes increasingly heterogeneous, the need to be cross-culturally competent is critical. There are three essential principles of cultural understanding. They are (1) acknowledgement of the importance of culture in people's lives, (2) respect for cultural differences, and (3) minimization of any negative associations or consequences of cultural differences.[19]

In the diverse United States, health care professionals have the opportunity to serve patients and clients from many different cultures. Thus, it is important that counselors recognize the influence of cultural factors on dietary patterns among various ethnic groups. Specifically, they must learn about each cultural group's traditional foods and food practices.[17] Transmission of this learning requires effective communication between the dietetics professional and the patient. To eliminate disparities in the nutritional status of people from different cultural backgrounds, dietetics professionals must recognize, respect, understand, and acknowledge the cultural differences or variations. Otherwise, nutrition counseling and education will be ineffective.[20]

As someone who serves diverse clients, it is also imperative that the dietetics professional not stereotype people based on their national origin or their appearance. India, for example, includes several cultural groups who practice different religions, have different customs, and speak different languages. Although a health care professional may assume that all people from India practice Hinduism, he or she must recognize that this narrow-minded assumption is not true. Similarly, practitioners must recognize that all Arab people are not Muslim, while all Irish people are not Catholic.

It is also important that health care professionals recognize the cultural divide that exists among the various generations within each culture. Individuals are unique in the degree to which they adhere to cultural patterns, with some identifying with the dominant culture more strongly than others.[15] Generally, most first-generation immigrants cling closely to their cultural ways. Over time, the second- and third-generation offspring of these immigrants tend to assimilate more completely into the dominant culture. They are more likely to adopt American customs and ideologies, yet they also keep some of their native cultural practices and food choices. Children, for example, adapt to new cultural patterns more easily than adults because they often interact with people of different cultures at school or in social activities.

Health care professionals must also be prepared to combat and prevent ethnocentrism. Although culture creates harmony within ethnic groups, it can also create disharmony. Ethnocentrism is the innate belief that one's own values and practices are absolute truths. Ethnocentric people, in turn, have a tendency to judge all others based on their own established belief system.[16] They believe that the norms and values of other cultures or ethnic populations are secondary to the norms and values of their own culture. To prevent ethnocentricity from penetrating the workplace, dietetics professionals need to know that their opinions, viewpoints, and ideologies may differ from those of their colleagues or clients. They also must understand that their own culture and world views may not be inherently "right."[15] This realization requires that one know one's own culture, its origins, its history, and its beliefs.

Cultural Competence

Dietetics professionals need to develop cultural competence in order to treat patients with care and efficiency.[21] Although cultural competence is similar to cultural understanding, there are key differences. Cultural competence consists of "ways of thinking and behaving that enable members of one cultural, ethnic, or linguistic group to work effectively with members of another."[15] It is a "unique category of awareness, knowledge, and skills" that enables a professional to succeed in cross-cultural counseling.[19] Although dietetics professionals cannot be culturally competent in every culture, they must be culturally competent about the various cultures they encounter on a regular basis. They also need to recognize and investigate unique differences within particular cultures so that they can determine the best way to treat their patients.

Understanding Health Practices

Culture determines how a person defines health, recognizes illness, and seeks treatment.[14] Each culture holds values, beliefs, and practices about good health and disease prevention, the care and treatment of the sick, whom to consult when ill, and the social roles and relationships between patient and health care provider. Most Americans, for example, believe in scientific medicine, individual decision through informed consent, the health care provider as the manager of care, and the separation of body, mind, and spirit in treatment programs. However, the health care orientation of other cultures may differ. For example, in non-American cultures, a family member or the community as a whole may have decision-making responsibility rather than the individual; emotional and psychological remedies may supersede scientific medicine; and body, mind, and spirit may be seen not as separate, but as joined.[16]

In Mexico, health is believed to be a matter of fate or God's will. Rather than believe in the power of science, medicine, or doctors to heal, many Mexicans believe that illnesses can be cured by folk healers or herbal remedies and teas. Similarly, they believe that particular medical conditions should be accompanied by particular food choices. These food choices are categorized as "hot" or "cold."[16] Specifically, pregnancy is considered to be a "hot" condition. As a result, pregnant Mexican women are urged to avoid foods that are classified as "hot," such as garlic, grains, expensive meats, and alcohol. Instead, they are urged to eat "cold" foods, such as vegetables, dairy, inexpensive meats, and tropical fruits. In reviewing this list of "hot" versus "cold" foods, it is interesting to note that this health concept has nothing to do with the temperature or spiciness of the food (after all, breads or grains are not actually hot); instead food are labeled according to traditions within the Mexican culture.[22] In addition, in Mexican culture, men are considered the dominant group, and the husband or his family is consulted and included in all decisions relating to a woman's pregnancy. Thus, a dietetics professional who is working with a pregnant woman may need to involve the man and his family in the decision-making sessions.

Many other cultures also believe that diseases are caused by factors other than those identified by western scientific medicine. In India, disease is believed to be caused by an upset in the balance of the body. Additionally, the husband's ownership of his wife is quite pervasive, and unquestioned obedience to elders is expected. Conversely, Haitians believe that some illnesses originate supernaturally or magically and may be treated with voodoo medicine.

Understanding Nonverbal Behavior

Nonverbal behaviors also differ among cultural groups and have different connotations. Customs concerning personal contact, body gestures, eye contact, interpersonal space, public displays of affection, and punctuality vary greatly.[14] In terms of personal contact, norms about touching another person are culturally determined. For example, in many Muslin communities it is considered illicit to hug a married woman. Similar notions also apply to eye contact.

In American culture it is considered disrespectful or suspicious to avoid meeting someone's eye. In some cultures, however, looking into a person's eyes is deemed disrespectful. Rules about touching and space are also culturally determined. Some cultures keep short distances between people, while others expect longer distances.[18] These spatial relationships also extend to signs of affection between men and women. In the United States it is culturally acceptable to see partners exchange romantic gestures or tokens of affection, yet in other parts of the world intimate partners do not even hold one another's hands.[15]

Last, punctuality is culturally determined. In the fast-paced United States, emphasis is placed on being on time and tardiness is frowned upon. Conversely, in parts of Asia as well as South and Central America, it is socially acceptable for a client to be late or miss an appointment without contacting the service provider. In these parts of the world, people's personal use of their own time is often considered to be a more important priority than the clock. Dietetics practitioner need to be aware of these different customs so they can better serve and understand clients' behaviors and choices.

Understanding Verbal Behaviors

In addition to understanding nonverbal behaviors, dietetics professionals must also be privy to how verbal behaviors vary among different cultures. Slang is a verbal behavior that American dietetics professionals should be cautious about using in the workplace with employees or clients. Although in American culture people often greet each other informally by asking "How's it going?" or ask others to repeat what they just said by interjecting "What?", in many cultures this level of familiarity would be considered improper and even disrespectful. Instead, dietetics professionals should greet clients by saying "Welcome." When they would like a client to repeat a statement, they should say "Excuse me" and then ask for a restatement.

Similarly, American dietetics professionals should pay attention to how they address their clients. Americans are among the most informal people worldwide and frequently call both friends and strangers by their first names. Nearly all other cultures expect a more formal and respectful approach, using the person's surname.[18] For example, if a client's full name is Diana Morales, the dietetics professional should refer to her as Ms. Morales, not Diana.

Dietetics professionals should carefully craft the types of questions they ask their clients. Americans tend to be fairly direct and ask somewhat personal questions, yet in many cultures, direct questions are deemed inappropriate. They may even cause people to feel uncomfortable.[15] Moreover, asking personal questions of a patient in order to obtain personal health and nutrition data may be perceived as intrusive and disrespectful.[18] Therefore, health professionals may want to try a formal approach rather than a quick, direct approach.[15]

Dietary managers and staff should try to understand the relationship that the patient expects from them as a service provider. In many cultures throughout the world, professionals are held in high regard for their expertise. Expecting individuals and families to be talkative and assertive may be unrealistic if they expect to have a dependent role in which they are told what types of foods they should be eating.

Understanding Family Relations

Another factor that nutrition specialists must learn and understand is the various types of family compositions. Families may be patriarchal, matriarchal, nuclear, or extended. Because one's own culture generally determines the interactions and composition of one's family, the roles of each family member may vary by age or gender. In some non-American cultures, a woman may not be allowed to speak openly, may not be allowed to work outside the home, and may have to defer to her husband or mother-in-law. In these cultures, a woman may have an insignificant role in making decisions for both herself and her family. As a result, counseling sessions may need to include the woman's father, husband, or whoever is the family decision maker.[15]

Nutrition specialists must also identify whether the family is monocultural or bicultural. Monocultural families identify with one primary ethnic group; those that are bicultural identify with two or more groups. More highly educated, middle-class clients may move back and forth among cultural groups easily.[15] Consequently, the food choices made by clients may depend on situational factors or a diverse cultural identity.

Models of Multicultural Nutrition Counseling

Several models of multicultural competence are found in the literature.[15,23,24] One model for multicultural nutrition counseling competencies identified 28 competencies within the following three factors: (1) multicultural awareness, (2) multicultural food and nutrition counseling knowledge, and (3) multicultural nutrition counseling skills.[22]

According to the American Dietetic Association (ADA), multicultural competence "is not a luxury or a specialty, but a requirement for every registered dietitian."[25] Cultural competence is essential for rendering effective nutrition services to clients. Campinha-Bacote describes multicultural competence as a "continuing journey."[24] She maintains that every client needs a "cultural assessment."

Multicultural Awareness

To achieve multicultural competence in nutrition counseling, dietetics professionals must first strive for multicultural awareness.[23] A personal awareness of the various cultures within the United States first requires that the individual become aware of his or her own culture or heritage. Each individual has a cultural, ethnic, linguistic, and racial identity.[16] Awareness of personal values, beliefs, assumptions, biases, and prejudices must be brought to the level of conscious awareness before one can become cross-culturally competent. Therefore, professionals should learn about the customs and traditions of their own culture, identify the historical connections between their culture and those of others, and examine their world views and cultural assumptions.

Second, individuals who strive to become aware of various cultures must identify whether they are a member of the dominant culture or a minority group. Those in the dominant culture may not be at the same level of self-awareness as those in a minority group. They may be unaware of the ways in which their culture influences other people's behaviors, reactions, and interactions. This examination might begin by assessing all of the values, beliefs or behaviors that shape one's self, including family and heritage, socioeconomic factors, politics, religion, educational level, occupation, gestures, terms of endearment, and the like.[26]

There are three key proficiencies that health care professionals must develop in order to be multiculturally competent.[27] First, dietetics professionals must develop a multiculturally competent attitude, that is, a mindset that respects cultural differences and similarities, while tolerating unclear intercultural communication due to language barriers. This attitude requires that health care professionals maintain a high level of patience for the additional time needed for effective communication. Second, dietetics professionals must develop multiculturally competent practices. These practices should ensure that clients' traditional health beliefs and diet are being balanced with healthy American food choices. Third, dietetics professionals must develop multicultural counseling skills. These skills may include listening skills, bilingual communication skills, diet modification skills, or evaluation skills.

Food and Nutrition Counseling Knowledge

To provide clients with effective counseling, dietetics professionals must have knowledge of multicultural foods and the cultural food practices of various groups. Dietetics professionals should gather information regarding cultural food choices, food preparation methods within a cultural context, knowledge of cultural eating patterns, family dynamics, typical meal patterns, and traditions during celebrations.[23] Information specific to each culture and community in which clients live is also needed. The counselor may determine the degree to which the family or each individual within the family follows these cultural traditions by consulting with each family member separately.[23,25]

How can we learn about patients' cultures? One suggestion is to visit their neighborhoods and go to the various ethnic food stores, ethnic restaurants, and, if possible, religious ceremonies in their places of worship or other neighborhood events.[16] Another suggestion is to attend workshops or training sessions on cultural food practices.[23] Dietetics professionals can also learn about various cultures by consulting the media, novels, newspapers, music, and some television shows. Reading about the role of foods in health and illness, approaches to health promotion, and treatment of disease and illness as well as beliefs about care and caregivers is another possibility.[16] Dietetics professionals can also examine authentic recipe books and try cooking the characteristic foods of various cultures.

Focus groups can help dietetics professionals learn about their patients' culture and dietary habits. During these sessions, the professional should explore the differences within cultural groups by talking about food preferences, recipes, ingredients, portion sizes, and how certain food items are prepared. If unfamiliar with eating a particular food, such as horse meat, Korean kimchee, Indian ghee, or hummus, the counselor should ask for a description of the food and cooking methods. It is important to gather all of this information so that one can respectfully incorporate family foods and cultural practices into proposed dietary changes.

When counseling people of different ethnic backgrounds, dietetics professionals must realize that the MyPyramid nutritional guidelines published by the U.S. Department of Agriculture (USDA) may not meet the cultural and ethnic needs of their target population. However, food pyramids designed for use with other cultures are available on the Internet. In addition, the Internet is a valuable resource providing vast amounts of other information about culture and diversity. Selected web sites are listed at the end of the chapter.

EXAMPLE: The following phrases may be helpful in eliciting information about a client's cultural food practices:

"I am not familiar with the way you cook _____ (name of food). Will you please tell me about it?"

"When you celebrate a cultural holiday, what food items do you prepare? What types of snacks do you prefer?" (widens the focus to the whole group)

"That dinner dish you mentioned sounds interesting. Can you tell me how you prepare it?"

"You are the expert on your food choices. You can teach me a lot."

You should reinforce any client response with one of the following statements:

"Thank you for that information."

"You are helping me to understand."

"I appreciate your taking the time to explain your cultural foods to me"

Avoid saying:

"I had a Mexican client last week and he told me . . . ."

"Those foods you mentioned are strange to me"

"I heard all Hispanics eat . . . . ."

Nutrition Counseling Skills

Multicultural nutrition counseling skills demonstrate one's ability to handle culturally appropriate interactions. These include conducting nutrition and cultural assessments, identifying nutrition-related problems, and planning and implementing relevant interventions.[14,15] Effective counseling skills require one to be aware of and knowledgeable about various cultures.[23]

Trust is an important counseling skill that all dietetics professionals must develop. One must be credible in the eyes of the client. Although the counselor may find that trust is difficult to develop, it is a necessary key to success.[17,18,20] The gap between the professional and the client must be bridged whether the client comes voluntarily or by referral. One way to achieve this is to develop rapport through conversation on neutral subjects that are unrelated to health or nutrition. For example, you may want to develop a personal relationship with your clients first by asking them questions such as, "Where did you grow up?" In providing counseling, you may want to first inform clients of what you will be doing by saying, "You are probably wondering what we are going to do. Let me explain." Then, you can explain the purpose, process, and the client's role as your cultural guide.

Clients may have also have problems with spoken and written English. In an effort to address the natural language barrier, the counselor may take some preliminary measures. First, the counselor can determine the native language spoken in the home. Second, the counselor can determine if the native language spoken is different from the language in which the client reads or writes. For example, some Spanish speakers may speak one dialect of Spanish, yet read or write Spanish in a different dialect. Third, counselors should try to learn some key words or phrases in the client's language, such as a greeting and the names of commonly eaten foods or ingredients. Learning some key words that describe tastes, smells, or cooking techniques is also useful.

Finally, a counselor may want to call upon the services of a translator to assist with transmitting nutrition information. The translator may help by rewriting written handouts or transmitting oral information into the client's language. An experienced translator should always be the first option. Although often the translating skills of the client's son or daughter are sufficient for these purposes, dietetics professionals must be cautious about using a family member in this role. In many cultures, having a child act as the interpreter presents the problem of role reversal, which can lead to resentment and can change the family dynamics at home.[15] Regardless of the type of translator, remember to address questions directly to the client, not the interpreter, and focus on the client as answers are provided.

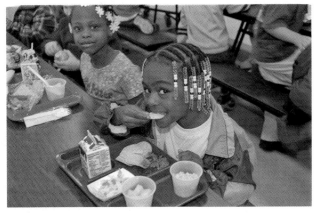

Food served at school lunch programs contributes to total nutrition.
Source: United States Department of Agriculture.

COUNSELING THROUGHOUT THE LIFE SPAN

Besides counseling patients with different cultural and ethnic backgrounds, dietetics professionals also counsel people of diverse ages. Nutrition is a fundamental pillar of health and development across the entire life span. At all ages, the goal of dietetics professionals is to promote good nutritional practices to meet age-specific nutrient needs for optimum health and well-being, normal development, and prevention of disease. Although many of the communication and education principles and strategies in other chapters of this book are appropriate for people of all ages, this section focuses specifically on preschool-aged children, school-aged children, adolescents, and older adults[28]

Promoting nutritional health across the life span is a cooperative goal of many public and private agencies.[29] Many agencies have a nutrition education component; examples of such components include the Special Supplement Food Program for Women, Infants, and Children (WIC); the Food Stamp program; the School Breakfast and National School Lunch programs; the Nutrition Education and Training (NET) program; and the Commodity Supplemental Food Program (CSFP).[30] The USDA funds Team Nutrition to develop and disseminate nutrition education materials to schools. For school nutrition education programs to produce changes in food attitudes and behaviors, at least 50 hours of instruction time is recommended.[30] Federal, state, and local public health agencies employ nutritionists. As members of a collaborative health care team, they assess the community nutrition needs as well as provide services, such as maternal and child health. Other organizations, such as the American Heart Association and the ADA, also provide educational materials. However, the $10 million budget for Team Nutrition and $1 million for the National Cancer Institute's Five A Day for Better Health Campaign are dwarfed in comparison with the $11 billion spent annually by the food industry on advertising.[30]

Preschool-Aged Children (2 to 5 Years)

Health care professionals should work with parents and other caregivers to healthfully influence preschool-aged children's eating behaviors. For the purpose of this chapter, preschool-aged children are defined as children between the ages of 2 and 5 years. The goal of health and nutrition education for these children is to promote healthful development and to prevent chronic diseases of adulthood, such as obesity.[26] Children's food habits are learned through family food experiences, personal experiences, and education.

Influences on Eating Habits

In the preschool years, family and cultural practices are a major influence on what children eat.[28] Since young children are unable to make cognizant decisions, vocalize their likes or dislikes, or determine appropriate behaviors, preschool-aged children's eating habits are often determined by their parents, guardians, or caregivers. Most young children tend to eat the same food as their parents or the types of food their parents believe are healthy.[28,31] For example, if parents routinely eat fruits and vegetables, it is more likely that their children will eat them; whereas if parents routinely eat cake and cookies for dessert, it is more likely that their children will eat these sweets. As previously mentioned, many preschool-aged children also eat the foods that their caregivers believe are healthy. For example, if a mother believes that Cheerios are a healthy breakfast because they are full of soluble fiber, her child will eat Cheerios for breakfast. On the other hand, if a mother thinks that two eggs are a healthy breakfast because they are full of protein, her child will eat eggs for breakfast. Thus, parents, siblings, and caregivers must explore their own nutritional beliefs and try to model and choose appropriate eating behaviors and choices.

Another dietary influence on preschool-aged children comes from watching television and the media.[28,29] Young children watch approximately 22 to 25 hours of television per week. Their still-developing minds are unable to distinguish between Saturday morning cartoon programs and commercials that advertise specific products that companies are trying to sell.[28] A study of 2- to 6-year-old children found that even brief exposures to televised food commercials could influence preschool children's food preferences, leading them to pressure parents to buy particular food items at the grocery store.[32]

The dietary behaviors of many children are formed away from the home, particularly in school or day-care programs. In modern society, many young children are enrolled in preschool, Head Start, or other day-care programs. About 60% of children 5 years of age or younger attend some type of child care program where they are supervised by adults other than their mother, father, or family members.[33] As a result, many preschool-aged children consume a large portion of their nutrients away from home and without parental influence. Therefore, parents, families, and guardians must work together with teachers to mutually reinforce learning about nutrition and making proper eating choices.[34] Parents may also want to provide their child's teacher with information about specific dietary restrictions they impose to ensure that the child's diet consists of similar foods both at home and in school.[35]

Counseling Challenges

Dietetics professionals are often faced with challenges when counseling preschool-aged children. One challenge they may face is the changing diet pattern of the child. Young children tend to change their behaviors rather quickly; for example, a child who is a good eater as an infant may be a fair to poor eater as a toddler. Children may also neglect to eat a particular food for weeks to months without any explanation. A child may love to eat whole-wheat toast for breakfast and then may suddenly stop eating whole-wheat toast for 2 months.

In addressing these challenges, dietetics professionals should provide the child and his or her caregivers with suggested diets that offer a variety of food choices. The Dietary Guidelines for Americans and the National Cholesterol Education and Prevention Programs recommend that children over the age of 2 years follow a diet in which only 30% of calories come from fat and less than 10% come from saturated fat.[36,37] The American Academy of Pediatrics Committee on Nutrition supports these goals.[29] As such, the recommended diets should enforce these guidelines. The MyPyramid for Kids offers a colorful food guide of food to include as well as servings for children **(Figure 8-1)**. Dietetics professionals should also recommend that the child refrain from eating the same type of food repeatedly and alternate different types of food choices. For example, dietetics professionals should advise parents of preschool-aged children to avoid too many juice boxes and alternate beverage consumption at lunch between juice, water, and 2% milk.

Another strategy to address a fickle preschool-aged eater is to let the child determine the quantity and frequency of his or her eating patterns. Dietetics professionals may want to make young children accountable for their dietary habits and allow them to decide how much and how often they should eat. However, this method must be approached with caution because children may be unable to make informed or logical decisions. In these situations, the dietetics professional should advise the caregiver to provide the child with only nutritious foods for meals and snacks. After a period of time, the caregiver can allow the child to make limited choices from the nutritious food available to them. Counselors should also provide nutritional learning activities for the child. Recommended strategies for teaching nutrition to young children include action stories, songs, videotapes, tasting parties, visiting vegetable and fruit gardens, puzzles, art projects, and field trips.

Nutrition assessment with a diet history, when needed, may take longer to accomplish at these ages. As preschool-aged children tend to be fickle, it may be difficult to determine the quantity or frequency of particular food consumption. To rectify this challenge, a dietetics professional may recommend that the child's parents, guardians, or caregiver keep a 7-day food record or journal that lists the type and amount of food consumed by the child. To make this activity fun for the child, you may suggest that older preschool-aged children draw pictures of what they eat.[28,38]

School-Aged Children (6 to 12 Years)

The ADA takes the position that "all children and adolescents should have access to adequate food and nutrition programs," including "nutrition education, screening, assessment, and intervention."[39] For the purpose of this chapter, school-aged children are defined as children between the ages of 6 and 12 years. As childhood is the optimal stage of human development, where lifestyle choices can affect later development and behaviors, it is essential that children be provided with guidance and advice to assist them in establishing healthy dietary and exercise habits.[3] Partnerships of children, schools, and families can promote health and well-being and influence these necessary lifetime food habits.[34]

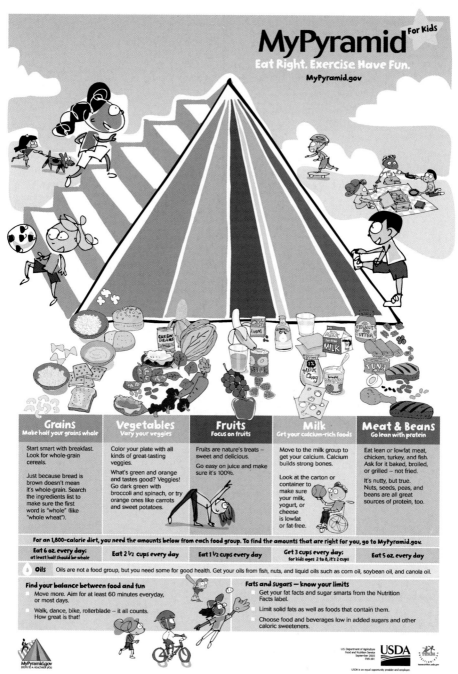

FIGURE **8-1**   MyPyramid for Kids. (Source: U.S. Department of Agriculture.)

Goals of Nutrition Education

During this stage of the life span, nutrition education seeks to provide children with the knowledge needed to select healthy foods. Dietetics professionals seek to facilitate the development of children's analytical and evaluative skills so that they may be better able to understand food and nutrition information.[40] Because risk factors for some chronic diseases begin in youth, behaviorally focused nutrition education is appropriate. This type of education encompasses cognitive learning, in which children learn how to select a healthful diet; affective teaching, in which children and counselors address motivation for dietary change; and behavioral components, such as selecting new food choices and lifestyle behaviors. Studies show that these types of interventions, which focus on specific behavior changes, result in more effective changes than a general nutrition education approach.[41] (**Box 8-2** lists topics considered essential at the elementary, middle, junior high, and senior high school levels.)

For example, a study assessed the effects of a home-based, parent–child autotutorial (PCAT) program for 4- to 10-year-old children with elevated low-density lipoprotein cholesterol (LDL-C).[42] The PCAT program, based on social cognitive theory, included

---

B O X 8-2

Nutrition Education Topics for Children and Adolescents

Essential topics to teach at the elementary through senior high school level

MyPyramid Food Guide
Benefits of healthful eating
Making healthful food choices for meals and snacks
Preparing healthy meals and snacks
Using food labels
Eating a variety of foods
Eating more fruits, vegetables, and grains
Eating foods low in saturated fat and total fat more often
Eating more calcium-rich foods
Balancing food intake and physical activity
Accepting body size differences
Following food safety practices

Additional topics appropriate at the middle, junior high, and senior high school level

Dietary Guidelines for Americans
Eating disorders
Healthy weight maintenance
Influences on food choices such as families, culture, and media
Goals for dietary improvement

Adapted from the U.S. Department of Health and Human Services, Healthy People 2010. Available at: http://www.healthypeople.gov/document.

10 talking book lessons (audiotaped stories with accompanying picture books) and follow-up paper-and-pencil games for the children. A manual for parents was provided. The program was effective in helping children gain knowledge of "heart-healthy eating" and in reducing their dietary fat consumption and their plasma LDL-C levels. This study demonstrates how behaviorally focused nutrition education effectively promotes healthy dietary practices.

During the school years, family, culture, and the body's physical composition greatly influence what children eat.[28] Therefore, dietetics professionals need to spend time assessing the child's social, physical, and psychological environment as well as his or her overall health when counseling children and their caregivers on the types of dietary changes that they should make to ensure a well-balanced diet and a healthy lifestyle. Since a 6-year-old is very different from a 9-year-old, an evaluation of the developmental stage of the child according to theories of child psychology and of the child's cognitive level must also be done before a health care professional can plan any nutrition intervention.[29] In addition, a nutrition professional should make reference to scientific studies that specifically focus on the behaviors within this age cohort. For example, studies have shown that in the earlier grades (ages 6 to 8 years) family-based programs are an effective and successful method for nutrition intervention.[39,43] In these types of programs, worksheets, games, and other activities are often mailed to homes so that the child and family can collaboratively discuss nutrition and healthy eating habits. Yet, in the later grades (ages 9 to 12 years) school-based programs, where students collaboratively discuss nutrition and healthy behaviors with their peers, tend to be more effective.

The dietary behaviors of many school-aged children, like those of preschool-aged children, are often formed away from the home, particularly in school or at after-school programs. Thus, a dietetics professional should collaborate with members of the school faculty, school lunch program, athletic department, and local community so that together they can teach children about nutrition and assess children's dietary trends.[34] Although studies indicate that teachers spend about 10 to 15 hours per year on nutrition education, this short amount of time is not sufficient to promote necessary behavioral changes.[39,43] To devote the recommended 50 hours per year, dietetics professionals can suggest that teachers partner with the school lunch program to provide nutritional knowledge to students during lunch time. They can have children create colorful posters of the food pyramid and then hang them throughout the lunch room.[39] Dietetics professionals can also assist teachers to incorporate nutrition principles into academic coursework, such as portion sizes in math classes.

Activity and School Challenges

Dietetics professionals should assess and note the child activity patterns, including number of hours spent exercising, participating in athletic events, watching television, or playing video games. During the school-aged years, children tend to be heavily influenced by peers and classmates. In addition, they are more exposed to the various forms of technology, such as television, the media and the Internet. Studies indicate that school-aged children watch approximately 23 to 24 hours of television weekly[29] and spend numerous hours playing computer games. This large amount of time spent watching television has various negative effects on children that have an impact on their overall health. In particular, there appears to be a strong relationship between obesity or weight gain and time spent watching television. This correlation may be a result of a child's inactivity; that is, a child is sedentary while watching television when instead he or she could be playing outside with friends or riding a bike through the neighborhood.

The American Medical Association states that this negative relationship between hours spent watching television and weight gain may cause the "couch-potato" syndrome—the unconscious consumption of high-caloric foods, labeled "junk food," while idling watching a television program. This unconscious action has been said to be a result of television commercials that attractively market junk food, snacks, and treats.[29] Some critics of these commercials have even suggested that they exploit unknowing school-aged children by appealing to their emotional and psychological needs, not their nutritional needs. Although some older children may be able to understand that the purpose of food commercials is to sell a product (not to provide sound nutritional information and choices), younger school-aged children must be advised by dietetics professionals on how to best evaluate and assess these ads. In a national study of 8,459 kindergarten-aged children, those children who watched more television and ate fewer family meals were more likely to be overweight. In addition, when the child's parent reported that the family lived in an unsafe neighborhood that did not allow for outdoor play, the child was more likely to be persistently overweight.[44] Dietetics professionals must be aware of these factors when counseling families.

As with preschool-aged children, health care professionals must address various challenges when counseling school-aged children and their caregivers about healthy nutrition plans. One challenge that the dietetics professional will encounter is a child's busy, and often unpredictable, schedule. In modern American society, many adults and their children do not eat breakfast because they are in a rush to get to work or catch the bus to get to school. Yet,

breakfast is essential for children and adolescents. According to the ADA, children who eat a healthy breakfast are more likely to have lower cholesterol levels, maintain a healthy weight, maintain a higher level of awareness and concentration in school, and have better problem-solving skills and hand–eye coordination.[40,45] Dietetics professionals should advise school-aged children and their parents or guardians to eat breakfast and provide quick breakfast options.

Another problem with scheduling that the dietetics professional must address is that the noon meal for many children may be a bag lunch from home or the school lunch program. If a child participates in a lunch program,

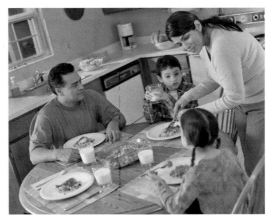

At all ages, parents should set a good example.
Source: United States Department of Agriculture.

he or she should be advised to make healthy choices for the beverage and snack option.

Lastly, the dietetics professional must address the time challenge of extracurricular activities, that is, activities that occur outside of school and generally after 3 PM. In a study of African-American children who participated in a 12-week after-school program that included physical activity and parental involvement, body weight, fat, dietary intake, and other health indicators all showed improvement for both the child and parents.[46] After-school snacks are required to meet the child's energy needs. Children who become involved in competitive sports, such as Little League baseball or soccer, may need additional nutrients or have an increased appetite.[29] Again, the dietetics professional should advise caregivers and coaches to provide healthy snacks to the children so they do not choose unhealthy ones.

Managing Medical Problems

Children who have medical problems present a counseling challenge to dietetics professionals. In the management of children and adolescents with type 1 or type 2 diabetes mellitus, involvement of families is essential. Parents can serve as resources for other families through participation in support groups. Needs can be assessed through telephone contacts, formal questionnaires, or informal information supplied at clinic visits. Games for use with diabetic children are found in the literature.[47,48]

Dietetics professionals should be aware of the nutritional trends and patterns among school-aged children. The number of school-aged children who are overweight is of concern because it has more than doubled in the past decade. Approximately 11% of children are overweight.[40,49] Inactivity, parental overweight, and skipping meals may contribute to overweight in children. Although chronic undernutrition is rare among children in the United States, approximately 8% of 12-year-olds are estimated to experience food insecurity, that is, limited access to nutritious food. School-aged children also have many concerns about their body image and appearance. It is during these years that many children become preoccupied with their weight and start dieting. About one third of children think they weigh too much. Many children also believe that their weight is above average cultural and societal standards. As a result, nearly half of all children have attempted to lose weight or have engaged in a diet plan within the previous year.[38,49]

Nutrition Education Activities

Based on these current dietary trends, health educators should create nutrition activities programs that seek to educate children about appropriate and healthy food choices and nutrition behaviors. Children want learning to be fun.[50,51] Childhood is a time for play exploration that offers opportunities for learning. The play approach to learning has been recommended as an alternative to the social learning theory and behavioral approaches. The play approach, based on the theory of Jean Piaget, focuses on internal transaction, intrinsic motivation, and fun rather than on external transaction and motivation.[50,51] In school-based nutrition education programs, intrinsic motivation was defined as performing a behavior for its own pleasure or purpose and was linked to an advanced stage of readiness to change. In contrast, extrinsic motivation was defined as performing a behavior to receive external rewards or pleasures, such as losing 5 pounds to receive a desired reward.

In the play approach, children actively explore and experiment with objects, materials, and knowledge. Active experimentation, hands-on experiences, and self-directed activities are recommended. For example, dietetics professionals can have children actively measure quantities or amounts of food by providing them with actual ingredients, scales, and measuring cups. Specifically, if they are trying to demonstrate to children how much sugar is in a can of soda, they may provide the children with a measuring cup and a bag of sugar and then allow them to measure the amount of sugar as indicated on the soda can label. If they are trying to have students compare how much sugar is in two different types of cereal, one high-sugar, the other low-sugar and high-fiber, they can provide groups of students with the food labels and measuring cups and ask them to read the food label, measure the amount of sugar, and record and chart the data (the amount of sugar in each cereal). Then they can have the children discuss in small groups which cereal is the better nutritional choice. For homework, they can ask the children to provide a list of cereal choices they should make based on this exercise.

Experiments with new foods and methods of preparing them are appropriate activities for children.[50] For example, in teaching the diabetic exchange system, children can use cultural food exchange playing cards, play nutrition bingo, or participate in scavenger hunts where they must locate exotic food.[52]

Dietetics professionals should also use visual aids and materials to appeal to conceptual learners. For example, while discussing the basic food groups, they may show students the MyPyramid (see Figure 8-1); or, when teaching children the importance of understanding serving size, they may provide each child with nutrition food labels from everyday, popular foods. In an effort to appeal to the oratory learner, one can encourage students to vocally discuss and compare the amount of nutrients, fats, protein, or fiber in particular food items based on an oral description of the food provided. Dietetics professionals may also engage students in written activities, such as writing in a food diary.

Dietetics professionals and teachers should also use technology and the Internet to provide students with self-directed activities. For example, they can introduce students to an electronic program called "5 a Day Virtual Classroom," which gives students the opportunity to counsel then-President Clinton about how to motivate children to eat five servings of fruits and vegetables daily (5 a Day).[53]

When dietary modifications are needed in a child's diet, the dietetics professional should try to choose words that children understand. Avoid medical terms, such as "lipids" and "polyunsaturated," and define difficult-to-understand words with flash cards. Choose words that have a positive connotation, rather than a negative one. For example, many children and adults consider the word "diet" to be negatively associated with weight and being fat. Therefore, use words such "food plan," "food choices," "meal plan," or "menu" to indicate the type of foods the child should eat.

Dietitians who counsel children in an office can avoid a "cold," unwelcoming feeling by using color and visual images to create an inviting space. The office environment can be made attractive with colorful food models, magazine pictures, posters, food packages of commonly eaten foods, and beverage glasses of various sizes and shapes.

National objectives for the nutrition education of children have been identified by government agencies, including the Department of Health and Human Services, the Department of Education, and the NET program, referred to earlier.[30] Objectives, priorities, and strategies for promoting healthy eating in children are recommended by NET. All states mandate or have initiatives to promote nutrition education in schools as a component of the curriculum. Examples of other agencies that commit resources to nutrition education of youth and adults include the National Cancer Institute (NCI) and the National Heart, Lung, and Blood Institute (NHLBI). The USDA's Team Nutrition web site and others mentioned at the end of the chapter offer recommendations and activities for children.

Family Counseling for Children

Family is the most prominent influence on preschool-aged and school-aged children's early eating patterns. As mentioned throughout the preceding sections, dietetics professionals must include parents, family members, or guardians in the child's nutrition counseling sessions.[34] The goal of effective family nutrition counseling is to use the shared environment to influence positive nutrition and health patterns and to foster healthy food consumption practices.

To provide effective nutrition guidance, dietetics professionals must be aware of the client's family composition and family roles and responsibilities as they relate to food production. Family nutrition counseling involves providing guidance and advice to people who live in the same household. In many U.S. households, families are composed of "nuclear" relatives, such as parents and siblings, as well as "extended" relatives, such as grandparents, aunts, uncles, or cousins.[26] In others, children may be raised by only one parent. Many children of divorced parents spend certain days in one household and other days in another.

Because changes in family food buying and food preparation influence the child's adherence to the regimen, it is essential that the dietetics professional know which family member primarily engages in these activities.[54] Historically, in many typical U.S. households, a child's mother was the person responsible for food shopping and food preparation. In modern-day U.S. society, this is no longer true of all households. Many women work outside the home, and other members of the family (fathers, grandparents, older siblings) may have the primary responsibility for menu planning, purchasing food, and preparation of food. In some households, none of the family members has time for these responsibilities. As such, nannies or babysitters may be responsible for menu planning. In other circumstances, older children may be responsible for preparing their own breakfasts, bag lunches, and after-school snacks. When only nutritious food is brought into or made within the home, children are given environmental cues that enhance their healthy dietary regimen and reduce their intake of high-fat, high-calorie foods.[54,55]

Members of a household share common biological, social, cultural, psychological, or environmental spheres, and it is the task of the dietetics professional to provide a food program that addresses each of these spheres. When family members cooperate and provide the child with social, psychological, and environmental support, they greatly assist in fostering the child's dietary changes and help other family members improve their diet habits, as well. For example, in families dealing with childhood obesity, diabetes mellitus, or hyperlipidemia, dietary changes often benefit everyone in the family.

Preschool-aged and school-aged children, and even adolescents, are highly dependent on their parents or guardians to model appropriate, and sometimes inappropriate, eating behaviors. Family members can serve as good role models by eating healthy food and rewarding healthful habits in the child.[28,56] Children frequently mimic their parents' food habits. For example, if a boy sees that his father refuses to eat broccoli, he will be more likely to refuse broccoli. Thus, parents need to set a good example. The counselor must help parents and guardians to be the role models by helping them negotiate changes in what is purchased, prepared, and eaten by members of the family.

Dietetics professionals may face some challenges while providing nutrition counseling to families. Some clients do not wish to involve certain family members; step-parents may refuse to participate; spouses and parents may be overly controlling and negative in dealing with the child; and mutually acceptable times for appointments may be difficult to arrange for several people.[57,58] In these cases, other sources of social support may have to be located.

Other concerns may be present. Parents may not be good role models or supportive of their children. They may use sweets and desserts as a reward or bribe: "Eat this and you can have dessert," for example. Siblings may tempt and tease a brother or sister who is not supposed to eat certain foods. Parents who take a food plan too literally may create a stressful environment in the family, leading to food battles and conflicts. Nagging, criticism, and policing about food and weight issues should be replaced with positive reinforcement and praise when correct dietary behaviors are observed.[26]

Adolescents (13 to 19 Years)

Adolescence is a period of cognitive, physical, and psychosocial change. As teenagers experience these rapid and unknown changes, they need to adjust their nutritional behaviors by increasing their healthy dietary habits and decreasing those that are unhealthy.

Before a dietetics professional can plan a teenager's nutrition counseling, the adolescent's overall health must first be assessed. This includes, but is not limited to, assessing the young person's weight, weight fluctuation, physical growth, timing of growth spurt, physiological maturation, and activity level. Dietetics professionals and adolescents may engage in either one-on-one counseling or group counseling sessions. In one-on-one counseling, personal decisions related to self-care can be explored between the counselor and the adolescent. In working with groups, the counselor may ask teens to discuss and share how they handle particular situations.[57]

Teenagers vary in rates of physical growth, in the timing of the growth spurt, and in physical activity patterns. Although the growth spurt of most adolescent girls occurs between 10 and 12 years of age, and 2 years later for adolescent boys, rates of growth may vary among both sexes because of external influences, such as poor diet, prenatal health conditions, or chronic illnesses.[29] Moreover, physical activity patterns may vary because of external factors. For example, teenagers who participate in sports engage in high levels of physical activity, whereas those who frequently watch television or play video games are considered to engage in minimal to moderate activity.

The dietetics professional must be familiar with the characteristics and external pressures that are associated with the teenage years. Adolescence is a time of awkwardness, self-awareness, and experimentation. Take a moment to recall your teenage years: suddenly, you are given more accountability and responsibility, yet you are unable to fully exercise your new freedoms because you are still under the jurisdiction of your parents and teachers. As you try to exert your independence and search for your identity, you are faced with the challenge of balancing freedom with responsibility and personal preferences with authority. Do these thoughts sound familiar? Well, many teens that dietetics professionals treat will be experiencing these internal conflicts and emotions.[54,55] In addition, they will be balancing the demands of their quasi-adult, yet quasi-child, environment which includes school, friends, family, and even work.[55] As a health care professional it is imperative to keep these factors in mind when counseling adolescents.

Influences on Food Practices

Why do adolescents make the food choices they do? A study of adolescents assessed their perceptions of factors influencing their food choices.[58] These factors included hunger and food cravings, appeal of the food, taste of the food, time considerations, convenience of the food, food availability, parental influences on eating behaviors (such as culture or religion), health benefits of foods, situation-specific factors, mood, body image, habit, cost, media influences, and vegetarian beliefs. However, the most influential factor was the adolescent's desire to fit the social norms of the peer group; that is, teenagers' food choices were most likely influenced by what their best friend was eating.[58]

Food is often a social experience and eating often occurs when one is surrounded by one's friends or peers. In a given week, approximately 25% of preteens and 61% of teens eat with friends in fast-food eateries.[56] Because adolescents are uncomfortable with anything that makes them seem different from their peer group, they may tend to eat whatever snacks or meals their friends are eating.[55] Sometimes this may be a positive experience, as when adolescents mimic the healthy eating habits of their friends. But it may have a negative effect if adolescents choose to mimic the unhealthy dietary choices of their peers. Peer interaction can also affect food choices at parties and sporting events, entice after-school snacking, and induce consumption of alcohol or cigarettes. Thus, the challenge for the counselor is to help individual adolescents incorporate healthful eating habits into their lifestyle, rather than mimic the unhealthy eating habits or their peers.[58,59]

In a study that examined adolescent barriers to healthy food choices, eating healthy food was a low priority for teens, while the taste of food was of great importance.[58] Adolescents perceived healthy food choices to be less tasty than unhealthy food choices. The study also found that approximately one third of adolescents eat outside the home, in such places as school and restaurants. When eating away from home, many teens ate out of vending machines, or at convenience stores or fast-food restaurants.[58] In these places, healthy food choices were generally unavailable. Although almost all public schools participate in the school lunch programs, many high schools raise money by giving vending companies contracts to sell soft drinks, candy, chips, and other high-fat foods.[58–60] In addition, many convenience food items are high in fat and energy and low in nutrients.[61] Currently, initiatives are being made by local governments and school boards to ban unhealthy snacks and sodas from school cafeterias and vending machines, yet the fact remains that adolescents will continue to crave salty, fatty snacks. Thus, effective dietary interventions and counseling requires that dietetics professionals explore the external factors influencing food choices so that healthy changes can be made.[62]

Dietary intakes of teens tend to be high in fat, sugar, salt, and fast foods but low in vegetables, fruits, fiber, and foods rich in calcium and iron.[58,59] The connection between food choices and health may be discussed, but it is not a primary influence on food practices in this age group.[57] Cognitive-behavioral therapy intervention strategies should target the affective domain, or feelings and attitudes, not just give information to increase knowledge.[28] Adolescent attitudes and patterns related to food choices and physical activity should be explored, since they may persist into adulthood.[3]

Counseling for Special Needs

Adopting a healthy lifestyle in adolescence and young adulthood is important in the prevention of future health problems, such as heart disease and osteoporosis.[58] For example, obesity is increasing in the teenage years and is associated with the risk of type 2 diabetes, discrimination and rejection by peers, and low self-esteem.[60]

Dietetics professionals should be knowledgeable of the specialized nutritional trends of adolescents (refer to Box 8-2 for essential topics). One particular trend, dieting, is a common practice among teenagers. Dissatisfied with their weight and body, many adolescents reduce their caloric and fat intake through dieting. By cutting calories without thought to the nutritional value of foods, adolescents may eliminate important nutrients from their diet, leading eventually to marginal nutritional status.[29]

Dieting is generally a result of a poor body image. As such, professionals have to be aware of how an adolescent's negative body image can affect his or her nutritional habits. The obsession with body image and weight is more prevalent among girls than boys.[28,29] Studies have found that approximately 50 to 70% of adolescent girls are dissatisfied with their weight and body image.[58,60] This obsession with body image may be attributable to a young person's desire for a thin body similar to popular peers or fashion models or their unfamiliarity with their changing bodies. For example, during the adolescent years, girls go through puberty and suddenly see their hips begin to widen and their breasts begin to develop. Uncomfortable with these changing features, young girls may develop a poor body image because they do not realize that this change is "natural" and will balance out as they get older.

The depiction of extremely thin actresses and models by the media tends to enforce unrealistic, idealized standards of weight; yet many adolescents strive to look like them and resort to drastic dieting, refuse to eat food, take diet pills, or overexercise. The National Eating Disorders Association estimates that 81% of young adolescents are afraid of being fat and between "5 [and] 10 million girls and women and 1 million boys and men are struggling with eating disorders including anorexia, bulimia, binge eating disorder, or borderline conditions." Of this total, it is estimated that 85% of these eating disorders begin during adolescence.[63] According to a 2006 study, conducted by the University of Minnesota's "Project EAT" (Eating Among Teens), the use of diet pills by adolescent girls nearly doubled over a 5-year period from 7.5% to 14.2%.[64]

Dietitians must realize that they cannot treat these serious eating disorders alone. Although they must provide nutrition counseling, they must also provide a nutrition intervention for the young girls and boys who are suffering from these disorders. Often, eating disorders occur because of a young person's dissatisfaction with his or her personal life or because weight appears to be the one area of life that he or she can control.[61] Thus, effective treatment requires an interprofessional "team" approach in which psychologists and medical specialists collaborate with the nutritionist to assess and treat patients across a continuum of care.[63]

Dietetics professionals also provide nutrition counseling and prenatal care to pregnant teenagers. Although the teenage birth rate has fallen 33% since 1991, many adolescent girls continue to get pregnant. Adolescent pregnancies are at greater risks than adult pregnancies because many teenage girls have yet to complete their growth spurt. Pregnant teens are at a greater risk of having premature, low-birth-weight babies and developing personal conditions, such as anemia and hypertensive disorders.[3]

In an effort to promote a healthy pregnancy for both the mother and the baby, dietetics professionals should advise pregnant adolescents to eat healthy foods and achieve the recommended weight gain.[28] Pregnant teens require significant caloric intake in order to support the growth and development of the fetus, as well as to support their own personal growth.[29] It is recommended that pregnant teens who weigh within the recommended weight range for their height should gain between 28 and 40 pounds during their pregnancy.

High caloric intake is especially important for adolescents who recently began menstruation and became pregnant. Since adolescents have a tendency to be vulnerable to poor nutritional practices, dietetics professionals should advice pregnant teens to eat a diet high in fluids, fiber, vitamins, and minerals.[65]

Another adolescent diet trend that professionals must be aware of is vegetarianism. Those who become vegetarians may be vulnerable to nutritional deficiencies if their food intake is not balanced properly.[66] Adolescents who are vegetarians need to be assessed for essential nutritional deficiencies as well as signs of potential eating disorders. For example, studies have found that some young women engage in vegetarianism in an effort to lose weight or restrain their caloric and fat intake. As a result, dietetics professionals particularly need to watch their vegetarian clients and ensure that they are not abusing their bodies or becoming preoccupied with weight loss or body image.[66,67]

In treating adolescents, dietetics professionals must be knowledgeable about the importance of exercise and sports. Many teens are involved in competitive sports activities. Athletic participation can have both a positive and a negative impact on healthy adolescents. Positively, in some sports, such as wrestling, adolescent boys may be highly motivated to learn about nutrition to improve their athletic performance. On the other hand, boys may be trying to lose weight by inappropriate means so that they may wrestle within a lower weight class. Thus, athletic coaches should look for nutrition misinformation and fads with this group and be privy to the positive and negative effects of athletic participation.[29]

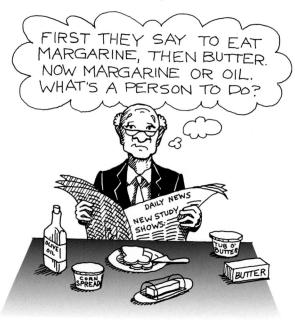

Many people are confused by conflicting media reports about food.

Older Adults

The aging of the U.S. population presents challenges to families, policy makers, and health care providers. Although many older adults enjoy a standard of living and increased life span unknown a century ago, this is not true of everyone. Because of immigration, the elderly population is becoming more ethnically and racially diverse.[68] While the majority of elderly today are Caucasian (84%), this number is expected to shift downward to 52.8% by 2050, as the number of ethically diverse elderly increases.[69]

Since there can be vast differences among older adults, the U.S. census uses three age categories:[1]

Ages 65 to 74—the young-old
Ages 75 to 84—the old
Ages 85 and older—the oldest-old and fastest-growing segment of older adults

In general, older Americans are living longer after age 65 and living better than they did in the past. Although the young-old may still be working part-time and may be in relatively good health, the oldest-old may be living with limited independence, serious health problems, or disabilities. In 2001, an estimated 35 million people—almost 13% of the population (one in eight people)—were 65 years or older, and these numbers are expected to continue increasing.[1] Within the population of individuals aged 65 years and older, those over 80 years of age constitute the fastest-growing segment. The number of people 80 years old or older is projected to reach 19.5 million by 2030, more than double the 2000 figure of 9.3 million.[69]

Today's older Americans are generally better educated than previous generations. This factor can influence socioeconomic status, health, and quality of life. Many continue to live independently. A large majority enjoy social contacts with friends and relatives, including activities such as going to restaurants for meals. Although economic resources are sufficient for many, there are significant disparities in income and wealth, and some elderly adults live in poverty.

Challenges of Aging

When asked to rate their health, most older adults aged 65 to 75 report it as "very good to excellent." But at more advanced ages (75-plus years), only 33% have a self-reported health status of "good to excellent."[69] Health and quality of life can be threatened by chronic diseases, depression, disability, and memory impairments. Hypertension, heart disease, diabetes, stroke, cancer, arthritis, and osteoporosis are examples of chronic health problems, and many older people have multiple health problems. A comprehensive nutrition assessment of any older adult should be performed that considers the economic, psychosocial, cultural, health, physiological and lifestyle factors influencing food intake before planning a nutrition intervention.[70]

People aged 85 years and older are the most likely individuals to live in nursing homes. Those in nursing homes tend to be more impaired functionally and may need assistance with eating. Malnutrition affects about two of every five elderly nursing home residents.[71]

The Gerontological Nutritionist (GN) dietetics practice group has developed practice standards for working with older adults.[72] More than half of the GN members work in nursing homes, and others are employed in community nutrition programs and hospitals. The members of GN "work with and through others while using their unique knowledge of food, human nutrition, and management as well as skills in providing services," including providing quality nutrition care, counseling, and services for older adults. Members of the Consultant Dietitians in Health Care Facilities (CD-HCF) dietetics practice group work in long-term care and other settings. They also have published standards of professional practice.[73]

Food and Nutrition Challenges

Achieving and maintaining optimal nutritional status of the older population is a goal for nutrition counselors. However, obtaining the proper amount of nutrients can be a challenge, and the counselor needs to explore several issues for those undergoing economic, physiological, social, and family changes, including the following:[28,74]

- Although protein, vitamin, and mineral needs do not decrease and in some cases may increase, caloric needs decrease owing to changes in resting energy expenditure and decreased levels of physical activity, thus requiring a smaller quantity of food to be eaten that needs to be nutrient-dense.[75]
- Senses of taste and smell decline, making food less appealing and influencing appetite and what people choose to eat. About 50% of older adults between ages 65 and 80 and 75% of those over age 80 have major loss of taste buds. Declining vision and hearing are other sensory changes.[28]
- The fact that many older adults lack healthy diets and do not engage in physical activity is of concern. A study using the Healthy Eating Index showed that 21% had diets rated as "good," 67% needed improvement, and 13% were "poor." Scores were low on daily servings of fruit and milk products.[68]
- Chronic diseases may require costly medications that may affect appetite and result in drug–nutrient interactions. Older adults use 35% of all prescription drugs and many over-the-counter drugs as well.[28,76]
- Income may be limited or fixed while health care and other expenses increase, resulting in food insecurity and economic problems.[75]
- Social isolation, loneliness, and bereavement due to loss of spouse decrease interest in cooking and eating.[77]
- Physical disability and cognitive impairments (depression and dementia) may make shopping and cooking difficult. Lack of physical activity decreases muscle mass, which can affect mobility and strength. Approximately two thirds of older adults do not exercise regularly.[75]
- Dental problems, dentures, or swallowing problems may limit food choices and intake.
- Physiological changes in digestion and absorption increase with age.[28]

Good nutrition is essential to the health, self-sufficiency, and quality of life of older adults. Enjoying food and maintaining the desire to eat reduce the risk of weight loss and undernutrition. The nutrition counselor should assess and identify potential problems and their effects on nutritional status. The counselor should establish individualized plans for intervention. Interventions need to be culturally and age sensitive.

It may be necessary to go slowly, listening carefully and observing the

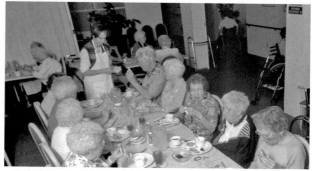

Older adults dine together at a community site.
Source: United States Department of Agriculture.

spoken and unspoken needs. Health problems can vary by ethnic group; African Americans, Hispanics, and Asians have different problems.[77] For example, minorities generally come to old age with fewer economic resources. At present, 42% of U.S. adults say they take daily vitamins, and 23% report they use herbal supplements; this is something to inquire about with all clients.[78]

Nutrition counselors should be aware of community programs to recommend to older adults. Examples are the Food Stamp program and the Congregate/Group Meal program funded under the Older Americans Act, which funds meals at little or no cost in a social setting such as community or recreational centers, senior citizen centers, and churches. The program also funds Meals on Wheels, home-delivered meals to the frail elderly.[75]

LIMITED LITERACY

About 40 to 44 million people, or approximately 25% of the U.S. adult population, cannot understand materials written at a basic proficiency level.[79] Although individuals with limited literacy skills vary, most are of lower socioeconomic status, have dropped out of school, are learning disabled, are older, or are immigrants who do not yet know much English and may not read even in their native language.[79,80] It is important to identify these individuals, because poor reading skills are associated with poor health.[3,81]

Practitioners probably encounter illiterate clients more often than they realize, as such individuals hide the fact that they cannot read. The dietetics professional should be aware of the following excuses expressed by clients in an effort to hide their illiteracy: "I don't have my glasses with me and will read this later," or "I broke my glasses." Another technique to identify such individuals is to hand them written materials upside down. Readers normally turn the paper right-side up, whereas nonreaders may not. Another approach is to ask the person to select a food from a list on the paper and read the word aloud. If the client cannot read the word, then it is unlikely that he or she knows how to read.

The average reading level of U.S. adults is around eighth-grade level, but among enrollees in Medicaid, it is only at the fifth-grade level. Typically, health education print materials are written at the 10th grade level or higher instead of an appropriate level for the audience—generally fifth-grade level.[3,81] To rectify this imbalance, dietetics professionals may need to test written materials for readability and incorporate more visuals (graphics, pictures) when educating people with low literacy. They should also keep language simple and repeat important information. "Dietary cholesterol" and "blood glucose," for example, are challenging terms to understand and are inappropriate for this audience. Another suggestion is to keep sentences short (10 to 15 words) and use one- and two-syllable words when possible.[79] Paragraphs should also be limited to three or four sentences. To ensure that clients understand the words, the counselor should ask them to repeat what was said. Actual practice, such as planning a menu or a grocery shopping list, and role-playing are helpful activities in helping clients connect words to language.

The Joint Commission on Accreditation of Healthcare Organizations (JCAHO) requires that steps be taken to ensure that patients and clients understand the oral and written information they receive.[82] Several readability formulas exist, including SMOG (Simplified Measure of Gobbledygook), Flesch, Fry, and others.[83] These and other tools can help dietetics professionals promote nutritional literacy among their clients who are illiterate or have limited literacy. The principle to remember is to be sensitive to the fact that many clients may have literacy problems that they may attempt to hide during the assessment process. If the issue of literacy is not properly diagnosed, addressed, and remedied, the chances of successfully counseling the individual will be greatly reduced.

This chapter examined the challenges of dealing with a diverse workforce as well as counseling and educating culturally diverse clients. Food and nutrition professionals need to develop awareness, knowledge, and communication skills in order to counsel individuals from cultures other than their own.

Practitioners also need to acquire the knowledge and skills necessary to counsel and educate people of all ages with a variety of food and nutrition problems and challenges. It is particularly important to identify those with limited literacy, as this will have a significant impact on nutrition teaching.

CASE STUDY 1

Julia is a health care professional within the food industry who was recently promoted to lead and manage a team of 15 workers. Of these workers, three people are white, one is an African-American woman, seven are second-generation immigrants from Central and South American countries, and four are first-generation immigrants from Central and South American countries who speak little English. While most of her staff is between 21 and 45 years of age, one staff member is 62 years old. Julia is extremely knowledgeable about her profession; however, she is having difficulty managing, directing, and communicating with her staff. One of the biggest problems is the language and cultural barrier between her and the four non–English-speaking staff members. This barrier is also causing problems among members of the team, who seem to be naturally divided by their race and ethnicity. As a result, the team is not working together and sharing ideas. In addition to these problems, Julia was recently informed that she must recruit and hire two new employees to add to her team. It has been specified that these new hires should add more diversity into the company.

1. What are the problems that Julia is experiencing in managing her team?
2. What are three suggestions that would help Julia to help her rectify these problems?
3. How can Julia effectively deal with the language barrier that exists within her team?
4. How can she utilize the talents of her team to help her with these issues?
5. What strategy should Julia use to successfully recruit and hire two new employees from diverse racial and ethnic backgrounds?

CASE STUDY 2

Judy R. is a new registered dietitian whose responsibilities at the medical center frequently involve nutrition interviewing, counseling, and community education. Many of her patients are from cultural and ethnic groups other than her own. They are mainly Mexican,

CASE STUDY **2**

Puerto Rican, Thai, and Korean. She is finding it somewhat overwhelming to understand the variety of unfamiliar foods that they eat. This also inhibits her ability to provide appropriate food alternatives as she counsels them on modifying their diets. She wants to increase her effectiveness as a counselor.

1. List three strategies Judy could use to improve her interviewing and counseling with patients from other cultural and ethnic groups.
2. What resources can you suggest for Judy to assist her in counseling? Where might she find them?
3. What activities can she plan in the community to educate these diverse groups?

CASE STUDY **3**

Mrs. Smith, a widow, is 76 years old. She is 5'3" tall and weighs 150 pounds. She lives alone in an apartment. The arthritis in her knees and hands for which she takes aspirin or Tylenol tends to limit her mobility. She lives on a small pension and on Social Security. She mentions that her pension money does not go as far as it did 10 years ago, and her rent continues to increase annually.

Mrs. Smith walks to a small private grocery store three blocks from her apartment or to a convenience store two blocks away for food once or twice a week. During snowy winters, a daughter who lives an hour away takes Mrs. Smith to a larger store every 2 weeks. She eats cereal for breakfast and a sandwich or soup for lunch; she may do a small amount of cooking at the evening meal. She snacks on candy during the day. She comes to your office for advice on her diet.

1. What socioeconomic and lifestyle factors influence Mrs. Smith's food intake?
2. What physiological factors may influence her food intake that you would inquire about?
3. List at least two key nutrition issues you might discuss with Mrs. Smith.
4. What other questions could you address in the interview to gather a more precise diet history as a basis for an implementation plan?
5. What are your recommendations for Mrs. Smith's nutrition intervention? What federally funded programs would you explore with her?
6. Develop written documentation for your session with this client, incorporating the Nutrition Care Process (NCP) model as applicable.

REVIEW AND DISCUSSION QUESTIONS

1. What is diversity? What are some of the ways in which people differ?
2. As a manager, what would you see as the goals and benefits of workplace diversity?
3. What activities can be planned to address workplace diversity? How can they be evaluated?
4. What is culture?

5. Define assimilation, ethnocentrism, enculturation, and acculturation.
6. How does culture influence people's daily practices, including food choices?
7. What is cultural competence? What can a dietetics professional do to develop it?
8. In counseling preschool-aged and school-aged children, what factors should be assessed? What educational and intervention strategies are recommended for children?
9. In dealing with adolescent boys and girls, what factors should be assessed?
10. What factors may have an impact on the diet and nutrition of older adults?
11. What strategies are helpful in educating older adults?
12. What strategies are helpful when counseling a client with a low literacy level?

SUGGESTED ACTIVITIES

1. At your place of employment, identify which cultural and ethnic groups are represented. Do you believe that the talents of the diverse workers are being recognized?
2. List the cultural and traditional foods that you and your family members prepare. Share your cultural foods with neighbors and friends and inform them about your cultural customs.
3. Select one cultural or ethnic group with which you are unfamiliar. Research the food choices and practices of this culture.
4. Find someone from a culture you would like to learn more about. Ask the person to be your cultural guide or teacher. After developing a list of questions to ask in advance, interview the person to gather information on their food choices, practices, recipes, cooking methods, and foods for special occasions such as holidays. Include spiritual beliefs and practices that influence food choices and overall health.
5. Watch a child's television program. While doing so, note the number of food advertisements. Did these commercials make you want to consume the food item? Do they promote healthy eating?
6. Interview a dietetics professional who works with children or adolescents. Ask questions about the nutritional challenges encountered when counseling diverse populations.
7. Interview the mother or caregiver of a child. Ask what strategies she or he uses to encourage healthy eating habits and introduce new foods into the child's diet.
8. Plan a 15-minute presentation on nutritious snacks for fifth graders. What types of materials would you use? Why?
9. Interview a teenager about his or her eating practices. Ask the person about food preferences. What factors influence food choices? How does the type of food the teen chooses to eat compare with what friends eat? Are foods chosen for health or weight reasons?
10. Buy a magazine read by teens. Assess the content of any articles on nutrition, food ads, weight control supplements, and the like.
11. Interview an older adult (aged 65 or older) about his or her food choices and eating practices. Ask about how the person purchases and prepares food, the number of meals eaten daily, and the intake of water and other beverages.
13. Evaluate a patient education handout that is distributed in a public health community program. Does the information in the handout give correct information? Is it written at the correct level for the population targeted?

WEB SITES

Many sites devoted to diversity and multicultural issues can be found on the Internet, along with links to other sites. A few suggestions follow:

http://www.aarp.org/health/healthguide/   American Association of Retired Persons (AARP) site with information on health living

http://www.actionforhealthykids.org/   Includes resources, program design information, and tools to develop school wellness sites

http://www.aoa.gov/   U.S. Department of Health and Human Services, Administration on Aging; can be viewed in more than seven languages

http://www.diversityresources.com/   Information on diversity issues in the workplace, including a yearly multicultural calendar to plan culturally appropriate workplace events

http://www.diversityrx.org/   Promotes language and cultural competence to improve the quality of health care for minority, immigrant, and ethnically diverse communities

http://www.doi.gov/diversity/   U.S. Department of the Interior web page with information on workforce diversity and statistics

http://www.dole5aday.com/   Educational activities relating to fruits and vegetables for school-aged children, with resources for professionals

http://www.fda.gov/oc/opacom/kids/   Food and Drug Administration site for children; includes interactive games on food safety and other health issues

http://www.fitness.gov/   President's Council on Physical Fitness and sports site with links

http://www.fns.usda.gov/tn/   Team Nutrition site designed to empower children to make healthy food and activity choices

http://www.foodsafety.gov/   Food safety information, including resources in more than 14 languages

http://www.girlpower.gov/girlarea/index.htm   U.S. Department of Health and Human Services site that focuses on empowering girls to make positive lifestyle choices

http://www.hhs.gov/kids/   U.S. Department of Health and Human Services web page devoted to children's activities

http://www.healthypeople.gov/document/   Contains the Healthy People 2010 on-line documents, including the leading health indicators for the nation, nutrition objectives, and baseline data for target population groups

http://www.justmove.org/   Fitness advice for all age groups, affiliated with the American Heart Association; includes an exercise diary and exercise resources

http://kidshealth.org/index.html   Access to government web pages related to health of children from elementary through high school

http://www.nal.usda.gov/fnic/etext/000023.html   Food and Nutrition Information Center of the U.S. Department of Agriculture; has cultural and ethnic food guide pyramids with links to other sites, including resource lists for educators

http://www.nal.usda.gov/fnic/etext/000023.html   USDA Food and Nutrition Information Center

http://ohioline.osu.edu/hyg-fact/5000/   Information on eight cultural groups found under "Cultural Diversity" as well as information on nutrition in the life cycle

http://oregonstate.edu/dept/ehe/nu_diverse.htm/   Oregon State University site with information on cultural diversity

http://www.semda.org/info/   Southeast Michigan Dietetic Association site; has 16 or more food pyramids, which are copyrighted and may not be copied for commercial purposes without consent

http://www.surgeongeneral.gov/publichealthpriorities.html   U.S. Department of Health and Human Services, Office of the Surgeon General; addresses priorities for public health issues for diverse populations

http://www.usa.gov/Topics/Seniors.shtml   Health information for seniors with links to other resources

http://www.3aday.org/3aDay/   Educational activities and resources for moms, kids and health professionals, designed to encourage three servings of dairy each day

REFERENCES

1. Profiles of General Demographic Characteristics, 2000. Washington, DC: U.S. Department of Commerce, U.S. Census Bureau, 2001.
2. The Hispanic Population, 2000. Census 2000 Brief. Washington, DC: U.S. Department of Commerce, U.S. Census Bureau, 2001.
3. U.S. Department of Health and Human Services. Healthy People 2010. McLean, VA: International Medical Publishing, 2000.
4. Arthur D. Recruiting, Interviewing, Selecting, & Orienting New Employees. 4th Ed. New York: American Management Association, 2005.
5. Alfred MV. Immigration as a context for learning: What do we know about immigrant students in adult education? In: Clover EE, ed: Proceedings of the Joint International Conference of the 45th Annual Adult Education Research Conference and the Canadian Association for the Study of Adult Education. Victoria, Canada: University of Victoria, 2004:13–18.
6. Keeping your edge. Managing a diverse corporate culture. Fortune 2001;143:S2–S6.
7. Cabrera A, LaNasa SM. On the path to college. Res Higher Educ 2001;42:119–149.
8. Hudson NL. Management Practice in Dietetics. 2nd Ed Belmont, CA: Wadsworth, 2005.
9. Griffin B, Dunn JM, Irvin J, et al. Standards of professional practice for dietetics professionals in management and foodservice settings. J Am Diet Assoc 2001;101:944–946.
10. Wilson JP. Workplace diversity and training: more than fine words. In: Wilson JP, ed: Human Resource Development: Learning & Training for Individuals & Organizations. 2nd Ed. Sterling, VA: Kogan Page, 2005:252–275.
11. Rasmussen T. Diversity Mosaic: The Complete Resource for Establishing a Successful Diversity Initiative. Hoboken, NJ: Jossey-Bass, 2006.
12. Brown C, Lane J. Studying Diverse Institutions: Contexts, Challenges and Considerations: New Directions for Institutional Research. Hoboken, NJ: Jossey-Bass, 2003.
13. Healthy People 2000. Washington, DC: U.S. Department of Health and Human Services, Office of Disease Prevention and Health Promotion, 1990.
14. Kittler PG, Sucher KP. Food and Culture. 4th Ed. Belmont, CA: Wadsworth, 2003.
15. Lynch EW, Hanson MJ. Developing Cross-Cultural Competence. 3rd Ed. Baltimore: Brookes, 2004.
16. D'Avanzo C, Geissler DM. Pocket Guide to Cultural Assessment. 3rd Ed. St. Louis: Mosby, 2003.
17. Archer SL. Acculturation and dietary intake. J Am Diet Assoc 2005;105:411–412.
18. Gordon L. Multicultural competence: Beyond the basics, J Am Diet Assoc 2001;101:520.
19. Paasche-Orlow M. The ethics of cultural competence. Acad Med 2004;79:347–350.

20. National Center for Cultural Competence. Policy Brief 1. Available at: http://www11.georgetown. edu/research/gucchd/nccc/documents/policy brief 1 200.3/pdf. Accessed March 15, 2007.

21. Fong R, Furuto S B. Culturally Competent Practice: Skills, Interventions, and Evaluations. Boston: Allyn & Bacon, 2001.

22. Ayoob KT, Duyff RL, Quagliani D. Position of the American Dietetic Association: food and nutrition misinformation. J Am Diet Assoc 2002;102:260–266.

23. Harris-Davis E, Haughton B. Model for multicultural nutrition counseling competencies. J Am Diet Assoc 2000;100:1178–1185.

24. Campinha-Bacote J. Cultural desire: The key to unlocking cultural competence. J Nurs Educ 2003;42:239–240.

25. Curry KR. Multicultural competence in dietetics and nutrition. J Am Diet Assoc 2000;100:1142–1143.

26. Bronner YL. Nutritional status outcomes for children: ethnic, cultural, and environmental context. J Am Diet Assoc 1996;96:891–903.

27. Kittler PG, Sucher KP. Accent on taste: an applied approach to multicultural competency. Diabetes Spectrum 2004;17:200–204.

28. Worthington-Roberts BS, Williams SR. Nutrition Throughout the Life Cycle. 4th Ed. New York: McGraw-Hill, 2000.

29. Committee on Nutrition. Pediatric Nutrition Handbook. 5th Ed. Elk Grove Village, IL: American Academy of Pediatrics, 2003.

30. U.S. Department of Agriculture Food Assistance and FANRP Nutrition Projects. Available at: http://www.ers.usda.gov/Briefing/FoodNutritionAssistance/projects/long.asp?Project=Food+ and+Nutrition+Information+Center+%28FNIC%29. Accessed March 15, 2007.

31. Skinner JD, Carruth BR, Bounds W, et al. Children's food preferences: a longitudinal analysis. J Am Diet Assoc 2002;102:1638–1647.

32. Borzekowski DLG, Robinson TN. The 30-second effect: an experiment revealing the impact of television commercials on food preferences of preschoolers. J Am Diet Assoc 2001:101:42–46.

33. Briley ME, Roberts-Grey C. Position of the American Dietetic Association: nutrition standards for child-care programs. J Am Diet Assoc 1999:99:981–988.

34. Briley ME, Roberts-Grey C. Position of the American Dietetic Association: benchmarks for nutrition programs in child care settings. J Am Diet Assoc 2005;106:979–986.

35. Stang J, Bayerl CT, Flatt MM. Position of the American Dietetic Association: child and adolescent food and nutrition programs. J Am Diet Assoc 2006;106:1467–1475.

36. U.S. Department of Agriculture Dietary Guidelines for Americans. Available at: http://www. health.gov/dietaryguidelines/dga2005/document/2005. Accessed March 15, 2007.

37. National Cholesterol Education Program of the National Heart, Lung, and Blood Institute. Available at: http://www.nhlbi.nih.gov/about/ncep/. Accessed March 15, 2007.

38. Resnicow KD, Davis R, Rollick S. Motivational interviewing for pediatric obesity: conceptual issues and evidence review. J Am Diet Assoc 2006;106:2024–2033.

39. Brigg SM, Safaii S, Beall DL. Position of the American Dietetic Association: nutrition services: an essential component of comprehensive school health programs—Joint Position of ADA, Society for Nutrition Education and American School Food Service Association. J Am Diet Assoc 2003;103:505–514.

40. Nicklas T, Johnson R. Position of the American Dietetic Association: dietary guidance for children: aged 2 to 11 years. J Am Diet Assoc 2004;104:660–677.

41. Cullen KW, Hartstein MS, Reynolds KM, et al. Improving the school environment: results from a pilot study in middle schools. J Am Diet Assoc 2007;107:484–489.

42. McKenzie J, Dixon L, Smiciklas-Wright H, et al. Change in nutrition intakes, number of servings and contributions of total fat from food groups in 4- to 10-year-old children enrolled in a nutrition education study. J Am Diet Assoc 1996;96:865–873.

43. Ritchie LD, Crawford PB, Hoelscher DM, et al. Position of the American Dietetic Association: individual-, family, school, and community-based interventions for pediatric overweight. J Am Diet Assoc 2006;106:925–945.

44. Gable S, Chang Y, Krull JL. Television watching and frequency of family meals are predictive of overweight onset and persistence in a national sample of school-aged children. J Am Diet Assoc 2007;107,53–61.

45. Mayo Clinic Food and Nutrition Center. Healthy breakfast: The best way to begin your day. Available at: http://www.mayoclinic.com/health/food-and-nutrition/NU00197. Accessed March 15, 2007.

46. Engels HJ, Gretebeck RJ, Gretebeck KA, et al. Promoting healthful diets and exercise: efficacy of a 12-week-after-school-program in urban African Americans. J Am Diet Assoc 2005;105,455–459.

47. Patton SR, Dolan LM, Powers SW. Dietary adherence and associated glycemic control in families of young children with type 1 diabetes. J Am Diet Assoc 2007;107,46–52.

48. Mackner LM, McGrath AM, Stark LJ. Dietary recommendations to prevent and manage chronic pediatric health conditions: Adherence, intervention, and future directions. J Dev Behav Pediatr 2001;22:130–143.

49. Dwyer JT, Stone EJ, Yang M, et al. Prevalence of marked overweight and obesity in a multiethnic pediatric population: findings from the child and adolescent trial for cardiovascular health (CATCH) study. J Am Diet Assoc 2000;100:1149–1154.

50. Rickard KA, Gallahue DL, Gruen GE, et al. The play approach to learning in the context of families and schools: an alternative paradigm for nutrition and fitness education in the 21st century. J Am Diet Assoc 1995;95:1121–1126.

51. Johnson SR, Mellin LM. Just for Kids! San Francisco: Balboa Publishing, 2001.

52. Matheson D, Spanger K. Content analysis of the use of fantasy, challenge, and curiosity in school-based nutrition education programs. J Nutr Educ 2001;33:10–16.

53. DiSogra L, Glanz K. The 5 a day virtual classroom: an on-line strategy to promote healthful eating. J Am Diet Assoc 2000;100:349–352.

54. Neumark-Sztainer D, Story M, Ackard D, et al. The "family meal": views of adolescents. J Nutr Educ 2000;32:329–334.

55. Sturdevant MS, Spear BA. Adolescent psychosocial development. J Am Diet Assoc 2002;102:S30–S31.

56. Patton S. Connecting with overweight kids. Today's Dietitian 2001;3:34–36.

57. Sigman-Grant M. Strategies for counseling adolescents. J Am Diet Assoc 2002;102:S32–S39.

58. Story M, Neumark-Sztainer D, French S. Individual and environmental influences on adolescent eating behaviors. J Am Diet Assoc 2002;102:S40–S51.

59. Hoelscher DM, Evans A, Parcel GS, et al. Designing effective nutrition interventions for adolescents. J Am Diet Assoc 2002;102,S52–S63.

60. Lytle LA. Nutritional issues for adolescents. J Am Diet Assoc 2002;102:S8–S12.

61. Calderon L. Promoting a healthful lifestyle and encouraging advocacy among university and high school students. J Am Diet Assoc 2002;102:S71–S72.

62. Neumark-Sztainer D, Story M, Perry C, et al. Factors influencing food choices of adolescents: findings from focus-group discussions with adolescents. J Am Diet Assoc 1999;99:929–937.

63. Henry BW, Ozier AD. Position of the American Dietetic Association: nutrition intervention in the treatment of anorexia nervosa, bulimia nervosa and other eating disorders J Am Diet Assoc 2006;106:2073–2082.

64. Neumark-Sztainer D, Wall M, Haines J, et al. Why does dieting predict weight gain in adolescents? Findings from Project EAT-II: a five year longitudinal study. J Am Diet Assoc 2007;107:448–455.

65. Trissler RJ. The child within: a guide to nutrition counseling for pregnant teens. J Am Diet Assoc 1999;99:916–917.

66. Klopp SA, Heiss CJ, Smith HS. Self-reported vegetarianism may be a marker for college women at risk for disordered eating J Am Diet Assoc 2003;103:745–747.

67. Mangels AR, Messina V, Melina V. Position of the American Dietetic Association and Dietitians of Canada: vegetarian diets J Am Diet Assoc 2003;103:748–765.

68. Older Americans 2000: Key Indicators of Well-Being. Federal Interagency Forum on Aging Related Statistics. Washington, DC: U.S. Government Printing Office, 2000.

69. Kuczmarski MF, Weddle DO. Position of the American Dietetic Association: nutrition across the spectrum of aging. J Am Diet Assoc 2005;105:616–633.

70. Niedert KC. Position of the American Dietetic Association: liberalization of the diet prescription improves quality of life for older adults in long term care J Am Diet Assoc 2005;105:1955–1965.

71. HCFA launches national nutrition and hydration awareness campaign. J Am Diet Assoc 2000;100:1305.

72. Shoaf LR, Bishirjian RO, Schlender ED. The Gerontological Nutritionists standards of professional practice for dietetics professionals working with older adults. J Am Diet Assoc 1999;99:863–867.

73. Vogelzang JL, Roth-Yousey LL. Standards of professional practice: measuring the beliefs and realities of consultant dietitians in health care facilities. J Am Diet Assoc 2001;101:473–480.

74. Guthrie JF, Lin BH. Overview of the diets of lower and higher income elderly and their food assistance options. J Nutr Educ Behav 2002;34:S31–S41.

75. Kuczmarski MF, Weddle DO. Position of the American Dietetic Association: nutrition, aging, and the continuum of care. J Am Diet Assoc 2000;100:580–595.

76. Blumberg J, Couris R. Pharmacology, nutrition, and the elderly: interactions and implications. In: Chernoff R, ed. Geriatric Nutrition: The Health Professional's Handbook, 3rd Ed. Gaithersburg, MD: Aspen, 2006.

77. Amarantos E, Martinez A, Dwyer J. Nutrition and quality of life in older adults. J Gerontol Biol Sci Med Sci 2001;56A:54–64.

78. Diet & health: Ten megatrends. Nutrition Action Health Letter 2001;28:3.

79. Unsworth L. Teaching Multiliteracies Across the Curriculum. New York: McGraw–Hill, 2001.

80. Fidalgo G, Chapman-Novakofski K. Teaching nutrition to Hispanics at an English as a second language (ESL) center: overcoming barriers. J Extension 2001;39:1. Available at: http://www.joe.org/joe/2001december/a3.html. Accessed December 12, 2007.

81. Boehl T. Linguistic issues and literacy barriers in nutrition. J Am Diet Assoc 2007;107,380–383.

82. Kalista-Richards M. The dynamics of education: making a match. J Renal Nutr 1998;8:88–94.

83. Harvard School of Public Health, Health Literacy Studies, Department of Society, Human Development and Health. Available at: http://www.hsph.harvard.edu/healthliteracy/materials.html. Accessed March 15, 2007.

Motivating Clients and Employees

OBJECTIVES

- Define motivation and differentiate between intrinsic and extrinsic motivators.
- Compare classic models of the motivational process with contemporary theories.
- Describe motivation principles as they apply to clients, including variables motivating and maintaining changes in food and lifestyle choices.
- Identify actions and strategies to motivate employees from a management perspective.

"I think I can. I think I can. I will."

Professionals in food, nutrition, and dietetics need to know how to enhance and maintain the motivation of their clients and employees. This can be a challenging task. Before people can do things differently, make changes in their dietary practices, or work efficiently, they must have the motivation to do so.

Applying what is currently known regarding human motivation is vitally important in setting goals, planning behavior modification strategies, designing and executing educational programs and seminars, and counseling others individually or in groups. Professionals who understand motivational concepts and theories and have the skills to adapt them to particular situations significantly increase their chances of being instrumental and influential in helping others.

Because the exact nature of motivation cannot be scientifically validated, myriad differing opinions and definitions of motivation currently exist. Motivation can be defined as something that causes a person to act or the process of stimulating a person to action. It is concerned with the questions of why human behavior occurs. The word "motivation" is frequently used to describe processes that (1) arouse and instigate behavior, (2) give direction and purpose to behavior, (3) continue to allow behavior to persist, and (4) lead to choosing or preferring a particular behavior. Motivation concerns not only what people can do but also what they will do. Recent studies appearing in the medical literature indicate continuous and ongoing study into the applications of motivation to health care.[1–8]

Motivation is complex, and many factors or variables influence the process at any one moment in time. Today's motivational influences may differ from tomorrow's, and short-term goals may take precedence over long-term ones. Having knowledge of how to work to get the most accomplished, of what to eat to become or remain healthy, or of what to do to cope with a current medical problem such as diabetes may easily be overpowered by other motivational factors. The problem is that being motivated to work, to make choices based on health, or to learn what one needs for appropriate cardiovascular or diabetes care involves long-term goals. Moreover, eating something such as chocolate cake or coming in late for work "just this once" meets a short-term goal of pleasure. Some people may delay the long-term for the immediate pleasure. Although there is a great deal of knowledge concerning motivation that is helpful, there are no miracle methods or universal answers to difficult motivational problems.[4,8]

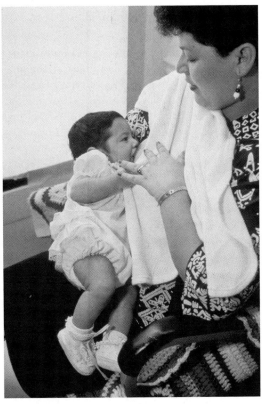

Parents may be motivated by concerns about child nutrition.
Source: United States Department of Agriculture.

Motivation can arise from factors that are either intrinsic (internal) or extrinsic (external), and these factors can affect the individual either positively or negatively. Intrinsic motivation arises from within people, according to their needs, desires, drives, or goals. People who desire to be promoted or clients who see recovery and better health as a personal priority after a heart attack have internal goals that motivate their behavior. External or extrinsic factors may supplement intrinsic motivation positively, or they may serve as barriers that have a negative impact on motivation. Examples of positive external factors enhancing motivation include support from others, praise, and material rewards. A person's motivation toward achieving lifestyle goals, however, may be hampered by social occasions or by family or friends who are not supportive and who offer improper foods.

A manager directly influences the motivation of employees who must learn the procedures necessary to work effectively, do their jobs conscientiously without close supervision, and grow to improve in the work environment. The clinical dietitian must motivate not only staff but also clients, who may need to learn about such things as the effects of diet on prenatal care or the problems of sodium, cholesterol, or sugar in the diet.

This chapter discusses motivation in two contexts: as an aid to client adherence and as an aid to managing staff. Although each area is treated separately, the same motivational principles and theories apply to both.

MOTIVATION OF CLIENTS

The goal of nutrition counseling and education is to change food and eating behaviors so that people select healthier diets. Food selection, however, is part of a complex behavioral system, which is shaped by a vast array of variables (see Chapter 1). The food choices of children are determined primarily by parents and by the cultural and ethnic practices in their environment. Other influences include the price of food, taste of food, religion, geography, peer and social influences, advertising in the media, facilities available, food preparation and storage, skills of the consumer in food preparation, time factors and convenience, and personal preferences and tolerances. Recent literature has focused on the role of environment and perception such as the effect of plate size on portion size and meal satisfaction. All these factors make food consumption a highly individual matter and resistant to change.[9,10]

As pointed out in other chapters, counselors hope to provide clients with interventions and strategies to motivate changes in health-promoting and disease-preventing behaviors that result in long-term lifestyle changes. However, no single theory or model is all-encompassing and ensures success. Instead, practitioners must be able to integrate a number of approaches and discern what may work with each individual. The motivational approaches referred to in this section have been discussed in more detail in other chapters of the book. This section combines the implications of the various approaches and models.

The purpose of most counseling is to enhance self-care and self-management. This, of course, depends on the person's readiness, willingness, and ability to undertake and maintain changes in eating practices.[8] Health-related decision making is influenced by many factors.[11,12]

Models to Enact Change

The Health Belief Model attempts to predict people's decisions about health behavioral change. Change is determined by the individual's belief (1) that he or she is susceptible to an illness or disease, (2) that it would be serious to contract the illness or leave it untreated, (3) that changing eating habits and practices will be beneficial in reducing the disease risk, and (4) that barriers to taking action can be overcome. The model is limited by the fact that behaviors such as eating are a matter of habit rather than decision making; that decisions to eat differently, such as to lose weight, may be made for reasons other than health; that health may not be a highly valued goal for some individuals; and that socioeconomic, psychological, and cultural factors may be more important to the person than health.[13,14]

The Transtheoretical Model or Stages of Change Model is helpful in pointing out that people are at one of several different stages of motivational readiness to change dietary practices from precontemplation (no intention of changing), to contemplation, preparation, action, and maintenance. At each stage, individuals use different processes or engage in various activities in making changes. Thus, the counselor can enhance motivation by recognizing the client's stage of change and using strategies appropriate to that stage. Decisions to change or move to a higher stage happen only when the pros outweigh the cons, or the benefits to the individual outweigh the costs and barriers.[6,7,15] An approach called motivational interviewing has been integrated into the Stages of Change Model discussed in Chapter 4.[16]

Self-Efficacy and Goal Setting

Albert Bandura's work on self-efficacy looks at people's beliefs about their capabilities to be successful at changing a behavior such as food choices to reach the health outcomes desired. People who believe they cannot do something (precontemplators) do not make any effort to change. If self-efficacy is low for a behavioral change or goal, another goal should be selected. Self-efficacy is more relevant in the preparation, action, and maintenance stages of change. Those with high levels of self-efficacy make a great deal of effort to change. Of four possible ways to increase self-efficacy in clients, the most effective is for the person to have small successes in reaching goals for change that can be followed by additional small successes.[17]

Goal setting can enhance motivation to change. People without specific goals are not motivated to make lifestyle changes. If you did not have a goal to obtain a college degree, for example, so that you were prepared for an interesting career that paid you well enough to sustain the lifestyle you wanted (note that motivational factors are multiple rather than singular), would you spend years of your life sitting in classes? Changes in food choices can be mutually negotiated into goals that are reasonable and measurable. The choices of goals should be selected by the client, not the counselor, and should be simple enough to promote success. People self-evaluate their own progress against the goals, and success increases self-efficacy.[18–20]

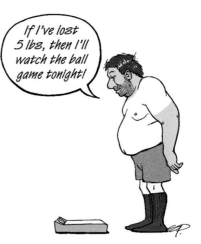

If I've lost 5 lbs, then I'll watch the ball game tonight!

Nonfood rewards are needed.

On the way to the goal, self-monitoring has been found to be helpful. Those who record food and exercise behaviors daily or for a period of time can see how well they are doing. They can note patterns of eating. Whether counting fat grams or recording changes in blood pressure or blood sugar, the client finds valuable information and increases self-understanding.[18,19]

When the goal is reached, clients need to reward themselves with nonfood items, which are external motivators. It is also helpful to decrease the stimuli or cues to eating in the environment and replace them with new and better cues. A behavioral program involves controlling the food and eating environment and rewarding oneself for successful change[21] (see Chapter 6).

No one is perfect, and there will be problems on the way to permanent change. James Prochaska notes that people may recycle to earlier stages of change more than once.[15] If so, the counselor changes strategies, matching them to the stage. Before that happens, however, clients can be counseled about the possibility of high-risk situations, slips, lapses, and ways to avoid total relapse.[22]

During a lapse, the person's cognitions or thoughts may turn negative. Instead of thinking "I can do this" (positive cognitions increase self-efficacy), the client may be thinking "This is too hard. I want to eat whatever I want" (negative thinking decreases self-efficacy).

SELF-ASSESSMENT

1. Compare your personal goals to the *Healthy People 2010* health objectives.
2. Do the pros outweigh the cons when reviewing barriers to accomplishing these objectives?
3. What is your stage of change for eating and for exercise?
4. What are key factors that motivate you?
5. List your short-term and long-term personal and professional goals. Analyze the factors that drive you to achieve these goals.

Most people greatly underestimate the influence of thoughts or self-talk on motivation and behavior. Counselors can ask clients to self-monitor their self-talk before and after eating and work on cognitive restructuring[22,23] (see Chapter 7).

Social support can have an impact on motivation and lifestyle changes as well. Is the family supportive of the change in food choices needed by one member? What are the cultural implications of the change? The support of significant others—family, friends, and the counselor—is helpful. Counselors may need to work with the family and within the cultural framework to ensure success. Recently, the term "nutritional gatekeeper" has been used to designate the person who controls the majority of food decisions in a client's life. This person, if not the client, needs to be included in the motivational plan as well.[9]

Nutrition education is important in letting people know what to do. Yet, it is over-rated as a way to motivate people to change. Many people already know what they should eat and how much they should exercise. But they are not doing it. Nutrition education is necessary, but it is not sufficient alone to motivate and promote change in food choices. Motivation to enact change is an essential part of the action process.

The preceding models and concepts should be combined and woven into counseling approaches and strategies to motivate change in eating behaviors. The client needs a combination of information, skills, and tools to address the continuum of challenges that each day brings. A comprehensive approach emphasizing internal over external motivators is more likely to be successful.

MOTIVATION OF EMPLOYEES

This section explores the concept of motivation as it relates to employees and examines theories of motivation and their behavioral implications for food and nutrition professionals. The reader should keep in mind that the forces instrumental in motivation are usually multiple rather than singular, that they differ in strength, and that more than one may be present at a given time.[24]

The foundation knowledge, skills, and competency requirements outlined by the Commission on Accreditation for Dietetics Education of the American Dietetic Association include several areas of human resource functions that include motivation. Motivation is also an integral element when participating in goal-setting processes as part of organizational change or business plan development.[25]

Classic Models of Maslow and Herzberg

Two early theorists who have made major contributions to the study of motivation are Abraham Maslow and Frederick Herzberg. Maslow correlated human motivation with individual desires. In his Hierarchy of Needs theory and "Need-Priority" Model, he lists five universal needs to explain human motivation: physiological needs, the need for safety and security, social needs, the need for esteem, and the need for self-realization. For each need to become active as a motivating factor, the desire immediately preceding the need must be fulfilled. In simplified terms, Maslow would say that the way to stimulate motivation in individuals is to determine which of their wants is most unsatisfied and then to structure their work so that in the accomplishment of the work goal, they satisfy their personal goals as well.[26]

The most basic human requirements are physiological (**Figure 9-1**). Sickness and hunger tend to take precedence over all other human needs. Only after they are satisfied does a person experience the desire to satisfy other needs. Indigent persons who are able to take care of only their physiological necessities may take a job regardless of the working conditions for their own and their families' sustenance and shelter. After they have enough money to satisfy these essentials, however, working merely for nourishment and shelter is no longer adequate. At that point, the motivation to work arises from a drive to maintain safety and security.

In most organizations today, security needs are satisfied through work contracts, unions, governmental regulations, and various insurance plans. With the fulfillment of biological and security needs, the individual's urge for social affiliation and activity becomes the dominant unsatisfied need and should therefore be considered in the design of work goals to motivate employees. Social needs can be experienced as a desire to

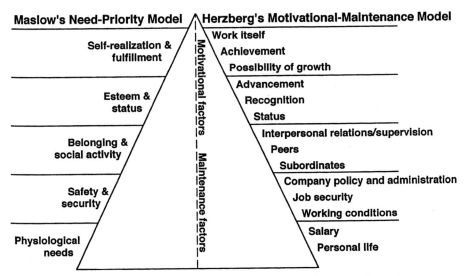

FIGURE **9-1**   A Comparison of Maslow's Need-Priority Model with Herzberg's Motivation–Maintenance Model. (Adapted from Herzberg F. Work and The Nature of Man. Cleveland, OH: World Publishing Co, 1966; and Maslow AH. Motivation and Personality. New York: Harper and Bros, 1954.)

become a member of, and participate in, a recognized group such as family, church, community, or work. If the social need becomes satiated, the employees' motivation is stimulated by a desire for esteem and status, which is commonly experienced as the need to attain recognition for accomplishments.

Although each of the five areas of needs becomes dominant at some time, the strongest motivator at a given moment is the one immediately above the last need satisfied. Once the requirement for esteem is no longer lacking, for example, the desire for self-realization becomes dominant. Self-realization is the highest human urge and the most self-centered. This drive for self-realization and the opportunity to grow as a person seems to be most effectively fulfilled only when most other needs are met. Now, during the 21st century, this need is commonly experienced as an urge for personal and professional growth that can best be satisfied through the work experience.[27]

It is difficult for dietetics practitioners to apply Maslow's theory with any degree of certainty, although social scientists still recognize his hierarchy of needs as fundamental. The task of getting to know subordinates well enough to infer their current need level accurately is unlikely unless a supervisor only has a small number of individuals reporting to him or her. Furthermore, need intensity at each level can vary from day to day and sometimes from hour to hour. One may be operating at the need level for increased esteem, suddenly have an accident, and become overwhelmingly concerned with the physiological needs of being able to feed one's family if incapacitated and unable to work. In spite of the limited applications of Maslow's theory, however, it does provide insight into the process of motivation and can often be useful in designing jobs, selecting staff, and developing strategies to maintain enthusiasm and interest among employees.

Frederick Herzberg, a contemporary of Maslow, is credited with the "two-factor theory of motivation" or the Motivation–Maintenance Model, which complements Maslow's theory and provides additional perspectives. Herzberg reviewed previous theories and studies and attempted to ascertain the essence of motivation by asking employees what they liked about their jobs and what they disliked about them. After examining the data, he determined that the answers to the first question ("What do you like about your job?") were "motivation factors," whereas the answers to the second question ("What do you dislike about your job?") were what he termed "maintenance factors."

The five motivators Herzberg compiled in response to the first question were (1) the work itself, being personally involved in the work, with a sense of responsibility and control; (2) achievement, feeling personal accomplishment for having done a job well; (3) growth, experiencing the opportunity for challenge in the job and the chance to learn skills and knowledge; (4) advancement, knowing that the experience and growth will lead to increased responsibility and control; and (5) recognition or being recognized for doing a job well, resulting in increased self-esteem.[28]

Herzberg called the answers to the second question maintenance factors because he found that they maintained but did not improve current levels of production. Maintenance factors were physical conditions, such as lighting in the office and food in the cafeteria; security—a feeling of certainty about the future and of contentment; economic factors—salary and fringe benefits; and social factors—relationships with fellow workers and the boss.

Herzberg found that when the maintenance factors were poor, productivity decreased. Inadequate maintenance factors, then, hindered production, whereas adequate maintenance factors only maintained the current level. Thus, maintenance factors merely "satisfy" workers; they do not motivate them. Although Herzberg's theory first gained prominence in the 1960s, it remains the basis for current research in the area of motivation.[29] As indicated in Figure 9-1, Herzberg's motivational factors are similar to those at the top of Maslow's Need-Priority Model, and his maintenance factors are toward the bottom of Maslow's model.

Contemporary Theories of Motivation

The theories of Maslow and Herzberg are well known but have not been consistently validated empirically. Several contemporary theories, however, do have a reasonable degree of valid supporting documentation. They are called contemporary theories not because they are only recently developed but because they represent the current state of the art in explaining employee motivation. Adult motivation has been classified into four broad categories: content theories, process theories, decision-making theories, and sustained-effort theories. Intrinsic motivation has been linked to a worker's own perception of competence as a direct link to accomplishment of goals.[30,31] Three specific contemporary theories are presented in more detail.

David McClelland's Theory of Needs

David McClelland's theory of needs focuses on three needs: achievement, power, and affiliation. Some people are driven by the need to excel, to achieve in relation to a set of standards, and to strive to succeed. Others are driven by a need for power, the desire to make others behave in a way that they would not otherwise have behaved. Still others are driven by a need for affiliation, the desire for friendly and close interpersonal relationships. McClelland suggests that determining an employee's major need structure is key to fitting that person into the right position. Although somewhat oversimplified, the theory posits that persons with high achievement needs might do particularly well managing themselves in sales, for example, but would not necessarily do well in management positions. Persons with high needs for power and recognition, however, would more likely be suited for management. Persons whose primary needs are in the affiliation area are best suited for the helping professions.

Although McClelland has conducted studies in the three need areas, most of the studies have focused on the area of achievement. McClelland has determined that high achievers prefer job situations with personal responsibility, feedback, and an intermediate degree of risk. When these characteristics are prevalent, high achievers are strongly motivated. A high need to achieve does not necessarily lead to being a good manager, especially in large organizations. People with high achievement needs are interested in how well they do personally and not in influencing others to do well.[32,33]

One promising phenomenon of McClelland's theory of needs is that employees have been successfully trained to stimulate their achievement need. Motivation specialists have been successful in teaching individuals to think in terms of accomplishments, winning, and success as well as helping them to alter behavior so as to act in a high achievement way by preferring situations in which they have personal responsibility, feedback, and moderate risks. Human resource professionals are hoping to learn that management can select a person with a high achievement need or develop its own candidate through achievement training.

Equity Theory

Equity theory is based on the belief that people compare their inputs and outcomes with those of others and then respond to eliminate any inequities. Employees might compare themselves with friends, neighbors, coworkers, colleagues in other organizations, or past jobs they themselves have had. Which referent an employee chooses is influenced by the information the employee holds about referents as well as by the attractiveness of the referent. If a registered dietitian, for example, was hired right out of college with a fair salary, challenging work, and an excellent opportunity to gain important experience, he or she would most likely be motivated to excel in the position until and unless someone he or she views as less competent is also hired to do the same work but for more money.

Based on equity theory, when employees perceive an inequity, they can be predicted to make one of six choices:

1. Change their inputs (i.e., stop exerting so much effort)
2. Change their outcomes (i.e., increase their pay if paid on a piece-rate basis by producing a higher quantity of units of lower quality)
3. Distort perceptions of self (e.g., "I used to think I worked at a moderate pace, but now I realize that I work a lot harder than everyone else.")
4. Distort perceptions of others (e.g., "Mary's job isn't as desirable as I previously thought it was.")
5. Choose a different referent (e.g., "I may not make as much as my brother-in-law, but I'm doing a lot better than my Dad did when he was my age.")
6. Leave the field (e.g., quit the job)

The primary distinction of equity theory is its contention that people are concerned not only with the absolute amount of rewards they receive for their efforts, but also with the relation of this amount to what others receive. They make judgments as to the relation between their inputs and outcomes and the inputs and outcomes of others. When people infer an imbalance in their outcome-input ratio compared with others, tension is created. This tension provides the basis for motivation, since people strive for what they perceive as equity and fairness.[34]

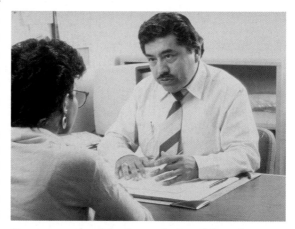

Managers can acknowledge the contributions of the employee.
Source: United States Department of Agriculture.

Expectancy Theory

The expectancy theory, formulated by Victor Vroom, is based on the belief that the strength of a tendency to act in a certain way depends on the strength of an expectation that the act will be followed by a given outcome and on the attractiveness of that outcome to the individual.[35] This theory is one of the most widely accepted explanations of motivation. Although it has its critics, research evidence is supportive of the theory.

Expectancy theory suggests that an employee is motivated to exert a high level of effort when he or she believes that effort will lead to a good performance appraisal; a good appraisal leads to organization rewards such as a bonus, a salary increase, or a promotion, and the rewards will satisfy the employee's personal goals.

This theory focuses on three relationships:

1. Effort–performance relationship: The probability perceived by the individual that exerting a given amount of effort will lead to performance.
2. Performance–reward relationship: The degree to which the individual believes that performing at a particular level will lead to the attainment of a desired outcome
3. Rewards–personal goals relationship: The degree to which organizational rewards satisfy an individual's personal goals or needs and the attractiveness of those potential rewards for the individual.[34]

Expectancy theory can be a useful tool in understanding why some dietetics employees are not motivated in their jobs and merely do the minimum necessary to get by. If, for example, an employee's motivation is to be maximized, an affirmative answer would be required for the three questions below:

1. "If I give a maximum effort, will it be recognized in my performance appraisal?"
2. "If I get a good performance appraisal, will it lead to organization rewards?"
3. "If I'm rewarded, are the rewards personally attractive to me?"

If the answer to any question is negative, less than maximum effort can be predicted according to the theory.[34–36]

Motivation Through Enhancement of Self-Esteem

Key issues of the early 21st century are the attraction and retention of skilled workers, with shortages of human talent rather than surpluses characterizing the United States during this period. Baby boomers, those born between 1945 and 1964, are now beginning to retire; with fewer offspring, they are the parents of the new generation of workers, the "baby-bust generation." Because of fewer entrants to the job market in the early 21st century, there may not be enough workers in the small cohort of people born after 1964 to fill the bottom level of the typical corporate pyramid. Increasingly, most of the workforce today is composed of post–baby boomers and recent immigrants. Both groups tend to define success in terms of power, prestige, and money. Senior management generally supports this definition as well. Managers face a challenge in responding creatively to these new demographics. A major concern of the contemporary manager is to understand the new workforce and how to adapt its needs to those of the organization.[37]

Another employment issue results from the fact that the number of highly qualified people in the workforce is growing at a much faster rate than is the number of senior-level jobs. Consequently, supervisors must understand how to spot the plateau problem and deal with it effectively before employees have no alternative but to quit the organization. The worker who has hit a career plateau often suffers from losses in productivity, self-esteem, or both. When employees' careers have reached a plateau and the company does not want to lose them, it can redefine success so that the sense of having reached a plateau does not arise.[38] Success can be redefined, for example, through various forms of public recognition, such as company awards, plaques, and other forms of recognition.

A third reality of the early 21st century, particularly in the health professions, is that organizations have to continue to maintain as lean and as motivated a staff as possible to compete and to comply with governmental regulations. In the process of becoming "lean," workers undergo changes such as "downsizing" and "right-sizing," which often involve merging of multiple existing positions. Those staff members who have survived may feel insecure, defensive, hostile, and fearful of losing their jobs. They may object to having had their former positions changed or enlarged without any monetary compensation. They may be unwilling to extend themselves because of the inference that the organization does not care about them. The manager or supervisor who is attempting to "motivate" staff under these conditions has a considerable challenge. While monetary increases are being kept to a minimum, the manager is expected to obtain more work from fewer people, who are already feeling unappreciated and overworked. Given this depressing but not unrealistic scenario, the manager needs to know and to exercise every motivational option available.

Generally, members of the current workforce differ considerably from their predecessors. The values of both post–baby boomers and recent immigrants, for example, are distinctly different from those of their parents. These younger employees generally are more affluent and educated and are less willing to rely on authority figures. They have different perceptions of themselves and are generally unwilling to tolerate a disrespectful supervisory style. Workers indicate that what they want most are a heightened sense of self-esteem, realization, recognition, autonomy, responsibility, and managers who recognize their capacity for these achievements.[39] Although some employees can always be motivated by the hope of merit salary increases, contemporary managers will benefit most from knowing how to enhance their staff's self-esteem and confidence, a vital methodology for increasing motivation of contemporary employees.[40–42]

There have been numerous studies of motivation among health care workers, and much is known about the relationship between motivation and increased self-esteem or recognition.[43–49] For more than half a century, social scientists have been aware of the phenomenon of the "self-fulfilling prophecy," which suggests that people perform and develop according to others' expectations of them. In one study, students and instructors were selected randomly, and some instructors were told that they had been selected to have all the brighter students in their classes. Later tests did verify that these instructors had students who performed statistically and significantly better than those in classes where instructors had no previous expectations.[50] People who are told that they are incompetent and will be unable to achieve a specific goal or task perform poorly compared with those who are told that they are competent and will be able to achieve the task, even though neither group has had previous experience with the task. A person's self-perceived ability, based on previous performance, is positively related to later performance. Success begets success, and failure begets failure.[47]

Unfortunately, an appreciation of the implications of this phenomenon for business and industry has only recently become apparent. Whenever supervisors acknowledge success in subordinates, they add to the likelihood that subsequent tasks will be performed successfully. For this reason, supervisors need to select carefully the right worker for the task, to provide adequate training to ensure employee success, and to assign work tasks that are manageable and accomplishable. Managers can enhance the self-esteem of employees by providing opportunities for their achievement, growth, recognition, responsibility, and control, which increase their motivation to improve or to continue to do well.

Empowerment is a concept that integrates autonomy with the ability to participate in decision making. Empowered individuals exhibit higher self-esteem. They often view their role as closer to that of their supervisor than their peers. Fostering empowerment in employees can increase performance and promote leadership traits.[51]

Motivation Through Setting Goals

Too often, subordinates believe that they are pleasing their supervisors only to learn that what they were doing was not what was desired or expected. Setting goals with subordinates as well as following up with subsequent periodic reviews provides feedback and promotes improved performance. Telling an employee, "Do your best," is useless. To the employee, who is faced with numerous alternatives for ways to spend his or her "working" time, this instruction can mean dozens of things. An effective way to assist others who wish to increase their esteem, growth, development, realization, and achievement is to teach them to be proactive in planning specific ways to accomplish more or to improve quality by setting goals. This sense of ownership also promotes empowerment and a feeling of inclusion in the goals of the organization.[49,51]

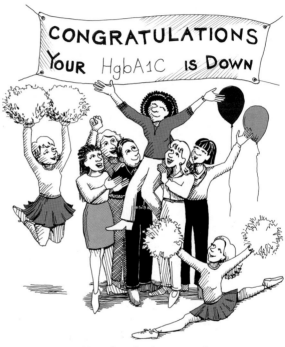

The counselor should reinforce the client positively.

The effect on individual performance of setting goals has been demonstrated. Theory and experiments support the proposition that supervisors should play an active role in setting goals with subordinates. Goals should be specific, clearly stated, and measurable.[34] When goals fulfill these conditions, they provide a criterion for feedback, accountability, and evaluation. A person can be highly motivated by knowing the objective and working on a plan with the dietetics manager to accomplish it. The three identifiable elements in goal setting are (1) an action verb, (2) a measurable result, and (3) the cost or date by which the objective will be accomplished. Both employee and manager must agree on their mutual expectations and clarify the difference, for example, between "I want you to get your work done soon," and "I want to see an increase of 10% by June 16th." Perhaps the single most significant advance in the field of management has been the growth of participative management. A major advantage of goal setting, a form of participative management, is that it directs work activities toward organizational goals and forces planning.

People who have specific and challenging goals tend to perform best. Goals seen as "sure things" may discourage motivation as much as those that are believed to be impossible. The best goals—those that inspire quality performance—are those that are perceived as difficult and challenging but attainable. A major proposition, supported experimentally, is that employees who set or accept harder goals perform at levels superior to those who set or accept easier goals.[52,53]

Regardless of whether the goal is set by the manager or the employee, the two parties need to agree. When staff members feel that they are actively participating in setting their own goals, even if the supervisor originally proposes the goals, they are more solidly motivated to perform with distinction than if they feel that they are merely being told what to do.

Motivation Through Reinforcement

Reinforcement, knowing how to encourage desirable behavior and to discourage undesirable behavior, is related to motivation. One way to increase the likelihood that a performance or behavior will recur is to follow the performance with a positive event, such as praise for a job well done. A positively reinforced response is more likely to recur simply because it pays off.

Another type of reinforcement is the removal of something negative after the performance. In this case, the persons are likely to repeat the behavior because something they dislike is taken away as a consequence of the behavior (see Chapter 6). This removal or elimination of adverse conditions is referred to as negative reinforcement. A hospital dishwasher, for example, who is constantly being checked by the manager and who has been able to decrease dish breakage by 30% from the previous month, will be motivated to continue improving if the manager not only praises the dishwasher but also checks this employee less often during the following week. The manager can then encourage the desired action by removing an unfavorable condition—the frequent inspections.

Two strategies that may discourage a given behavior are punishment and extinction. Reprimanding an employee for being late is an example of formal punishment. Although punishment is often used to eliminate undesirable behavior, its value is questionable because of its negative side effects. Punishment can make an employee hostile and prone to retaliation. If the punishment is perceived as unwarranted by employees, they may resume the undesirable behavior as soon as punishment stops. The way to overcome an employee's feelings of resentment when punished is to provide frequent constructive feedback each time an infraction occurs. In that way, when formal punitive action is taken, the employee perceives it as warranted and rational.[38,45]

The other basic technique for decreasing the likelihood of a behavior is extinction. With extinction, the undesirable performance is neither punished nor rewarded; it is simply ignored. Ignored behaviors tend to diminish and ultimately to become extinguished as a result of a consistent lack of reinforcement. For example, a manager who never acknowledges an employee's suggestions is actually encouraging the employee to stop sending them. Although its use may be unintentional, extinction is an effective technique for terminating behavior. A manager should be aware of the potentially negative consequences of ignoring desired behavior. Managers through carelessness can unintentionally extinguish motivated performances.

Managers should give recognition to employees in the presence of their peers. Recognition provides positive feedback and builds a worker's confidence and self-esteem. Organizations can benefit from involving their employees in the decision-making process. The more that employees are involved in decision making, the higher is the level of their performance and satisfaction. Employees who participate in making decisions feel a sense of ownership and commitment.

Managers at all levels reduce stress and increase efficiency and motivation when they negotiate with employees using clearly defined goals and objectives. The more employees understand what they are expected to do, the more highly motivated they become. Supervisors should give respect and dignity to their staff. The more they respect the rights and privileges of employees, the better the employees feel about themselves and the more they produce. Managers must become familiar with reinforcement techniques, training themselves to recognize and comment on good work to reinforce it. Ignoring good work may lead to extinction of desired behavior. Top management needs to instill in lower level management an appreciation of the human resources of the organization, supporting the development of increased self-esteem, recognition, and growth among all staff.[50]

This chapter emphasizes the complexity of motivation and discusses its behavior implications for professionals in food, nutrition, and dietetics. Practitioners are involved daily with motivation of both staff and clients. Understanding motivational concepts and being able to use the strategies and techniques associated with them can add immeasurably to the professional's effectiveness. The chapter provides a brief background on numerous theories of motivation. Attempts to validate most theories have been complicated by methodological, criterion, and measurement problems. As a result, many published studies that purport to support or negate a theory must be viewed with caution.

CASE STUDY 1

John, age 30, has been hired as an assistant cook at a small hospital. He has 1 year of previous experience cooking at a nursing home. The head cook and dietetics manager have participated in training John for the past 4 months.

1. What can the head cook and dietetics manager do to maintain and increase John's level of motivation?
2. Identify one specific strategy to increase John's sense of empowerment.

CASE STUDY 2

Martha M. was recently diagnosed with type 2 diabetes mellitus. She is 50 years old, 5'6", and 180 pounds. A homemaker, she is married to an electrician, and their only child is away at college. She is finding it increasingly difficult to motivate herself to get involved in outside activities now that the house is empty.

Martha describes her typical daily eating pattern as follows: She wakes in the morning with her husband, makes them both coffee, and prepares a warm breakfast for him

(continued)

CASE STUDY **2**

(continued from previous page)

before he leaves for work. She continues to drink her coffee but does not eat. She gathers her "to do" list and steps out to run errands. Around 11:00 AM she will grab a pastry and make another pot of coffee. For the rest of the afternoon she will clean house or work on crafts until about 5:30. She will than begin making dinner so that it will be prepared by about 7 PM, when her husband arrives home. Standard dinner dishes may include sausage lasagna and a small side salad; or fried chicken, mashed potatoes and gravy, and canned corn; or spaghetti and meatballs with toasted garlic bread and milk. Occasionally they will have dessert and share a bowl of ice cream or a brownie.

Now that the dietetics counselor has taken a nutrition history, he is considering alternative ways to motivate Martha to make changes in her food choices and eating practices.

1. Identify Martha's nutrition diagnosis, etiology, and signs and symptoms. What relevant information is available upon which to begin your session with this client?
2. What internal and external factors can you explore to motivate Martha to change her eating practices?
3. What nutrition interventions would you recommend for Martha?
4. Identify one specific strategy to motivate Martha to enact change.
5. Develop written documentation for your session with this client, incorporating the Nutrition Care Process (NCP) model as applicable

Note: Students may want to consult Emerson M, Kerr P, Soler MD, et al. American Dietetic Association Standards of practice and standards of professional performance for registered dietitians (generalist, speciality, and advanced) in behavioral health care. J Am Diet Assoc 2006:106:608–613.

REVIEW AND DISCUSSION QUESTIONS

1. What processes is the word "motivation" used to describe?
2. Give an example of positive external factors that enhance motivation.
3. Explain intrinsic motivation and give examples.
4. Discuss four ways to motivate clients.
5. List the factors in Maslow's Need-Priority Model.
6. Compare Maslow's and Herzberg's theories.
7. Compare and contrast two of the contemporary theories of motivation.
8. Describe four ways to enhance employee self-esteem.

SUGGESTED ACTIVITIES

1. List the factors that motivate a person to go to work or continue with his or her present job. Explain your response in terms of the Maslow and Herzberg models.
2. Interview someone who is interested in changing his or her eating habits, and determine the positive and negative influences on motivation.

3. Recall the last time you ate alone and you ate with others. Postulate what motivational factors affected your actions and choices. Sort them into categories as proposed under the theories discussed in the chapter.

4. Examine the forces that motivate you to learn something new. Are they related to your desire to remain physically well, secure, well-liked, and respected, or to your desire to prepare yourself for taking on additional responsibility, having more control, and achieving realization and actualization?

5. Indicate why the following statements would have a negative impact on an employee's motivation and how they might be amended so that they maintain the employee's self-esteem.
   A. "That job has been done incorrectly! What do I have to do to get you to understand?"
   B. "I'm tired of listening to you complain. Just keep still and do your job."
   C. "You will probably make a mess of this, but there isn't anyone else to do it."
   D. "If you would listen, you would understand."
   E. "You can't be serious about his order suggestion."

6. Interview someone about his or her current job or former job. Identify major factors that promote learning, achievement, or job retention.

7. For each of the following examples, list the reinforcement technique used and the feelings it might produce in the employee.
   A. Employee: "Mrs. Jones, since you told us to be on the lookout for problems with equipment, we have discovered two more."
      Manager: "Yes, but I'm looking for Helen now. Have you seen her?"
   B. Employee: "Mrs. Jones, I've finished all the work in the kitchen and have begun to rearrange the cabinets."
      Manager: "You mean it took you all this time just to do that?"
   C. Manager: "Mary, I am putting you on suspension for 3 days."
   D. Manager: "Mary, I want you to know that I appreciate how effectively you work with others. Several people have told me how thorough you are in using the new procedures."

WEB SITES

http://www.foodpsychology.cornell.edu   Motivation and food
http://www.mindlesseating.org   Motivation and behavior
http://www.mindtools.com   Goal setting
http://www.motivationalinterview.org   Motivational interviewing
http://www.motivation-tools.com   Motivation suggestions
http://www.prochange.com   Transtheoretical Model research and applications

REFERENCES

1. Newman VA, Thomson CA, Rock CL, et al. Achieving substantial changes in eating behavior among women previously treated for breast cancer—an overview of the intervention. J Am Diet Assoc 2005:105:382–391.

2. Hamman RF, Wing RR, Edelstein SL, et al. Effect of weight loss with lifestyle intervention on risk of diabetes. Diab Care 2006:29:2102–2107.

3. Snoek HM, van Strien T, Janssens JM, et al. The effect of television viewing on adolescents' snacking: individual differences explained by external, restrained and emotional eating. J Adol Health 2006:39:448–451.

4. Richards A, Kattelmann KK, Ren C. Motivating 18- to 24-year-olds to increase their fruit and vegetable intake. J Am Diet Assoc 2006:106:1405–1411.

5. Spencer EH, Frank E, Elon LK, et al. Predictors of nutrition counseling behaviors and attitudes of US medical students. Am J Clin Nutr 2006:84:655–662.

6. Johnson SS, Driskell MM, Johnson JL, et al. Transtheoretical model intervention for adherence to lipid-lowering drugs. Disease Man 2006:9:102–114.

7. Shepherd R. Influences on food choice and dietary behavior. Forum Nutr 2005:57:36–43.

8. Resnicow K, Davis R, Rollnick S. Motivational interviewing for pediatric obesity: conceptual issues and evidence review. J Am Diet Assoc 2006:16:2024–2033.

9. Wansick B. Mindless Eating: Why We Eat More Than We Think. New York: Bantam Books, 2006.

10. Wansink B, Chandon P. Meal size, not body size, explains errors in estimating the calorie content of meals. Ann Intern Med 2006:145:326–332.

11. Wee C, Davis RB, Phillips RS. Stage of readiness to control weight and adopt weight control behaviors in primary care. J Gen Int Med 2005:20:410–415.

12. Touyz S, Thornton C, Reiger E, et al. The incorporation of the state of change model in the day hospital treatment of patients with anorexia nervosa. Eur Child Adolesc Psychiatry 2003:12: 65–71.

13. Petrovici DA, Ritson C. Factors influencing consumer dietary health preventative behaviours. BMC Pub Health 2006:6:222–228.

14. Rosenstock IM. The health belief model and nutrition education. Can Dietet Assoc 1982:43:182–192.

15. Prochaska JO. Moving beyond the transtheoretical model. Addiction 2005 :101:768–774.

16. Di Noia J, Schinke SP, Prochaska JO, et al. Application of the transtheoretical model to fruit and vegetable consumption among economically disadvantaged African-American adolescents: preliminary findings. Am J Health Prom 2006:20:342–348.

17. Bandura A, Locke EA. Negative self-efficacy and goal effects revisited. J Appl Psychol 2003:88:87–99.

18. Schmitt JA, Benton D, Kallus KW. General methodological considerations for the assessment of nutritional influences on human cognitive functions. Eur J Nutr 2005:44:459–464.

19. Thorpe M. Motivational interviewing and dietary behavior change. J Am Diet Assoc 2003:103:150–151.

20. Diabetes Care and Education Dietetic Practice Group. ADA guide to diabetes medical nutrition therapy and education. Chicago: American Dietetic Association, 2005.

21. Robinson CH, Thomas SP. The interaction model of client health behavior as a conceptual guide in the explanation of children's health behaviors. Pub Health Nurs 2004:21:73–84.

22. Shepherd J, Harden A, Rees R, et al. Young people and healthy eating: a systematic review of research on barriers and facilitators. Health Educ Res 2006:21:239–257.

23. Schnoll R, Zimmerman BJ. Self-regulation training enhances dietary self-efficacy and dietary fiber consumption. J Am Diet Assoc 2001:101:1006–1011.

24. Thrash TM, Elliot AJ. Implicit and self-attributed motives: concordance and predictive validity. J Personality 2002:70:729–755.

25. Commission on Accreditation for Dietetics Education. Foundation Knowledge and Skills and Competency Requirements for Entry-Level Dietitians. American Dietetic Association, 2002.

26. Maslow AH. Motivation and Personality. 2nd Ed. New York: Harper & Row, 1970.

27. Maslow AH. Toward a Psychology of Being. 3rd Ed. New York: J. Wiley and Sons, 1999.

28. Herzberg F. Work and the Nature of Man. Cleveland: World Publishing Co, 1966.

29. Herzberg F. One more time: How do you motivate employees. Har Bus Rev 2003:81:86–96.

30. Barbuto JE. Four classification schemes of adult motivation: current views and measures. Perc Motor Skills 2006:102:563–575.
31. Cury F, Elliot AJ, Da Fonseca D, et al. The social-cognitive model of achievement motivation and the 2 × 2 achievement goal framework. J Pers Soc Psychol 2006:90:666–679.
32. McClelland DC, Winter DG. Motivating Economic Achievement. New York: Free Press, 1969.
33. McClelland DC. Toward a theory of motive acquisition. Am Psychol 1965:10:321.
34. Robbins SP, Judge TA. Organizational Behavior. 12th Ed. Englewood Cliffs, NJ: Prentice-Hall, 2006.
35. Vroom VH, Jago AG. The role of the situation in leadership. Am Psychol 2007:62:17–24.
36. Boverie PE. Transforming Work: The Five Keys to Achieving Trust, Commitment, and Passion in the Workplace. Cambridge, MA: Perseus Publishing, 2001.
37. Eccles JC, Wigfield A. Motivational beliefs, values, and goals. Annu Rev Psychol 2002:53:109–132.
38. Frey BS, Osterloh M. Successful Management by Motivation: Balancing Intrinsic and Extrinsic Incentives. New York: Springer, 2002.
39. Puckett RB. Practice paper of the American Dietetic Association: a systems approach to measuring productivity in health care foodservice operation. J Am Diet Assoc 2005:105:122–130.
40. Biesemeier CK. Achieving Excellence: Clinical Staffing for Today and Tomorrow. Chicago: American Dietetic Association, 2004.
41. Hanley GP, Owata BA, Roscoe EM. Some determinants of changes in preference over time. J App Beh Analysis 2006:39:189–202.
42. Crocker J, Park LE. The costly pursuit of self-esteem. Psychol Bull 2004:130:392–414.
43. Prochaska JM, Prochaska JO, Levesque DA. A transtheoretical approach to changing organizations. Adm Policy Men Health 2001:28:247–261.
44. Prochaska JO. Staging: a revolution in helping people change. Man Care 2003:12 (Suppl 9):6–9.
45. Dell DJ. Sustaining the Talent Quest: Getting and Keeping the Best People in Volatile Times. New York: New York Conference Board, 2002.
46. London M. Job feedback: Giving, Seeking, and Using Feedback for Performance Improvement. 2nd Ed. Mahwah NJ: Lawrence Erlbaum Associates, 2003.
47. Raj JD, Nelson JB, Rao KSP. A study of the effects of some reinforcers to improve performance of employees in a retail industry. Beh Mod 2006:30:848–866.
48. Petry NM, Alessi SM, Carroll KM et al. Contingency management treatments: reinforcing abstinence versus adherence with goal-related activities. J Consult Clin Psychol 2006:74:592–601.
49. Luthans F, Youssef CM, Avolio BJ. Psychological Capital: Developing the Human Competitive Edge. New York: Oxford University Press, 2007.
50. Hiam A. Motivational Management: Inspiring Your People for Maximum Performance. New York: American Management Association, 2003.
51. Buckley L, Maillet J, Decker RT, et al. Empowerment of registered dietitians who work in clinical positions. Top Clin Nutr 2007:22:9–19.
52. Senko C, Harackiewicz JM. Achievement goals, task performance, and interest: why perceived goal difficulty matters. Per Soc Psychol Bull 2005:31:1739–1753.
53. Bohlander G, Snell S. Managing Human Resources. 14th Ed. Cincinnati: South-Western Publishing Co, 2006.

Principles and Theories of Learning

OBJECTIVES

- Compare and contrast learning theories and strategies.
- Differentiate between types of behavioral consequences.
- Specify strategies that enhance long-term memory.
- Describe several learning and teaching styles.
- Define the stages involved in the innovation-decision process.
- Identify the role of technology in learning

To increase the effectiveness of nutrition education in promoting sensible food choices, food and nutrition professionals should utilize appropriate behavioral theory and evidence-based strategies[1].

The foundation for effective education efforts is based on theory. Theoretical concepts are used in the planning, implementation, and evaluation of education. Nutrition education focuses on health promotion, the prevention of chronic diseases, and intervention and treatment. Achieving healthier lifestyles is a challenge for many.

LEARNING

What is learning? Learning may be defined as a change in a person as a result of experience or the interaction of a person with his or her environment. The changes may be in knowledge, skills, attitudes, values, and behaviors, and there are relatively permanent outcomes. Cognitive psychologists view learning as an "active mental process of acquiring, remembering, and using knowledge."[2] As you read this chapter, for example, you are learning. Other than learning by reading, the practitioner's challenge is to determine how to present people with the right stimuli and experiences on which to focus their attention and mental effort so that they can acquire new knowledge, skills, attitudes, and behaviors.

How do people learn? How do they retain what they learn? The field of educational psychology studies questions about the process of learning, including learner preferences and teaching delivery methods. Its major focus is on the processes by which knowledge, skills, attitudes, and values are transmitted between teachers and learners. Teachers must "learn about learning" before they can effectively teach.[3]

In the workplace, food and nutrition professionals provide learning opportunities in a variety of ways. They train and educate new employees and retrain experienced workers. They also participate in the delivery of educational programs for other health professionals, students, interns, residents, and paraprofessionals. Practitioners are concerned with discovering the most effective methods of teaching to influence the dietary behaviors of clients and the work behaviors of employees. Although theory alone does not guarantee effective education, applying theories to planning and implementing interventions does.

A major emphasis is on the education of clients. Effective client education includes the process of influencing behavior, and producing changes in knowledge, attitudes, values, and skills required to improve and maintain health. Giving information (knowledge) or telling people what they should do is not sufficient to achieve changes in food practices. Counseling and education approaches that will promote changes in attitudes and behaviors benefitting health status are necessary.

Education takes place at different levels: the individual level, such as one-on-one or group classes; the social network, such as family; and the community level, such as society at large. The public health initiative "Fruits and Veggies—More Matters" produced by the Produce for Better Health Foundation is an example of a community-level educational program.[4]

Effective use of educational theory takes practice in helping people make changes in their eating practices and environments. Health behaviors are too complex to be explained by a single theory. To explain how people learn, psychologists have developed several learning theories. This chapter discusses behavioral learning theories and social cognitive theory, as well as memory, transfer of learning, adult learning or andragogy, learning and teaching styles, the adoption of innovations, and technology as a teaching tool. Many of these theories and strategies can be utilized together in the same intervention.[5]

The social and behavioral sciences provide many of the education models used by health professionals. These models can be found in other chapters of this book and include the Transtheoretical Model or Stages of Change Model and motivational interviewing in Chapter 4, behavior modification in Chapter 6, and social cognitive theory in Chapter 7. All of these can be applied to nutrition interventions. The educator must select the most appropriate strategies and methods for each situation.

BEHAVIORAL LEARNING THEORIES

Behavioral learning theories are explanations of learning that are limited almost exclusively to observable changes in behavior, with emphasis on the effects of external events on the individual.[2] Theorists are interested in the way in which pleasurable or painful consequences of behavior may change the person's behavior over time. This approach is based on the belief that what we learn has readily identifiable parts and that identifiable rewards and punishments can be given to produce the learning.[6] The teacher's role is to arrange the external environment to elicit the desired response.[7]

Behavioral learning theories evolved from the research of several individuals, including Ivan Pavlov on classical conditioning; Edward Thorndike, who noted that the connections between stimuli and subsequent responses or behaviors are strengthened or weakened by the consequences of behavior; and B.F. Skinner's work on operant conditioning.[2,8] Other information on their research may be found in Chapter 6.

Based on the Pavlovian approach, association theory suggests that a stimulus event cues or elicits a response in the learner. Teaching or conditioning, therefore, involves arranging the stimulus and response events. This is a teacher-centered approach with passive learners.

Skinner's work focused on the relationship between the behavior and its consequences. Skinner believed that many human behaviors are operants, not merely respondents. The use of pleasant and unpleasant consequences following a par-

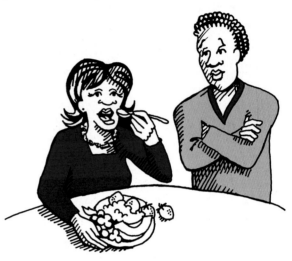

Pleasurable consequences reinforce eating behaviors.

ticular behavior is often referred to as operant conditioning.[2,8] Learning involves three related events: the stimulus, a response, and a reinforcer. The teacher must manage all three events. The desired target behavior must be followed by reinforcement for the behavior to continue. Thus, reinforcers, such as small objects, must be identified and given if the desired response is present. This is also a teacher-centered approach with a passive learner. Behaviorism does not explain every kind of learning as it disregards the activities of the mind.

In the following sections, four consequences of a behavior are discussed: positive reinforcement, negative reinforcement or escape, punishers, and extinction. In addition, shaping and the timing of reinforcement are examined.

Positive Reinforcers

One of the most important principles of behavioral learning theory is that behavior changes according to its immediate consequences. Pleasurable consequences are called "positive reinforcers" or rewards and may be defined as consequences that strengthen and increase the frequency of a behavior.[2] Examples are praise for a job well done, good grades received in school, money in the form of a salary increase, and token reinforcers such as stars or smiley-face stickers on a chart. When behaviors persist or increase over time, one may assume that the consequences are positively reinforcing them. The pleasure associated with eating, for example, is a positive reinforcer, ensuring that people will consume their favorite foods again and again.

These reinforcers are highly personal, however, and none can be assumed to be effective all the time. The behavior of an employee who has a poor relationship with a supervisor, for example, may not be affected by the supervisor's praise. And the professional's praise of a client who has followed a dietary regimen may not matter to that specific individual. The person must value the reinforcer to increase the frequency of a desired behavior. The professional can explore the items that an individual considers positive reinforcers and can help arrange such reinforcement in the person's environment. Knowledge of results is also an effective secondary positive reinforcer. Clients and employees should know their stage of progress. If they know they are doing something properly, that knowledge reinforces the response.

The way in which praise is given is also important, and the person doing the praising must be believable.[2] The praise should recognize a specific behavior, so the person clearly understands why he or she is being recognized. "Good job" as a praise is not as effective as saying specifically, "Thanks for completing the extra project on time. I appreciate it."

Negative Reinforcers/Escapes

Reinforcers that are escapes from unpleasant situations are called negative reinforcers. These also strengthen behaviors because they enable the individual to withdraw from unpleasant situations.[2] Overeating may be reinforcing if the individual escapes, for example, feelings of loneliness, unhappiness, fatigue, and the like. Or, an employee may escape the supervisor's wrath by behaving correctly. If some action stops, avoids, or escapes something unpleasant, the person is likely to repeat that action again when faced with a similar situation.

Punishers

Negative reinforcers, which strengthen behaviors, should not be confused with punishers, which weaken behaviors. Unpleasant consequences, punishers, decrease the frequency of or suppress a behavior.[2] Punishment may take one of two different forms. One form involves removal of positive reinforcers that the person already has, such as a privilege. A second form involves the use of unpleasant or adverse consequences, as when a person is scolded for improper behavior. Punishment can make a person avoid the situation in the future, so scolding a client who has not lost any weight is not appropriate.

Extinction

What happens when reinforcers are withdrawn? A behavior weakens and eventually disappears, a process called extinction of a behavior.[2] If a person starts an exercise program or dietary change, for example, and there are not continuous positive reinforcers, that person may decrease the new behavior and eventually end it.

When behaviors are undesirable and the reinforcers for it can be identified and removed, the behavior also may become extinct. An employee's boisterous behavior, for example, may change if the supervisor and other employees ignore the person and do not respond with the attention he or she is seeking. Instead, the supervisor will want to reinforce positively nonboisterous behavior in this person.

Shaping

The decision of what to reinforce in a client or employee, and when, is also important. Does one wait until the desired behavior is perfect? No! Most people need reinforcement along the way to something new. Reinforcing each step along the way to successful behavior is called shaping, or successive approximations.[2] It involves reinforcing progress rather than waiting for perfection. When client or employee goals can be broken down into a series of identified steps or subskills, positive feedback may be given as each step or subskill is mastered or accomplished.

Timing Reinforcement

An important principle is that positive consequences that are immediate are more effective than those that are delayed. The connection between the behavior and the consequences is better understood in the person's mind. As a result, the food and nutrition professional needs to identify with the client or employee not only what is positively reinforcing to that person, but also a time schedule for dispensing that reinforcement for proper behaviors. This concept explains why it is difficult for people to change their eating behaviors. Usually, the positive consequences of the change, such as weight loss or better health, are in the future, whereas eating disallowed foods is positively reinforcing immediately. It tastes good or hunger is reduced. Eating is intrinsically reinforcing, that is, a behavior that is pleasurable in itself.

The frequency of reinforcement has also been studied. In the early part of a behavior change, continuous reinforcement after every correct response helps learning. Later on, a variable or intermittent schedule of reinforcement is preferable. When rewards are overused, they lose their effect, so that after an individual has had some rewarded successes, rewards should be given less frequently. **Table 10-1** summarizes some of the implications of the theories discussed in this chapter.

SOCIAL COGNITIVE THEORY

Social cognitive theory expanded the behaviorist view. Since the 1970s, Albert Bandura has been considered the father of the modeling theory. He believed that the observation of and imitation of other people's behavior, that is, vicariously learning from another's successes and failures, had been ignored. He maintained that people learned not only from external cues, but also from observing models or "modeling." People who focus their attention on watching others are constructing mental images, analyzing, evaluating, remembering, and making decisions that affect their own learning. Professionals need to be aware of this and to be good role models. If we do not eat nutritiously and exercise regularly, for example, how can we expect others to do so?

When Oprah Winfrey lost weight the first time, many of her viewers started on the same diet to model after her success. It is preferable, of course, if the model is an attractive, successful, admired, and well-known individual. Then people will imitate the behavior, hoping to capture some of the same success.

In group learning situations, clients and employees can learn from good role models. In demonstrating the operation of kitchen equipment to a new employee, part of the learning comes from watching the trainer. Then the employee imitates what he or she has seen. In group classes for individuals making dietary modifications due to heart disease, for example, people may be influenced to make dietary changes by modeling after the success stories of others in the group.

T A B L E **10-1** | Implications of Learning Theories and Models

Theory/Model	Implications
Behavioral theory	Find out what reinforcers are valued
	Tell the person their stage of progress
	Use positive reinforcement
	Praise specific, not general, behaviors
	Reinforce progress on the way to mastery
	Use continuous reinforcement, then intermittent
	Ignore undesirable behaviors
	Avoid punishment
Social learning	Be a good role model
	Provide other good role models
	Avoid negative models
	Have new skills demonstrated and practiced
Cognitive theory	Explore prior knowledge
	Gain and maintain attention
	Ask questions
	Use goal setting
	Use repetition and review
	Make information meaningful
	Organize information
	Link new information to the memory network
Learning styles	Identify preferences for styles
	Offer several methods or techniques of learning
Adult learning	Adults are self-directed
	Recognize prior experience
	Use participatory methods
	Orient learning to problems and projects
	Use goal setting

Individuals also learn vicariously from watching negative models. When we see that something does not work or we disagree with it, we decide not to imitate it. Seeing an obese person can trigger this type of reaction in some people. "I'll never be like that" may be a response. People judge behaviors against their own standards and decide which models to follow. Sometimes, employees model after others who take shortcuts and do not follow proper procedures. If the supervisor takes extra-long breaks and lunches, for example, employees may conclude that this behavior is permissible.

When the professional wants people to model knowledge or skills they are acquiring, it is important to have them practice and demonstrate the skill, not just rehearse it mentally. This shows whether or not they are modeling correctly. For example, the practitioner may want a client who is learning to make different food choices to plan several menus to model the new knowledge and skill. A new employee who can demonstrate the proper use of equipment is modeling correctly. If the individual is correct, feedback and positive reinforcement such as praise should be given; self-efficacy and motivation are then enhanced. If the person is only partially correct, using "shaping," one may give positive reinforcement for the correct portion and then assist in altering the rest. Mentoring another person is another example of using these principles as the mentor models and guides new roles and behaviors.

Each learner is more effectively counseled by a professional who has a familiarity with the learner's unique circumstances, learning style, and context. Each person is at a different developmental life stage with degrees of motivation. Family and social contexts vary. The profes-

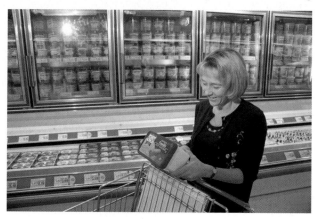

People learn through active involvement.
Source: United States Department of Agriculture.

sional can then personalize an intervention strategy for learning. A multicultural society requires the awareness of group customs, traditions, and acceptable counselor approaches (see Chapter 8, which discusses these aspects in detail).

COGNITIVE THEORIES

Cognitive psychologists studying learning focus on mental activities, such as thinking, remembering, and solving problems that cannot be seen directly. Rather than observable changes brought about by external events, cognitive learning theories are explanations of learning that focus on internal, unobservable mental processes that people use to learn and remember new knowledge or skills.[2]

Which is easier to learn—the formulas for the essential amino acids or the MyPyramid food guide? Which is easier to remember—a phone number used yesterday for the first time or the food that was eaten for dinner last evening? The difference is between rote learning, which requires memorizing facts not linked to a cognitive structure, and learning and remembering more meaningful information without deliberately memorizing it. Both are necessary.

The cognitive view sees learning as an active internal mental process of acquiring, remembering, and using knowledge rather than the passive process influenced by the external environmental stimuli of the behaviorists.[2] Individuals pursue goals, seek information, solve problems, and reorganize information and knowledge in their memories. In pondering a problem, the solution may come as a flash of insight as people reorganize what they know.

The cognitive approach suggests that an important influence on learning is what the individual brings to the learning situation, that is, what he or she already knows.[2] Prior

TABLE **10-2** | Learning Theories and Strategies

	Behavioral	Social Learning	Cognitive	Andragogy
Teacher's role	Arrange environment to get desired response Arrange reinforcement	Serve as role model Arrange for other role models	Structure content or problems with essential features Organize knowledge	Facilitator Plan, implement, evaluate jointly Provide resources
Management	Teacher-centered	Learner-centered	Learner-centered	Learner-centered
Learner participation	Passive/active	Active Imitate models	Active, solve problems Test hypotheses	Active
Motivation	Rewards motivate External	Both external and internal	Internal Use goal setting	Internal
View of learning	Rote learning Subject matter approach Practice in varied contexts	Observation of others	Insight learning Understanding Internal mental process	Performing tasks Solving problems Goal-oriented
Strategies	Stimulus-response Behavioral objectives Task analysis Competency-based Computer-assisted learning	Social roles Discussion Mentoring Role playing	Inquiry learning Discovery learning Simulation Learning to learn	Oriented to problem solving and task performance

knowledge is an important influence on what we learn, remember, and forget. Remembering and forgetting are other topics in cognitive psychology. **Table 10-2** compares the theories discussed in this chapter.

Discovery learning is an example of a cognitive instructional model. When people learn through their own active involvement, they discover things for themselves. This approach, using experimentation and problem solving, helps people to analyze and absorb information rather than merely memorize it.[2] The professional can provide problem situations that stimulate the client to question, explore, and experiment.

> EXAMPLE: What can you eat for breakfast? In a restaurant? On trips? What does the food label tell you?

MEMORY

There are many theories of memory that explain how the mind takes in information, processes it, stores it, retains it, and retrieves it for use when needed. Cognitive-perception theories see learning as an all-or-none event rather than an incremental process. Past perceptions already are stored in memory for future use. If the learner has no prior experience to draw upon (a perceptual deficit), a frame must be created with the help of the educator. With prior experience, a frame exists already. If the current frame is incorrect, a different frame must be created. Through the use of questions and listening, the food and nutrition professional can discover the learner's frame of reference and build on it. Strategies must fit the client's frame of reference. Teaching involves managing real or vicarious experiences until the learner develops insight, outlooks, or thought patterns.[9] This is a teacher–student-centered approach with cooperative and interactive inquiry and problem solving.[10]

Other interventions are based in cognition–rational/linguistic learning theory.[10] Experiences become encoded in memory. As a result, people can organize, modify, or combine memories, resulting in new knowledge or higher levels of thinking. Reasoning skills allow analysis of experiences and prediction of future outcomes. Most behavior results from the cognitive analysis of knowledge, so thoughts are believed to precede a person's actions.

The consumer information processing theory addresses processes by which a consumer takes in and uses information in decision making. The theory points out that people have a limited capacity to process, store, and retrieve information at any one time. In making decisions, they seek only enough information to make a choice quickly. Thus, information should be organized, limited, and matched to the comprehension level of the individual, who can then process it with little effort. For example, people may look for the frozen dessert with the lowest fat content, store the information about their satisfaction with the product, and decide whether or not to purchase it again.[11]

To enhance memory and reasoning, teaching requires providing labels for new experiences and structures. Problems may be treated as cognitive deficits requiring new structures. Clients with defeating self-statements and cognitive distortions, for example, require cognitive restructuring that rules out the current incorrect thought and introduces a new one (see Chapter 7).

The food and nutrition professional wants people not only to acquire information, skills, and attitudes, but also to remember and use them. Since people are bombarded with information all day long from family, friends, coworkers, supervisors, newspapers, magazines, television, radio, and the Internet, how do they remember it all? They don't. Much is immediately discarded.

Psychologists agree that people must make sense of new information to learn and remember it. Some information enters working or short-term memory until it is used, such as the time of an appointment; then it is forgotten. Of course, nothing even enters short-term memory until the person pays attention to it, that is, focuses on certain stimuli and screens out all others.[2] Therefore, the dietetics professional needs to think first of obtaining and then maintaining a client's or employee's attention and focus. Otherwise, the individual may be thinking about something else.

There are various ways to gain a learner's attention, such as the use of media, bright colors, raising or lowering one's voice, using gestures, starting a discussion with a question, explaining a purpose, repeating information more than once, and saying, "this is important." Gaining someone's interest in a topic at hand and indicating its importance to him or her as well as putting it in the context of what the person already knows are all helpful approaches. The professional should indicate how the information will be useful or important.[2]

Asking questions arouses curiosity and interest. The use of open-ended questions is an effective technique to solicit additional information. These questions typically begin with who, what, when, where, or why. Ask a new employee, "What do you know about the meat slicer?" Or, ask a new client with heart disease, "What do you know about saturated and trans-fats?" Ask why they think learning this information is important to them. This forces the person to focus attention.

Working Memory

The human mind is like a computer. It receives information, performs operations on it to change its form and content, stores it, and retrieves it when needed.[2] Not all information or stimuli are selected for further processing, but some is focused on at a given moment.

As a person attends to something new and thinks about it, it enters working memory. There are limits, however, to the amount of new information that can be retained at one time, perhaps five to nine items, and on the length of time it will be retained, probably 5 to 20 seconds.[2] Repeating something new over and over, such as the name of a person you have just met, helps to keep information in short-term memory longer. But if you meet five new people at once, this can be too much new information to handle.

Besides repetition, you may attempt to associate new information with information currently in long-term memory. Chunking, or grouping individual bits of information, also helps. For example, the telephone number 467-3652 becomes 467 36 52. Because of memory limits, it is helpful to give not only oral information, but also written dietary guidelines to a client or a written task analysis to an employee, since details are forgotten quickly.

Long-Term Memory

On a computer a person takes the input and "saves" it onto a memory-stick or hard drive to be retrieved later. To move new information from working memory to long-term memory, a person tries to organize it and integrate it with information already stored there in a network of interconnected neurons. Long-term memory involves three processes: encoding by attaching new information to other related memories, storage, and retrieval. Who cannot recognize the smell of a chocolate cake baking in the oven by retrieving the memory? Here, the professional needs to make clear to clients and employees what is important and probably repeat it more than once. It takes time and effort to reflect, to grasp the implications, to interpret and experience, and to guide an internal representation of new knowledge in the brain.[2]

The ability to recall rote information is limited, whereas meaningful information is retained more easily. The implication for planning educational sessions for clients and employees is to make the information meaningful to the individual, present it in a clear and organized manner, and relate it to what the individual already knows and has stored in memory. The person can then connect it to other known information and apply it if necessary.

Which is easier to store and later retrieve—something one hears, something one sees, or something one both sees and hears? People retain visual plus verbal images and messages better. Some people use imagery to aid retention by picturing something in the mind.[2,8] Can you picture the MyPyramid food guide, or a food product label, for example?

There are various strategies to help people remember. The professional can summarize in the middle and at the end of a presentation. Repetition and review are helpful for retention. You may put an outline on a handout or project an image to organize information. Get people involved in talking with active instead of passive learning activities. Present information in a clear, organized fashion, not as isolated bits of information. Then, ask the person to translate the information into his or her own words or solve a problem with it, such as plan a menu or summarize what was said so that material provides personal significance.

People also remember stories, metaphors, and examples better than isolated facts. In teaching employees about food sanitation, for example, stories of actual outbreaks of foodborne illness are helpful. When teaching about modified diets, examples of actual client cases may be used. In a discussion of fiber with a client, examples of whole-grain breads and cereals, fruits, and vegetables may be discussed. Learning requires people to make sense of information, to sort it in their minds, to fit it into a neat and orderly pattern, and to use current information to help assimilate the new.

Long-term memory requires connections of new knowledge to known information. Information is probably stored in networks of connected facts and concepts. Each piece of information in memory is connected to other pieces in some way. We remember things by association. The word "apple," for example, may be associated with fruits, red, or tree. You would be unlikely to associate it with a cat.

The following is an example of a partial knowledge network on water-soluble vitamins:

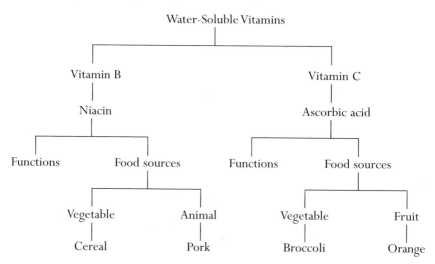

If a person already has this network and learns something new about vitamin C—for example, that raw cabbage is a good food source of vitamin C—it is easy to file it into the existing network by association. If, however, a person knows nothing about vitamin C, it would be much more difficult to file the new information into long-term memory. The result is that it may be forgotten.

The following is an example of a knowledge network on food sanitation:

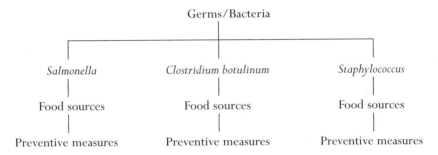

For food service workers, the term "germs" may be more meaningful and easier to store into memory than "pathogenic bacteria" since the latter term may be unfamiliar. It will be easier to add new information into an existing network if terms are recognizable and build upon previously learned concepts. Adding a new term such as "*E. coli*" (*Escherichia coli*) or "hepatitis A" will be more meaningful than a newer, broader term if a framework exists.

Food and nutrition professionals need to spend time finding out what a person already knows, actively listening to the words he or she uses, identifying the topics in the knowledge networks, probing with the use of questions, and assisting the person with integrating new information into the existing network. Material that is organized well is much easier to learn and remember than material that is poorly organized. Our motivation to learn is intrinsic or internal as we seek to make sense of what is happening in our world.[6]

Organizing around concepts also helps the learner to categorize vast amounts of information into meaningful units. The following is an example of organizing information around the concept of meals:

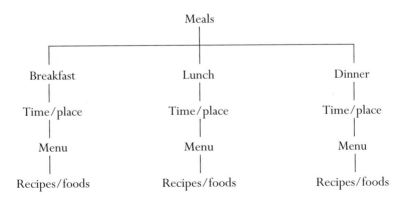

Posing questions helps people learn by asking them to examine what they are hearing or reading.

When teaching about concepts, one needs to use a lot of examples. What mental picture or ideas does the client or employee have if the professional discusses "cholesterol," "saturated fatty acids," "blood glucose," "microorganisms," "grams" as a weight, "ounces" of meat, "quality improvement," and the like. Finding out what words or terminology people use in the content of their current knowledge network helps when selecting examples to use with them.

TRANSFER OF LEARNING

In human resource management as well as in other situations, the question frequently asked is "Did the training transfer?" In other words, can an individual take the knowledge, skills, attitudes, and abilities learned in the training situation, remember them, and apply them effectively on the job in a new situation or in a dissimilar one.[2] Transfer of learning cannot be assumed. It depends partly on the degree of similarity between the situation in which the skill or concept was learned and the situation to which it is applied. The implication is that one should teach people to handle the range of situations that they are likely to encounter most frequently at work (employees) or at home (clients). The practitioner needs to give

many examples from the range of problems that the person may encounter in using the knowledge or skills learned.[12] When people actually use their new knowledge and skills to solve problems, transfer of training is confirmed.

For a client on a modified diet, for example, it is not enough to teach which foods to eat and avoid, but also how to transfer that information into planning menus, adapting current or using new recipes, choosing appropriate menu items in restaurants, and reading labels while shopping in the supermarket. Using knowledge or skills to solve problems, such as what to do in a restaurant, helps people apply what they learned. Can a person with diabetes, for example, convert the restaurant portion of a pasta serving into a serving from the exchange list or calculate the carbohydrate content? When grocery shopping, can the calories of a serving size be correctly identified?

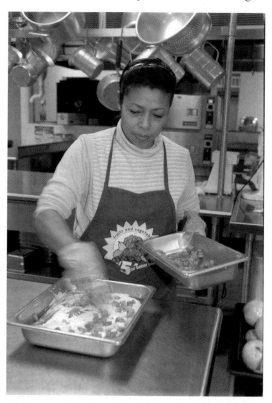

Adults are ready to learn when they have a need for learning.
Source: United States Department of Agriculture.

Learning does not transfer automatically. For employees, learning is enhanced when teaching takes place in an actual or simulated environment. Cashiers, for example, need to be trained on the equipment they will be using in handling all types of transactions. When training does not transfer to the job, possible reasons are that trainees found the training irrelevant, that they did not retain it, or that the work environment or supervisor does not support the newly learned behavior.[12]

Since most people consider that it is "bad" to be wrong, and "good" to be right, some people may avoid answering questions or solving problems for fear of being wrong, with the psychological discomfort this brings. The implication is that one should handle incorrect answers carefully, with every effort to preserve the person's self-image and avoid making the person feel embarrassed. If an answer is partially correct, concentrate on that part and encourage the person to elaborate more. If totally wrong, you may say, for example, "Perhaps I did not phrase my question well." Then you can rephrase it. Maintaining a relaxed atmosphere and demonstrating a nonjudgmental approach is desirable.

ANDRAGOGY

Besides behavioral and cognitive theories of learning, other theories have explored the differences between adults and children as learners. As a professional, understanding how adults learn will help you teach better. When you accept responsibility for teaching clients, patients, or employees, it is natural to think back to your own past experiences of being taught. Most educational experiences were the result of pedagogy, which may be defined as the art and science of teaching children.[13] The teacher was an authority figure, and students were dependents who complied with assignments and directions.

Adult education has challenged some of the basic ideas and approaches of pedagogy. Malcolm Knowles has focused attention on beliefs about educating adults, and instead of pedagogy, uses the term "andragogy." He maintains that the basic assumptions regarding adult learners differ from those regarding children. He sees adults as mutual partners in learning. Following are Knowles' major assumptions about adult learners:[13]

1. Adults become aware of a *need to know*. They seek to learn what they consider important, not what others think is important.
2. In adulthood, the *self-concept* changes from being a dependent learner to being a self-directed one. Adults have autonomy in the learning situation.
3. *Expanding experiences* are a growing resource for learning and can be shared with others.
4. *Readiness to learn* is based on the developmental issues in adults' lives. Learning should be relevant to their needs.
5. Adult learning is *problem-centered* rather than subject-centered, with a present-oriented focus not a future-oriented one. Adults pursue learning that can be applied immediately to solve a problem.
6. *Adult motivation* to learn comes more from internal than from external sources.

Need to Know

Before learning something new, adults must become aware of a *need to know* about it.[13] They need to understand where they are now and see a need to reach a higher level of knowledge or skill. This may, for example, improve the quality of a client's health and lifestyle. For employees, it may mean that they will work more eagerly and productively.

Self-Concept

Childhood is a period of dependency. As a person matures, the *self-concept* changes, and the individual becomes increasingly independent and self-directed. Eventually, people make their own decisions and manage their lives.[13] Once people become adults, they prefer to be independent and self-directing in learning experiences. Any educational experience in which a person is treated as a dependent child is a threat to the self-concept. Negative feelings may result, and resentment, resistance, or anxiety will interfere with learning.

Experience

Compared with children, adults have more experiences and different kinds of *experiences* that they bring to new learning situations. This background is a resource for learning. Ignoring the adult's quantity and quality of experiences may be misinterpreted as a sign of rejection. Employees may have had previous work experience that can be built upon.

A client who has had diabetes for 5 years, for example, has a wealth of experience that should be recognized when the food and nutrition professional discusses dietary changes. To ignore this prior experience and start from the beginning may annoy, bore, or possibly antagonize the client and may place obstacles in the way of the learning process. Teaching methods such as lectures are deemphasized in adult education in favor of more participatory methods that tap a person's wealth of experience, such as group discussion, problem-solving activities, role playing, simulation, and the like. Practical applications that apply learning to the individual's day-to-day life are appropriate and useful.

Readiness to Learn

Readiness to learn differs for children and adults. Children are assumed to be ready to learn because there are subjects they ought to know about and there are academic pressures from teachers and parents to perform. Adults have no such pressures and are assumed to be ready to learn things required to perform their social roles in life—as spouses, employees, parents, and the like—or to cope more effectively in some aspect of their lives.

Education of adults should be appropriate to the individual's readiness or need to know something, and the timing of learning experiences needs to coincide with readiness. People seek information and are ready to learn when they are confronted by problems that they must solve. For example, new employees may be ready to learn about their job responsibilities, but not necessarily about the history of the company. Clients may not be ready to learn about dietary changes until they have accepted the fact that their medical conditions and future health require it.

Problem-Centered Learning

A child's learning is oriented toward subjects, whereas an adult's learning is oriented toward performing tasks and *solving problems*. These different approaches involve different time perspectives. Because children learn about things that they will use some time in the future, the subject matter approach may be appropriate. Adults approach learning when they have an immediate need to learn because they have a problem to solve or a task to perform. The implication is that learning should be applied to problems or projects that the person is currently dealing with. Adults learn what they want to learn when they want to learn it, regardless of what others want them to learn.

Motivation

Children are motivated primarily by external pressures from parents and teachers, by competition for grades, and the like. The more potent *motivators* for adults are internal ones, such as recognition, promotion at work, self-esteem, and the desire for a better quality of health and life.

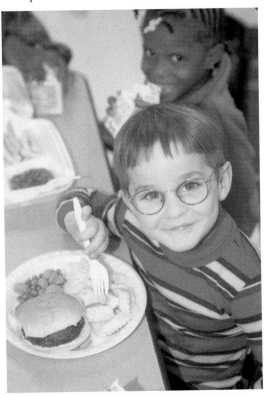

From an examination of various educational theories, Knowles describes the appropriate conditions for learning to take place.[13] He suggests that learners should feel the need to learn something and should perceive the goals of any learning experience as their own personal goals. Before undertaking new learning, adults need to know why they need to learn it. Adults should participate actively in planning, implementing, and evaluating learning experiences to increase their commitment to learning, and the process should make use of the person's life experiences. The physical and psychological environment needs to be comfortable, as discussed in Chapter 11. The relationship between the professional and the learner should be characterized by mutual trust, respect, and helpfulness, and the environment should

Children learn from family and peers.
Source: United States Department of Agriculture.

encourage freedom of expression and the acceptance of differences.[13]

The professional who accepts the assumptions of andragogy becomes a facilitator of learning or a change agent rather than a teacher. The practitioner involves the learner in the process of learning and provides resources for assisting learners to acquire knowledge, information, and skills, while maintaining a supportive climate for learning.

In summary, there is no single educational theory or model for dietetics practitioners to use to facilitate learning and behavioral change. However, the theory that the professional prefers will undoubtedly influence the way he or she teaches and the relationship with clients and employees. Individuals and groups are more likely to be motivated if the information presented emphasizes the personal consequences of behaviors, as mentioned in the Health Belief Model, and is appropriate to the individual's stage of change. Positive reinforcement appropriate to the needs and interests of the individual should be arranged.[2]

LEARNING STYLES AND TEACHING STYLES

Both teaching style and learning style affect the learning process for the client or the employee.

Learning Styles

People have preferred learning styles. People's learning styles play an important role in how effectively they deal with new information. Each of us has a unique learning style and teaching style. Think for a minute about the ways you learn best or how you process and remember new information. If you recall your own school experiences, you preferred some teaching methods to others and processed and retained for a longer period of time material presented in your preferred style.

A unique learning style differentiates people in terms of preferences for content, methods of delivery, learning environment, and teaching techniques. Learning-style preferences are defined as "preferred ways of studying and learning, such as using pictures instead of text, working with other people versus alone, learning in structured or in unstructured situations, and so on."[2] Emphasis is placed on the learner and the learning environment.

Different styles of learning reflect the fact that learners differ in their preferences for and ability to process the content of various instructional messages. We perceive things through our senses. Brilliant individuals who do well learning new information from reading (visual learners), for example, may be all thumbs in a hands-on activity or experience enjoyed by others (tactile/kinesthetic learners). Some people learn well by listening to lectures, participating in group discussions, or talking things through (auditory learners, for whom their own discussion enhances remembering). These preferences influence how easy or difficult learning is for the individual, and therefore they have important implications for educators. People have been described as "hear-learners," who are thinking about the topic at hand; "see-learners;" "feel-learners," who make judgments based on feelings; and "do-learners," who prefer active experimentation.[14]

Components of style that influence learning include cognitive, affective, and environmental factors. Cognitive factors are the person's preferences in thinking and problem solving. Those who think through an experience tend more to abstract dimensions of reality. They reason and analyze what is happening. Others who sense and feel (affective) tend

SELF-ASSESSMENT

What is your preferred way of learning? What atmosphere do you prefer for study?

to prefer learning by way of more concrete, actual, hands-on experiences and are more intuitive. Some learn best by thinking through ideas; others learn best by testing theories and learn through self-discovery or by listening and sharing ideas.

In addition to perceiving differently, people process information in different ways. Some are reflective, watching what is happening and thinking about it. Others are doers who prefer to jump right in and try. In learning to use a computer, for example, some prefer to read about it first and others just try different things. In a study environment, some require absolute silence to process information, others can block out sound, and still others prefer sound and turn on a radio or music when studying and learning. The learner's style preference may vary from situation to situation, affected by the subject matter or skill to be learned.

Learning styles are a function of personality.[15] One's personality can affect the preference for style of intervention. Extroverts, for example, enjoy a group environment for learning, whereas introverts prefer to listen, go away, and then try out the learning. Sensors need facts and details, whereas intuitives prefer the big picture and want to have a hand in getting there. Thinkers like brief, concise, logical information, and feelers want a way to change that will not affect themselves and others in a negative way. Judgers believe rules give structure to what they do, whereas perceivers find self-monitoring to be too structured.

Instruction can be improved and learners are likely to perform better if the professional identifies the learner's preferred learning style and makes the instructional environment compatible. Although people may have a mix of learning styles, many have a dominant style. To measure learning styles, researchers have developed a variety of inventories. Though perhaps helpful, they have been criticized for lacking reliability and validity.[2]

The instructor can attempt to diagnose learning style by observing how people learn or by asking them questions about their preferences, such as: "Do you prefer to read, to view, to listen, or to have actual experiences?" "Do you prefer to learn alone or in groups?" Whether training employees or designing adult nutrition education programs, professionals should offer new information in a variety of ways, since people learn in different ways—by thinking though ideas reflectively, by hands-on experiences, by solving problems, by experimentation, by trial-and-error, by viewing material, and by self-discovery. Since preferred style varies with the situation, offering alternative techniques and methods that reflect the variety of ways in which people acquire knowledge and skills allows the learners to learn in their preferred mode at least some of the time.

Teaching Style

Teaching style is a related matter that affects learning significantly. Teaching style refers to the sum of what one does as a teacher—the preferred instructional methods, activities, organization of material, interactions with learners, and the like. People may be categorized as either teacher-centered or learner-centered.[16] The teacher-centered approach is associated more with Skinner and assumes that learners are passive and that they respond to stimuli in the environment. It is currently the predominant approach to education. In the learner-centered approach, such as Knowles' andragogy, individuals are assumed to be proactive and to take responsibility for their actions. Focus is on the learners and their needs rather than on the subject matter.

BOX **10-1**

Habits of Mind

1. Persisting
2. Managing impulsivity
3. Listening with understanding and empathy
4. Thinking flexibly
5. Thinking about thinking (metacognition)
6. Striving for accuracy
7. Questioning and posing problems
8. Applying past knowledge to new situations
9. Thinking and communicating with clarity and precision
10. Gathering data through all senses
11. Creating, imagining, innovating
12. Responding with wonderment and awe
13. Taking responsible risk
14. Finding humor
15. Thinking interdependently
16. Remaining open to continuous learning

Some evidence suggests that teachers tend to select learning activities based on how they themselves prefer to learn, but instead they should be focusing on the learner's preferred style. Do you teach in the same way you were taught? Do you see yourself as the expert or as a facilitator? Good teachers seek to improve their styles through self-evaluation and adapt to the styles of learners.[17]

Educators Costa and Kallick encourage the use of "16 Habits of Mind" **(Box 10-1)**.[18] These habits can be used by teacher and learner alike to assist in problem solving and outcome-oriented behavior. Encouraging these habits in clients with chronic disease states can be an effective action-oriented tool.

DIFFUSION OF INNOVATIONS

The diffusion of innovations theory is important in the larger social environment of the community where people may, for example, rely on the mass media and the Internet as sources of information. This theory addresses how new ideas and practices are communicated and spread to members of the social system—in ways that may be either planned or spontaneous. The process by which adults adopt new ideas and practices, such as healthy eating patterns, involves five stages in the innovation-decision process:[19]

1. *Knowledge of the innovation.* A person becomes aware of a new idea, practice or procedure.
2. *Persuasion.* A person forms a favorable or unfavorable attitude toward the innovation based on perceived characteristics of the innovation.

3. *Decision to adopt or reject.* A person engages in activities that lead to a choice to adopt or reject the innovation based on trial.
4. *Implementation of the new idea.* The person puts it into use.
5. *Confirmation of the decision.* A person seeks reinforcement of the decision already made and evaluates it over time.

An individual's response to nutrition labeling on foods, for example, and the MyPyramid food guide requires that he or she progress through a series of steps from knowledge of their existence, to forming a viewpoint about them as a source of information, deciding to adopt or reject their use, implementing and using them, through confirmation that he or she will continue with their use. Nutrition education and employee education are incomplete until stage 5 is reached. People learn only what they want to learn and adopt new behaviors to satisfy the basic needs of survival or to achieve some personal goal.

The characteristics of the innovation influence whether or not someone is persuaded in stage 2. Innovations are more readily adopted if they provide a relative advantage over current practices; if they are compatible with current beliefs, values, habits, and practices; if they are simple (degree of complexity) to understand and to use; if they can be tried (trialability); and if results can be observed (observability).[19] It may be unrealistic to expect new behaviors to be adopted from short-term educational endeavors. Short-term intervention should aim at the achievement of one or two goals for change rather than total change. The importance of a positive self-image and "self-view" is being revisited in the literature.[20]

TECHNOLOGY AS A LEARNING TOOL

With new and emerging opportunities for dietetics practitioners and consumers to utilize various forms of technology, such as a PC, laptop, cell phone, or the like, it is important to examine their role as a learning tool. Quintana and colleagues believe that the use of technology should be learner-centered, allowing for interaction between learners and teachers.[21] The use of a "scaffolding framework" technique in the design of software applications includes a three-tiered approach to facilitate learning. The software should allow the learner to engage in (1) sense making, (2) process management, and (3) reflection and articulation.[21]

Effective education is based on theory. No single educational theory or model will facilitate learning and behavior change in all individuals; rather, an opportunity exists to adapt these theories to individual circumstances. This chapter focuses on several theories that seek to explain how people learn, including behavioral, social cognitive, and cognitive theories. These theories and the other topics explored in this chapter—andragogy, diffusion of innovations, technology as a learning aid, learning styles, teaching styles, and transfer of learning to new situations—provide dietetics practitioners with a variety of approaches to use in working with both clients and staff. A section on memory discusses how people remember new information.

CASE STUDY 1

"I am about ready to give up on this batch of new trainees," Ross said to his boss in frustration.

"I thought you liked training the entry-level employees, Ross," replied Bob, the Department Director.

"I do, but it seems as if this latest batch of trainees just is not retaining the information. Now they get two additional days of classroom training before going on-the-job, for a total of 5 days of instruction. Before I changed the program, they only got 3 days of classroom training and then 2 days on-the-job. They have 2 extra days of lecture now. I just don't understand what is wrong with these people."

1. Where is the problem: with the trainees, the trainer, or the training program?
2. What impact did changing the training schedule have on the trainees?
3. How should a training program be designed to provide more effective results?

CASE STUDY 2

John Richards has been referred for counseling because of his high blood pressure. He is 65 years old and of normal weight, with normal serum cholesterol levels. Six months ago, his wife died. Since her passing, he has lived alone in the family home and has relied more on prepackaged meals and convenience foods. His physician recommended a diet restricted in sodium, with an increase in fruits and vegetables. If dietary changes are successful, he may not need medication.

1. Identify the types of questions you would plan to ask Mr. Richards before educating him on the dietary changes he needs to make.
2. What is your assessment of both motivating and challenging issues facing this client?
3. What principles from the chapter would you use to enhance his memory of the changes you plan to tell him about?
4. What would be your recommendation for follow-up?
5. Develop written documentation for your session with this client, incorporating the Nutrition Care Process (NCP) model as applicable.

REVIEW AND DISCUSSION QUESTIONS

1. Compare and contrast the behavioral and cognitive theories of learning in terms of what is learned, the role of reinforcement, and the like.
2. Differentiate between the four types of consequences and their effect on behaviors.
3. What effect does the timing of reinforcement have?
4. How can you encourage persistence in a client's or employee's behavior?
5. What is modeling?
6. Can you remember today anything you learned yesterday?
7. What makes information easy for you to learn and remember?
8. What strategies enhance long-term memory?

9. How do adults differ from children as learners?
10. What steps are involved in adopting innovations?
11. What is meant by learning styles and teaching styles?

SUGGESTED ACTIVITIES

1. Match these types of consequences with the examples A through C following them:
    _____positive reinforcement
    _____negative reinforcement
    _____punishment
    A. "With the diet you are on, you should know better than to eat fried chicken and French fries."
    B. "Employees who learn the new procedures this afternoon will not have to take any work home to study this evening."
    C. "Congratulations on your success. I'm proud of you."
2. Extinction occurs as a result of which of the following?
    A. Not rewarding a response.
    B. Punishing a response.
3. According to cognitive learning theory, which of the following statements is true?
    A. Learning involves associations that are arbitrary.
    B. Learning involves specific information being organized into more generalized categories.
    C. Learning involves observing and modeling after others.
4. Cognitive educators believe that:
    A. New information and knowledge should be presented in an organized fashion that considers prior knowledge.
    B. New knowledge and information should be presented separately from prior knowledge.
    C. It does not matter how new knowledge is presented as long as rewards are given.
5. Discuss in small groups each person's examples of experiences with positive reinforcement, negative reinforcement, punishment, and extinction.
6. Discuss in groups the techniques or methods that individuals use in enhancing their memories of new information.
7. Discuss in groups the different learning styles and environments people prefer for learning.
8. Role-play with a partner. One person serves as the teaching professional and the other assumes the client role. Utilize the diffusion of innovations theory for a label-reading educational session.

WEB SITES

http://www.emtech.net/learning_theories.htm   Learning theories

http://www.learningstyles.org   Institute for Learning Styles Research

http://www.learningstyles.org/survey/index.html   Perceptual Modality Preference Survey

http://www.learning-styles-online.com/overview Learning styles

http://tip.psychology.org/theories.html Learning theory links

http://www.web-us.com/memory/human_memory.htm Memory

REFERENCES

1. Position of the American Dietetic Association. Total diet approach to communicating food and nutrition information. J Am Diet Assoc 2007;107:1224–1232.
2. Woolfolk A. Educational Psychology. 9th Ed. Boston: Pearson/Allyn & Bacon, 2004.
3. DiBartola L. Changes from within: improving lifestyle habits using personality type. J Allied Health 2006;35:238–245.
4. Produce for Better Health Foundation. Available at: http://www.fruitsandveggiesmatter.gov and http://www.pbhfoundation.org; http://fnic.nal.usda.gov/nal. Accessed July 3, 2007.
5. Glanz K, Lewis FM, Rimer BK, eds. Health Behavior and Health Education: Theory, Research, and Practice. 3rd Ed. San Francisco: Jossey-Bass, 2002.
6. Caine G, Caine RN. The Brain, Education, and the Competitive Edge. Latham, MD: Scarecrow Press, 2001.
7. Merriam SB, Caffarella RS, Baumgartner LM. Learning in Adulthood: A Comprehensive Guide. 3rd Ed. San Francisco: Jossey-Bass, 2007.
8. Elliott SN, Kratochwill TR, Cook JL, et al. Educational Psychology: Effective Teaching, Effective Learning. 3rd Ed. Boston, McGraw-Hill, 2000.
9. Gerber S. Where has our theory gone? Learning theory and intentional intervention. J Counsel Dev 2001;79:282–292.
10. Rankin SH, Stallings KD. Patient Education: Principles & Practice. Philadelphia: Lippincott Williams & Wilkins, 2001.
11. Glanz K. Current theoretical bases for nutrition intervention and their uses. In: Coulston AM, Rock CL, Monsen ER, eds. Nutrition in the Prevention and Treatment of Disease. San Diego: Academic Press, 2001.
12. Wexley KN, Latham GP. Developing and Training Human Resources in Organizations. Englewood Cliffs, NJ: Prentice-Hall, 2002.
13. Knowles MS, Holton EF, Swanson RA. The Adult Learner: The Definitive Classic in Adult Education and Human Resource Development. 5th Ed. Houston: Gulf Publishing Co, 1998.
14. Heffler B. Individual learning style and the learning style inventory. Educ Studies 2001;27: 307–316.
15. Wennick RS. Changes from within: improving lifestyle habits using personality type. J Am Diet Assoc 1999;99:666–667.
16. Conti GJ. Identifying your teaching style. In: MW Galbraith, ed. Adult Learning Methods: A Guide for Effective Instruction. 3rd Ed. Malabar, FL: Krieger, 2004.
17. Price P. Are You as Good a Teacher as You Think? NEA Higher Educ J. 2006;22(Fall):7–14.
18. Costa A, Kallick B. Habits of Mind: Discovering and Exploring. Alexandria, VA: Association for Supervision and Curriculum Development, 2000.
19. Oldenburg B, Parcel GS. Diffusion of innovations. In: Glanz K, Lewis FM, Rimer BK, eds. Health Behavior and Health Education: Theory, Research, and Practice. 3rd Ed. San Francisco: Jossey-Bass, 2002.
20. Swann NB, Chang-Schneider C. McCarty K. Self-concept and self-esteem in everyday life. Am Psychol 2007:62:84–94.
21. Quintana C, Shin N, et al. Learner-centered design. In Sawyer K, ed. The Cambridge Handbook of the Learning Sciences. New York: Cambridge University Press, 2006

CHAPTER 11

Planning Learning

OBJECTIVES

- Differentiate between teaching and learning.
- Describe the necessary steps to planning effective educational sessions.
- Discuss the process of developing performance objectives.
- Write performance objectives using Mager's three components.
- Compare the three domains of learning and write objectives.

> *"If you're not sure where you're going, you're liable to end up someplace else."*
> —ROBERT MAGER

The American Dietetic Association (ADA) requires accredited programs to include competencies in education to prepare future practitioners for their role in nutrition education, health promotion, and disease prevention. These include knowledge of educational theory and techniques, methods of teaching and learning, and the use of oral and written communications.[1] Teaching is a major job responsibility of most areas of nutrition including clinical, community, education, consultation, management, and private practice.[2] Health care facilities accredited by the Joint Commission on Accreditation of Healthcare Organizations (JCAHO), the largest health care accrediting body in the United States, are required to provide the patient, family, or significant others with education specific to their needs along with medical record documentation.[3]

The primary goal of teaching is to promote learning. Learning activities occur in both individual and group scenarios. Learning locations comprise a wide array of informal and formal settings that may include inpatient or outpatient, acute or long-term, assisted living and home care, public health and government programs, health fairs and community events. Other settings may include academia, work sites, schools, health clubs, supermarkets, wellness promotion, the Internet, or other media outreach.

The learning audience comprises a wide variety of learners. These may include patients, clients, employees, parents, caregivers and family members, nurses and physicians, students, interns and residents, teachers, paraprofessionals, therapists, health department personnel, athletes, consumers, food service personnel, and the public.[3]

Managers provide learning to employees through training, continuing education, and staff development. Human resource orientation enables employees to know their job responsibilities. An employee's on-the-job performance must meet standards acceptable to the organization and requires periodic updating of knowledge and skills. It is the responsibility of the manager to ensure that training needs are recognized and met. The fact that an employee knows proper procedures, but may not always follow them, is an indication of the difficulty involved in getting a person to change.[4]

Nutrition educators teach clients and patients about normal nutrition and preventive health strategies as well as diet modifications necessitated by such medical problems as cardiovascular disease and diabetes. One day an educator may be teaching a 50-year-old man about fatty acids and cholesterol in foods, the next day teaching an 18-year-old

pregnant woman about pre-natal nutrition, and the next day teaching an athlete about nutritional needs before, during, and after exercise. Nutrition education cannot improve a person's health unless the results influence the purchase and consumption of foods and beverages and change eating behaviors.

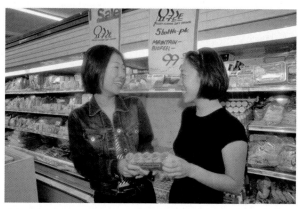

Cultural and ethnic groups may have different needs for learning.
Source: United States Department of Agriculture.

The terms "teaching" and "learning" have different meanings. Some people have the mistaken notion that if they teach something, the audience or individual learns automatically and will transfer the learning to appropriate situations. An educator may explain to a pregnant woman about the MyPyramid food guide, tell her why it is important to use in menu planning, and give her printed handouts. A passive learner may not participate in the learning. Individuals may be

unable to connect the content of the learning process as it does not use their own food choices or menu planning. Knowledge alone cannot guarantee a change in food choices.

Teaching factual information should not be mistaken for education. The term "teaching" suggests the educator's assessment of the need for knowledge and the use of techniques to transfer

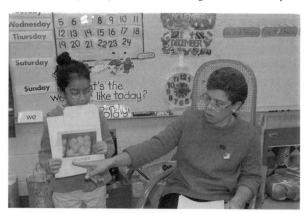

One should create an environment conducive to learning.
Source: United States Department of Agriculture.

knowledge to another person. Education is the process of imparting or acquiring knowledge or skills in the context of the person's total matrix of living. Education should assist people in coping with their problems and challenges as they adapt to circumstances.

Learning refers to the cognitive process through which people acquire and store knowledge, attitudes, or skills and change their behavior owing to an educational experience. The change in behavior may be related to knowledge, attitudes, beliefs, values, skills, or performance.[5,6]

The principles and theories of learning are covered in Chapter 10. The purpose of this chapter is to discuss the process of planning learning as a model or framework to promote effective education.

ENVIRONMENT FOR TEACHING AND LEARNING

An educational environment has two components: the psychological environment and the physical environment. Both are important to enhancing teaching and learning.

Psychological Environment

The psychological climate for learning is important. A supportive and friendly environment with a tolerance for mistakes and a respect for individual and cultural differences makes people feel secure and welcome. Openness and encouragement of questions create a climate for learning. Address learners by their names and show respect for their opinions.

In group teaching and learning, participants should be encouraged to introduce themselves and to get to know one another at the first session. This promotes the synergy experienced by a cohort of learners. Collaboration and mutual assistance should be promoted. To promote learning, competition should be minimized to reduce feelings of anxiety. The educator who creates this informal, supportive, and caring environment for adult learners can obtain better results than one who creates a formal, authoritative environment. Many adults may not have experienced a formal learning situation outside of their early classroom education.[7–10]

Physical Environment

The physical environment should provide appropriate temperature, good lighting, ventilation, and comfortable chairs to create conditions that promote learning rather than inhibit it. Noise from a radio, television, telephone, or people talking may be distracting and may interfere with a learner's attention. Everyone should be able to both see and hear each other. Facilitate interaction by seating groups of people in a circle or around a table where everyone has eye contact. Avoid seating people in rows of chairs where they only see the person's head in front of them.[11]

STEPS TO EFFECTIVE EDUCATION

Successful educational efforts that meet the needs of the adult learner include several interactive steps. The following seven steps comprise a framework or model for planning, implementing, and evaluating learning:

1. Assessing learning needs of the individual or group (preassessment)
2. Writing performance objectives that are measurable and feasible and can be accomplished in a stated period of time considering the domains of learning
3. Determining educational content based on the learner assessment and the performance objectives
4. Selecting methods, techniques, materials, and resources appropriate to the objectives and the individual or group
5. Implementing the learning experiences (intervention) and provision of opportunities for the person to practice new information
6. Evaluating progress and outcomes performed continuously and at stated intervals, including reassessment of learning needs (postassessment)
7. Documenting the outcomes and results of education

The first three steps (steps 1 to 3) of planning learning are discussed in this chapter: (1) learner needs assessment, (2) performance objectives, and (3) content determination. Chapter 12 discusses the four additional steps (steps 4 to 7) of implementing and evaluating learning.

CONDUCTING A NEEDS ASSESSMENT

The first step in education is to conduct a preassessment or needs assessment with the client or employee. Preassessment is a diagnostic evaluation performed by gathering data before instruction to establish a starting point. It serves to classify people regarding their current knowledge, skills, abilities, aptitudes, interests, personality, educational level, degree of literacy, age, gender, occupation, culture, lifestyle, health problem, and psychological readiness to learn (stage of change). Each person is unique.

A need for learning is the gap between what people know now and what they should know. This gap may also represent the difference between expectations of how employees should perform compared to how they actually function or perform.

| Desired knowledge, skill, attitude, or performance | − | Current knowledge, skill, attitude, or performance | = | Need for learning |

The goal is to assess the level of current knowledge and experience to match the beginning level of learning content. For example, an educator counseling a client with long-term diabetes who knows how to count carbohydrates would begin the learning process at a more advanced level compared with a newly diagnosed client. It is essential to determine in advance how much the person already knows since it would waste everyone's time to repeat known information and could lead to boredom or lack of attention on the part of the learner.

The basis for educational planning is the preassessment of the client's or employee's needs balanced with what they need to know or do. Preassessment data are often a compilation of multiple sources that may include activities such as oral interviewing or records review. The initial conversation assesses the learner's intellectual and reading skills to understand the instruction.

The line of questioning should be based on what the person needs to know or would like to know. It is important to ask a variety of questions that address both a learner's self-evaluation and the educator's objective perspective of his or her knowledge.

EXAMPLE: "Have you been on a diet before?"
"What foods are good sources of potassium?"
"What is the relationship between your diet and your health?"
"Have you ever used a meat slicer before?"
"Please show me how you set tables at the restaurant where you worked previously."

Psychological preassessment is also necessary to understand the client's or employee's attitudes toward health and nutrition, willingness to change, motivation, and readiness to learn, which influence his or her behavior. Attitudes are thought to be predispositions for action and change. Despite our efforts, people often do not make the changes recommended by health professionals. Problems may not be caused by deficits in knowledge. Rather the cause and solution may lie in the affective domain or in the individual's attitudes, values, and beliefs.[11,12]

Eating behaviors are the result of many motivations, and having nutrition information does not necessarily mean that it will be applied to better food choices. Motivation can enhance learning and behavior change as well as be a consequence of it. Extrinsic rewards—such as positive reinforcement or praise from peers, a promotion or salary increase for an employee, or a monetary incentive for participation—can influence learning. Intrinsic rewards for adults may be a better match to their learning interest. Adults tend to be highly pragmatic learners who want practical information leading to knowledge or skill about how to do something that *they* find important and valuable. The educator must identify the learner's environment, attitudes, values, and needs prior to delivering instruction.

For example, the hospitalized patient who has just learned of a confirmed diagnosis of chronic illness is likely to be more self-focused than knowledge-focused. The patient may be thinking: "Why me?" "What did I do to deserve this?" "How will this affect my job? My lifestyle? My marriage?" The patient is more likely to have a longer term rather immediate need for nutrition information.

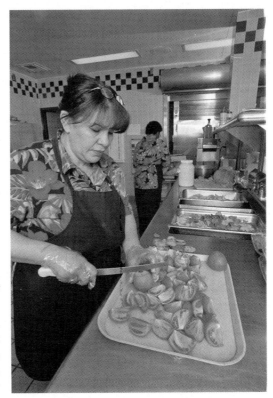

Objectives for learning should be planned around what the employee needs to know and do.
Source: United States Department of Agriculture.

A new employee may feel high levels of anxiety that may interfere with learning for the first few days on the job. Anxiety may arise whenever a superior trains a subordinate. "What does the superior think about me?" "I will appear to be dumb if I don't understand, so I had better pretend I do understand." Each of these feelings raises barriers to learning that must be recognized, reduced, or eliminated before teaching.[13–15]

In more formal situations, a preassessment questionnaire or test may be developed and administered to measure the knowledge gap. Pretest results are compared with posttest results after instruction has been completed. Preassessment is most necessary when the educator is unfamiliar with the knowledge, ability, and values of the learner. A survey questionnaire, a focus group, or a telephone interview survey may also be used.[16–19]

In the workplace, training and development programs are planned to meet current and future benchmarks of the organization. Training provides specific skills under the guidance of established personnel so that employees meet quality standards acceptable to the organization or as mandated by accreditation. Training is required on a continuous basis for both new and current employees accepting new assignments such as after a promotion or transfer.

Training needs assessment is the gap between current and desired performance: "What are the knowledge, skills, abilities, and attitudes that employees need to perform their jobs successfully?" Assessment data can be collected by directly observing the work, by structured interviewing of managers or employees about needs and problems, by seeing what is done correctly and especially what is not, by examining reports (accidents, incidents, grievances, turnover, productivity, and quality control and assurance), and by administering employee attitude surveys. This assessment deals with ends, not the means to the ends, which are determined later in the planning process.[12]

DEVELOPING PERFORMANCE OBJECTIVES

Developing performance objectives means writing precise statements about what will be learned. They define the purpose of instruction and are helpful tools in planning, implementing, and evaluating learning. The educator needs to decide what is to be learned before selecting the optimal methods, techniques, and tools to accomplish it. The term "performance objectives" is used in this chapter but the educational literature also interchangeably uses the terms "behavioral" and "measurable" objectives.

A well-stated performance objective communicates the intended outcome of instruction for the learner. It specifies the desired behavior or level of competence to be attained after instruction is complete. Writing performance objectives has many advantages. It results in less ambiguity regarding what is to be learned. Also, clear performance objectives make it possible to design and implement instruction, select appropriate instructional materials, and assess or evaluate whether or not the objectives are achieved. Both the teacher and the learner benefit from clearer instructions. When people know what they are supposed to learn, it does not come as a surprise. They should not be kept guessing about what should be learned or about what is important.

Objectives should focus on the person learning, not on the educator. The following objective is poorly stated: "The dietitian will teach the client about his diet." Note that this statement focuses on what the practitioner will do and not on what the client or learner will do. The following is preferred because it focuses on the client: "After instruction [when], the client [who] will be able to plan appropriate menus using the sodium-restricted diet as a reference [what]."

Mager wrote one of the most useful guides for writing performance objectives.[20] A key to writing measurable performance objectives is the selection of the verb that describes the desired outcome. Some verbs are vague and subject to misinterpretation, as in the following objectives:

- To know (is able to know which foods contain potassium)
- To understand (is able to understand that foods high in potassium should be consumed daily when certain medications are prescribed)
- To appreciate (is able to appreciate the importance of following the dietary instructions)

It is not clear when using "to know" whether "knowing" means that the client will purchase foods high in potassium, be able to tell a friend which foods are high in potassium, or recognize them on a list. "Understanding" could mean being able to recall reasons, being able to read an article about it, or being able to apply knowledge to one's own situation. The meanings of "know," "understand," and "appreciate" are vague and unclear.

Instead, select verbs that describe what the person is able to do *after* learning has taken place. Note that the phrase "after learning [when], the individual [who] is able to [do what]" is understood to precede the phrase since one is describing what the person will be capable of doing. Another method involves starting with the action verb. The first two examples are rewritten from the unsatisfactory objectives in the previous list. Better verbs to use are summarized in **Box 11-1** and include the following:

- To recall (is able to name five good food sources of potassium)
- To explain (is able to explain why foods high in potassium should be consumed)
- To write (is able to list the groups in the MyPyramid)
- To compare (is able to compare the nutrient needs of an adult woman with those of a pregnant woman)
- To identify (is able to identify on the menu those foods that are permitted)
- To solve or use (is able to plan menus that include five servings of fruits and vegetables daily)
- To demonstrate (is able to demonstrate the use of the mixer or is able to select low-fat foods at the grocery store)
- To operate (is able to slice meat on the meat slicer)

Mager noted that three characteristics improve written objectives: (1) performance, (2) conditions, and (3) criterion. The "performance" tells what the learner will be able to do after instruction is given. The second characteristic describes under what "conditions" the performance is to occur. Finally, a "criterion" tells how good the individual's performance must be to be acceptable. **Table 11-1** summarizes the three-part system for writing objectives. Conditions and criterion may not be included in all objectives. In general, detailed information is important. The more that can be specified, the better the objective and the more likely that the learner will learn what was planned.[20]

BOX 11-1

Verbs Describing Performance

Verbs to Use

analyze	discuss	prepare
apply	distinguish	produce
assemble	evaluate	recall
calculate	explain	recite
cite	identify	recognize
classify	illustrate	recommend
compare	interpret	repair
complete	list	select
construct	measure	solve
contrast	name	state
define	operate	summarize
demonstrate	plan	use
describe	practice	write

Vague Verbs to Avoid

appreciate	feel	learn
believe	grasp	like
comprehend	hope	realize
discern	know	understand

Performance Component

The performance component of an objective describes the activity that the individual will be doing. The performance may be visible or invisible. An overt or visible performance may be seen or heard such as listing, reciting, explaining, or operating equipment.

T A B L E 11-1 | Mager's Three-Part System for Objectives: Client and Employee Examples

Part	Question	Client Example
Learner behavior	Do what?	Plans a menu for a day
Conditions	Under what conditions?	Given a list of permitted foods
Criterion	How well?	With no errors

Part	Question	Employee Example
Learner behavior	Do what?	Measures sanitizer in a bucket
Conditions	Under what conditions?	When cleaning the work area
Criterion	How well?	Using the exact concentration recommended

A covert or invisible performance requires that the individual be asked to do something visible or audible to determine whether the objective is satisfied and learning has taken place. In invisible performance, an "indicator behavior" is added to the objective:

- Is able to identify the parts of the meat slicer (on a diagram or verbally)
- Is able to plan a day's menu based on the MyPyramid

Identifying is invisible until the learner is asked to identify the parts on a diagram or to recite them verbally, which are indicator behaviors. The major intent or performance should be stated using an active verb, and an indicator should be added if the performance cannot be seen or heard.

Conditions Component

Once the performance is clearly stated, it may be necessary to state whether there are specific circumstances or conditions under which the performance will be observed. The conditions describe the setting, equipment, or aids associated with the behavior. With what resources will the individual be provided? What will be withheld? Conditions are in parentheses in the following examples:

- (Given the disassembled parts of a meat slicer) is able to reassemble the parts in correct sequence.
- (Given a standard menu) is able to calculate the appropriate carbohydrate in the foods.
- (Given a list of foods including both good and poor sources of potassium) is able to identify the good sources.
- (Given a standard menu) is able to select low-sodium foods for a complete day.
- (Without looking at the diet instruction form) is able to describe an appropriate dinner menu.
- (Without the assistance of the practitioner) is able to explain the foods a pregnant woman should eat on a daily basis.

Although every objective may not have conditions, there should be enough information to make clear exactly what performance is expected.

Criterion Component

A criterion may be added once the end performance and the conditions, if any, under which it will be observed are described. The criterion describes a level of achievement measuring how well the individual should be able to perform. Possible standards for measuring performance include speed, accuracy, quality, and percentage of correct answers.[21] A time limit can be used to describe the speed criterion. The following are examples:

- Is able to set a table (in 8 minutes or less)
- Is able to reassemble the meat slicer (in 5 minutes or less)
- Is able to complete a diet history (in 20 minutes)

For objectives that require the development of skill over a period of time, you must determine how much time is reasonable in the initial learning period as opposed to the time when the skill is well developed. A new employee cannot be expected to perform a task as rapidly as an experienced person.

When the person is expected to perform with a degree of accuracy, include this in the objective. Accuracy should communicate how well the person needs to perform for his or her performance to be considered competent. Examples include:

- Is able to set five tables (with no errors)
- Is able to identify good sources of potassium (with 80% accuracy), when given a list of foods including both good and poor sources
- Is able to plan a menu for a complete day (with no errors) when given a copy of a sodium-restricted diet
- Is able to calculate the carbohydrate in the diabetic diet (within 5 grams)

Performance objectives should also indicate a quality indicator to assess what constitutes an acceptable performance. It is easier to communicate quality when objective standards are available to both the individual and the practitioner. Any acceptable deviation from the standards can then be determined. The following are examples of such standards:

- Is able to reassemble the meat slicer (according to the steps in the task analysis)
- Is able to measure the amount of sanitizer (according to the directions on the label of the container)
- Is able to substitute foods on a diabetic menu (using carbohydrate counting)
- Is able to pass the ADA registration examination (by attaining at or above the set criterion score)

Performance objectives are clear and measurable when they include the essential component of performance and optional components of condition and criterion to clarify quantity and quality.

DOMAINS OF LEARNING

Learning can be organized into domains, taxonomies, or classification systems to focus on precision in writing. There are three basic domains of objectives: (1) cognitive (knowledge), (2) affective (attitudes and values), and (3) psychomotor (skills). Each is a hierarchy from the simple to the complex. **Figure 11-1** shows their interrelationship.

Cognitive Domain

The cognitive domain involves the acquisition and utilization of knowledge or information and the development of intellectual skills and abilities. A taxonomy of educational performance objectives in the cognitive domain, published by Bloom and colleagues, includes six major levels or categories and a number of subcategories:[21–23]

SELF-ASSESSMENT

Plan several performance objectives for clients or employees, including some with conditions and criteria.

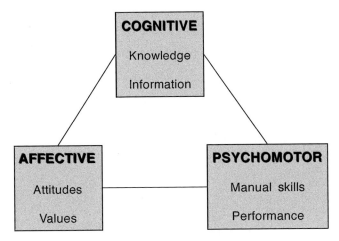

FIGURE **11-1**   The Interrelationship of Objectives.

1.0 KNOWLEDGE
   1.1 Knowledge of specifics
   1.2 Knowledge of ways and means of dealing with specifics
   1.3 Knowledge of the universals and abstractions in a field

2.0 COMPREHENSION
   2.1 Translation
   2.2 Interpretation
   2.3 Extrapolation

3.0 APPLICATION
4.0 ANALYSIS
   4.1 Analysis of elements
   4.2 Analysis of relationships
   4.3 Analysis of organizational principles

5.0 SYNTHESIS
   5.1 Production of a unique communication
   5.2 Production of a plan, or proposed set of operations
   5.3 Derivation of a set of abstract relations

6.0 EVALUATION
   6.1 Judgments in terms of internal evidence
   6.2 Judgments in terms of external criteria

   The levels or categories are arranged in a hierarchy from simple to complex, from concrete to more abstract. The objectives in any one level are likely to be built on the behaviors in the previous level. The subcategories help to define further the major headings and make them more specific.

The educator needs to think beyond the simplest levels of knowledge and strive to write objectives at higher, more complex levels. Without examining the possibility of writing higher level objectives, educators may tend to think only in terms of knowledge and comprehension, which are the easiest objectives to write (and learn). The learner may then be denied the opportunity of applying knowledge or using it in problem solving and will be reduced to memorizing facts. In nutrition education, for example, knowing facts is necessary at the lowest level (knowledge). Higher level objectives will include the ability to analyze food labels, to synthesize all information learned so knowledge can be shared, and to evaluate nutrition information in making wise food choices. In the following discussion of the six levels in the taxonomy, examples of objectives are given.

Knowledge

At the lowest levels in the cognitive domain, knowledge involves remembering information without necessarily understanding it. This includes the recall of specific bits of information, terminology, and facts, such as dates, events, and places, chronological sequences, methods of inquiry, trends over time, processes, classification systems, criteria, principles, and theories. **Table 11-2** suggests verbs describing performance in the cognitive domain.

EXAMPLE: Is able to list foods high in sodium.

Comprehension

The second level, comprehension, is the lowest level of understanding. It involves knowing what is communicated by another person and being able to use the information

TABLE **11-2** | Verbs Describing Performance—Cognitive

Level	Verbs to Use
Knowledge	cites, defines, describes, identifies, labels, lists, matches, memorizes, names, outlines, recalls, recites, repeats, reproduces, selects, states
Comprehension	converts, defends, discusses, distinguishes, estimates, explains, generalizes, gives examples, paraphrases, predicts, recognizes, rewrites, selects, summarizes, translates
Application	applies, assembles, calculates, changes, computes, demonstrates, designs, manipulates, modifies, operates, plans, practices, prepares, produces, shows, solves, translates, uses
Analysis	analyzes, compares, differentiates, discriminates, distinguishes, identifies, illustrates, interprets, investigates, outlines, relates, researches, separates, solves, studies
Synthesis	assembles, categorizes, classifies, combines, compiles, composes, creates, designs, diagnoses, explains, formulates, generates, manages, organizes, plans, recommends, revises, rewrites, summarizes, writes
Evaluation	assesses, appraises, compares, concludes, contrasts, criticizes, critiques, discriminates, evaluates, judges, justifies

communicated. The use of information may include restatement or paraphrase, interpretation, summarization or rearrangement of the information, and extrapolation or
extension of the given information to determine implications or consequences.

EXAMPLE: Is able to explain (verbally or in writing) why certain foods
are not recommended on the diabetic diet.

Application

At the level of application, a person is able to use information, principles, concepts, or
ideas in concrete situations. Knowledge is understood sufficiently to be able to apply it to
solve a problem.

EXAMPLE: Is able to plan a sodium-restricted menu for the day.

Analysis

Analysis entails the breakdown of information into its parts to identify the elements, the
interaction between elements, and the organizing principles or structure. Relationships
may be made among ideas.

EXAMPLE: Is able to analyze the nutrition labeling on a food product for fat
content.

Synthesis

Synthesis requires the reassembling of elements or parts to form something new. You may
assemble a unique verbal or written communication, a plan of operation, or a set of
abstract relations to explain data.

EXAMPLE: Is able to explain the low-cholesterol diet accurately to a friend.

Evaluation

At the highest level in the cognitive taxonomy, evaluation is the ability to judge the value
of materials or methods in a particular situation. Such judgment requires the use of criteria, which may be internal criteria, such as logical accuracy or consistency, or external
criteria, such as external standards.

EXAMPLE: Is able to evaluate a nutrition article from the daily newspaper.

Affective Domain

The affective domain deals with changes in attitudes, feelings, values, beliefs, appreciation, and interests. Often, the educator wants the learner not only to comprehend what
to do, but also to value it, accept it, and find it important. Attitudes and beliefs about food
are widely recognized as important determinants of a person's food choices. We want

SELF-ASSESSMENT

Plan several performance objectives in the cognitive domain on a similar topic.

people to value good nutrition and select healthful foods. When imparting information fails to bring about behavior change, the common response is to redouble efforts to teach facts and explain why something should be done. Instead, an examination of the person's attitudes and values should be pursued.

The affective domain involves a process of internalization from least committed to most committed. It categorizes the inner growth that occurs as people become aware of, and later adopt, the attitudes and principles that assist in forming the value judgments that guide their conduct. A learning goal for a pregnant woman would be to attain a level of basic knowledge (cognitive domain) about the proper foods to eat during pregnancy, but also to value the knowledge so much (affective domain) that she eats nutritious foods and practices good nutrition. Note that an objective in one domain may have a component in another. Cognitive objectives may have an affective component, and affective objectives may have a cognitive one.

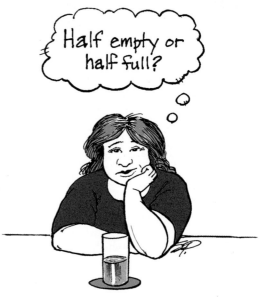

Affective objectives are more nebulous and resist precise definition; therefore, evaluation of their achievement is more difficult. The

One's outlook may be positive or negative.

practitioner may find it a formidable task to describe affective behaviors involving internal feelings and emotions, but they are as important as overt behaviors. Because affective objectives are more difficult to express, most written objectives express cognitive behaviors.

Krathwohl and colleagues have published a taxonomy of educational objectives in the affective domain.[24] It includes five major levels with subcategories:

1.0 RECEIVING (ATTENDING)
    1.1 Awareness
    1.2 Willingness to receive
    1.3 Controlled or selected attention

2.0 RESPONDING
    2.1 Acquiescence in responding
    2.2 Willingness to respond
    2.3 Satisfaction in response

3.0 VALUING
    3.1 Acceptance of a value
    3.2 Preference for a value
    3.3 Commitment

4.0 ORGANIZATION
4.1 Conceptualization
4.2 Organization of a value system

5.0 CHARACTERIZATION BY A VALUE OR VALUE COMPLEX
5.1 Generalized set
5.2 Characterization

The ordering of levels describes a process by which a value progresses from a state of mere awareness or perception to the status of greater complexity until it becomes an internal part of one's outlook on life that guides or controls behavior. This internalization may occur in varying degrees and may involve conformity and high commitment or nonconformity. At higher levels, behavior may be so ingrained that it is unconscious rather than a conscious response. Responses may be produced consistently in the absence of external authorities and in spite of barriers. Thus, a client may eventually select healthful foods, or an employee may wash his or her hands without thinking about it at the conscious level. **Table 11-3** suggests verbs describing performance in the affective domain.

Receiving

At the lowest level of the affective domain, the learner is willing to receive certain phenomena or stimuli. Receiving represents a willingness to attend to what the teacher is presenting. The person may move from a passive level of awareness or consciousness to a neutral willingness to tolerate the situation rather than to avoid it and then to an active level of controlled or selected attention despite distractions.

E X A M P L E : Is able to focus attention on instructions on a diabetic diet.

T A B L E **11-3** | Verbs Describing Performance—Affective

Level	Verbs to Use
Receiving	asks, attends, chooses, describes, follows, gives, identifies, listens, replies, selects, uses
Responding	answers, assists, complies, conforms, cooperates, discusses, helps, participates, performs, practices, presents, reads, recites, reports, responds, selects, tells, writes
Valuing	completes, describes, differentiates, explains, follows, imitates, joins, justifies, participates, proposes, reads, selects, shares, supports
Organization	accepts, adheres, alters, arranges, combines, compares, defends, discusses, explains, generalizes, identifies, integrates, modifies, organizes, prefers, relates, synthesizes
Characterization	acts, advocates, communicates, discriminates, displays, exemplifies, influences, performs, practices, proposes, questions, selects, serves, supports, uses, verifies

Responding

The second level is responding, which indicates a desire on the part of the learner to become involved in, or committed to, a subject or activity. At the lowest level of responding, the client or employee may passively acquiesce, or at least comply, in response to the professional or manager. At a higher level, a willingness to respond or voluntarily make a commitment to a chosen response is evident. Finally, a feeling of satisfaction or pleasure in response involves internalization on the part of the learner.

E X A M P L E : Is willing to read diet materials with interest and ask questions.

Valuing

At the third level, valuing, the learner believes that the information or behavior has worth. The person values it based on a personal assessment. When the value has been slowly internalized or accepted, the client or employee displays a behavior consistent with the value. When something is valued, motivation is not based on external authorities or the desire to obey, but on an internal commitment. The learner will then demonstrate acceptance of a value, preference for a value, or commitment and conviction.

E X A M P L E : Is able to select a nutritious meal from the cafeteria line.

Organization

At the level of organization, the learner discovers situations in which more than one value is appropriate. Individual values are incorporated into a total network of values, and at the level of conceptualization, a person relates new values to those he or she already holds. New values must be organized into an ordered relationship with the current value system. Perhaps a client has previously valued eating whatever he or she wants. Now the client has to learn a new value (different foods) and change an old one (some of the current eating choices).

E X A M P L E : Is able to discuss plans for making different, healthful food choices.

Characterization

The highest level, characterization, indicates that the learner has internalized the values for a sufficient time to control behavior and acts consistently over time. A generalized set is a predisposition to act or perceive events in a certain way. At the highest level of internalization, beliefs or ideas are integrated with internal consistency.

E X A M P L E : Is able to select only those foods permitted on the diet at almost all times.

Behavioral change in the affective domain takes place gradually over a period of time, whereas cognitive change may occur more rapidly. Affective change may take days, weeks, months or years at the higher levels.

S E L F - A S S E S S M E N T

Plan a performance objective for each level in the affective domain on a similar topic.

T A B L E **11-4** | Verbs Describing Performance—Psychomotor

Level	Verbs to Use
Perception	attends, observes, perceives, recognizes, watches
Set	demonstrates, positions, prepares, senses, touches, uses
Guided response	calculates, computes, cuts, imitates, performs, practices, repeats, replicates, tries
Mechanism	assembles, calibrates, cleans, disassembles, operates, performs, practices, prepares, repairs, uses, washes
Complex overt response	cooks, demonstrates, executes, interviews, masters, performs
Adaptation	adapts, changes, develops, modifies, organizes, produces, solves
Origination	instructs, operates, originates, uses

Psychomotor Domain

The psychomotor domain involves the development of physical abilities and skills. Knowledge and attitudes are interrelated and may be necessary to perform these skills. For example, a person cannot drive a car or operate a meat slicer (tasks requiring manual skills) without some basic knowledge of the equipment. **Table11-4** suggests verbs describing performance at the various levels of the psychomotor domain. The performance of physical ability proceeds to increasingly complex steps. Following are Simpson's seven levels and selected subcategories; there are other similar psychomotor domain category systems:[25,26]

1.0 PERCEPTION
    1.1 Sensory stimulation
        1.1.1 Auditory
        1.1.2 Visual
        1.1.3 Tactile
        1.1.4 Taste
        1.1.5 Smell
        1.1.6 Kinesthetic
    1.2 Cue selection
    1.3 Translation

2.0 SET
    2.1 Mental set
    2.2 Physical set
    2.3 Emotional set

3.0 GUIDED RESPONSE
    3.1 Imitation
    3.2 Trial and error

4.0 MECHANISM
5.0 COMPLEX OVERT RESPONSE
    5.1 Resolution of uncertainty
    5.2 Automatic performance

6.0 ADAPTATION
7.0 ORIGINATION

Perception

The lowest level of the psychomotor domain is perception. It involves becoming aware of objects by means of the senses—hearing, seeing, touching, tasting, and smelling—and by muscle sensations or activation. The learner must select which cues to respond to in order to perform a task and then must mentally translate the cues received for action.

    EXAMPLE: Is able to recognize a need to learn how to use the meat slicer.

Set

Set is the second level and suggests a readiness for performing a task. This may involve mental readiness to start the task, physical readiness to correct body positioning to accomplish the task, and emotional readiness by having a favorable attitude or willingness to learn the task.

    EXAMPLE: Is able to position oneself to use the meat slicer.

Guided Response

The third level of the psychomotor domain is guided response. The professional or trainer guides the employee during the activity by emphasizing the individual components of a more complex skill. The subcategories include imitation of the practitioner, trial and error, and feedback until the task can be performed accurately. Performance at this level may initially be crude and imperfect.

    EXAMPLE: Is able to practice the steps in using the meat slicer under supervision.

Mechanism

Mechanism, the fourth level, refers to habitual response. At this stage, the learner demonstrates an initial degree of proficiency in performing the task which results from some practice.

    EXAMPLE: Is able to use the meat slicer properly.

Complex Overt Response

The fifth level, complex overt response, suggests that a level of skill has been attained over time in performing the task. Work is performed smoothly and efficiently without error. Two subcategories are resolution of uncertainty, in which a task is performed without hesitation, and automatic performance. Performance is characterized by accuracy, control, and speed.

    EXAMPLE: Is able to demonstrate considerable skill in using the meat slicer with a variety of foods.

Adaptation and Origination

Adaptation requires altering manual skills in new but similar situations, such as in adapting slicing procedures to a variety of different foods on the meat slicer. The final level, origination, refers to the creation of a new physical act, such as slicing something that has not been done before.

In understanding the psychomotor domain, it may be helpful to recall the process of learning to drive an automobile: responding to the physical and visual stimulation, feeling mentally and emotionally ready to drive, learning parallel parking by trial and error under the guidance of an instructor, developing a degree of skill, and finally starting the car and driving without having to think of the steps. With time, sufficient skill is developed so that the person can adapt quickly to new situations on the road and create new responses automatically.

DETERMINING THE CONTENT OF LEARNING PLANS

A close examination of the learning objectives helps to identify the content of the learning plan. Each objective states what the learner will be able to do when instruction is complete and defines the content to be taught. The preassessment may have eliminated certain objectives as unnecessary; those that remain are used in planning content.

Using the taxonomies ensures that the objectives of learning are applied to the needs of the learner. Some people may need to start at the lowest level in the taxonomy, whereas those who have already mastered the lower level objectives are ready for those at higher levels. The taxonomies assist the educator in thinking of higher levels of knowledge that may be more appropriate for the learner. They also serve to remind the educator that there are interrelationships among the three domains. Although clients can plan menus using their diets, it is also important they think that the food choices are important enough to their health to follow them. Employees need not only to know proper sanitation procedures but also to value them if they are going to practice optimum sanitary procedures regularly.

ORGANIZING LEARNING GROUPS

Learning may take place individually or in groups. Groups are advantageous in that they save time and money and provide opportunities for people to share experiences. Those who are successful in making dietary changes can model behaviors and discuss information with those who have been unsuccessful in coping. The more complex the information to be learned, the greater is the need to discuss it in groups. However, an experienced

SELF-ASSESSMENT

Plan a performance objective for each level in the psychomotor domain in a similar subject area.

employee who needs to be trained in a new technique would derive greater benefit from an individual non–group-focused learning plan that does not waste time reviewing steps he or she has already mastered.

Even when a single learner is involved, the educator should consider whether or not other learners should also be present. In nutrition counseling and education, the individual responsible for purchasing the food and preparing the meals should be present. When a child is placed on a modified diet, such as a diabetic diet, usually the mother or caregiver requires instruction as well, since her cooperation is essential to the child's successful adherence to the diet and management of the disease.

The preassessment should show differences in knowledge levels and should assist in making grouping decisions. Frequently, all new employees are grouped together for initial orientation and training. This is an example of grouping by similar learning needs rather than by age, educational level, amount of experience, or job title. Grouping by general learning content often requires division into more than one learning group based on employees' job content and application. Wait staff, for example, may require sessions on sanitary dish and utensil handling while cooks may need classes on sanitary food handling.

Another consideration is whether supervisors should be taught in the same classes as their employees. One disadvantage of such a grouping is that the employees may be reluctant to participate by asking questions when the superior is present. Setting the size of the group will affect the learning plan. Larger groups of 30 to 50 or more will decrease the ability for individual participation compared with small groups of 10 to 15.[11,12,27]

This chapter has explored the initial steps in planning learning. After needs assessment has been completed, performance objectives should be written in the cognitive, affective, and psychomotor domains. Decisions need to be made about whether learning should be organized by individuals or groups. The content of instruction is determined from an examination of the objectives. The steps taken to plan learning will increase the effectiveness of the learning process. Chapter 12 explores the remaining steps in the framework for education.

CASE STUDY 1

Kathy Smith is the dietetics professional responsible for employee education at a work site. She moderated a focus group interview consisting of 10 employees. The purpose was to determine the employees' concerns about nutrition and health. At the top of the list of concerns was the relation of diet and fats to heart disease.

1. The follow-up focus group will determine more precisely the employees' needs and interests related to the topic. What questions would you ask the focus group?
2. What objectives could you write for an educational presentation to employees on the topic?
3. Create an outline for an educational program emphasizing social support and rewards or reinforcement techniques in counseling.

CASE STUDY 2

Paul Fisher is responsible for the school lunch program at a large urban high school with over 3,000 students. In the first 6 months on the job, he noted that some students did not eat a well-balanced diet and discarded portions of their meals, leading to a waste of food.

Before planning any nutrition education, he decides to identify what seems to be influencing students to select less healthful food choices.

1. List some initial methods to direct the planning and establishing of goals and objectives?
2. What approaches can he consider to assess the reasons why high school students are not eating nutritiously?
3. What information should he collect?
4. What nutrition problems can he ascertain from what he has observed and gathered?
5. What approaches to nutrition education might he try with high school students eating lunch in the cafeteria?

REVIEW AND DISCUSSION QUESTIONS

1. How do you define teaching and learning?
2. What are the three parts of Mager's learning objectives? What question does each answer?
3. What are the three domains of learning objectives? What are the levels in each domain?
4. How are the objectives in the three domains interrelated?
5. What training topics would be appropriate for food service employees in the three domains? For health care educators?
6. What are some guidelines for arranging physical and psychological environments?
7. What are the steps to education?
8. What are the reasons for conducting a preassessment or needs assessment?

SUGGESTED ACTIVITIES

1. Make a list of questions you would ask in the preassessment of knowledge of some subject with which you are familiar.
2. Write three performance objectives using active verbs to describe behavior.
3. Write examples of performance objectives containing conditions and a criterion.
4. Write examples of objectives in various levels of the cognitive, affective, and psychomotor domain. Note overlap from one domain to another.
5. Decide which of the following performance objectives are measurable.
   A. Presented with a menu, the client will be able to circle appropriate food selections according to his or her diet.
   B. At the close of the series of classes, the clients will be more positively disposed toward following their diets.
   C. After counseling, the client will know which foods he or she should eat and which not to eat.
   D. The client will be able to explain the diabetic diet to her husband.

6. Examine the following objectives and decide whether each concerns primarily the cognitive, affective, or psychomotor domain.
   A. All dishwashing staff will be able to complete the meal service clean-up within 1 hour of close of service.
   B. Given a series of objectives, the student will be able to classify them according to the taxonomies in the chapter.
   C. At the end of the session, clients will request more weight control classes.

WEB SITES

www.amanet.org   American Management Association

www.astd.org   American Society of Training and Development

www.compstrategies.com/staffdevelopment   Professional Teacher Development

www.eatright.org   American Dietetic Association

http://en.wikipedia.org/wiki/Learning_Plan   Wikipedia

www.igpe.edu   Institute for General Practice Education

www.nraef.org   National Restaurant Association Education Foundation

www.usda.org   U.S. Department of Agriculture

REFERENCES

1. Commission on Accreditation for Dietetics Education. Foundation Knowledge and Skills and Competency Requirements for Entry-Level Dietitians. Chicago: American Dietetic Association, 2002.
2. American Dietetic Association. Position of the American Dietetic Association: the roles of registered dietitians and dietetic technicians, registered in health promotion and disease prevention. J Am Diet Assoc 2006:106:1875–1884.
3. Joint Commission on Accreditation of Health Care Organizations. 2007 Comprehensive Accreditation Manual for Hospitals: The Official Handbook. Oak Brook, IL: Joint Commission Resources, 2007.
4. Puckett RB. Practice paper of the American Dietetic Association: a systems approach to measuring productivity in health care foodservice operation. J Am Diet Assoc 2005:105: 122–130.
5. Boroditsky L. Comparison and development of knowledge. Cognition 2007:102:118–128.
6. Newman VA, Thomson CA, Rock CL, et al. Achieving substantial changes in eating behavior among women previously treated for breast cancer-an overview of the intervention. J Am Diet Assoc 2005:105:382–391.
7. Schmitt JA, Benton D, Kallus KW. General methodological considerations for the assessment of nutritional influences on human cognitive functions. Eur J Nutr 2005:44:459–464.
8. Diabetes Care and Education Dietetic Practice Group. ADA Guide to Diabetes Medical Nutrition Therapy and Education. Chicago: American Dietetic Association, 2005.
9. Sweet M, Michaelsen LK. How group dynamics research can inform the theory and practice of postsecondary small group learning. Educ Psychol Rev 2007:19:31–47.
10. Johnson DW, Johnson RT, Smith K. The state of cooperative learning in postsecondary and professional settings. Educ Psychol Rev 2007:19:15–29.
11. Lucas RW. People Strategies for Trainers. New York: American Management Association, 2005.

12. Kirkpatrick DL. Improving Employee Performance Through Appraisal and Coaching. 2nd Ed. New York: American Management Association, 2005.

13. Ebbeling CB, Garcia-Lago E, Leidig MM, et al. Altering portion sizes and eating rate to attenuate gorging during a fast food meal: effects on energy intake. Pediatrics 2007:119:869–875.

14. Frey BS, Osterloh M. Successful Management by Motivation: Balancing Intrinsic and Extrinsic Incentives. New York: Springer, 2002.

15. Senko C, Harackiewicz JM. Achievement goals, task performance, and interest: why perceived goal difficulty matters. Pers Soc Psychol Bull 2005:31:1739–1753.

16. Arthur D. Recruiting, Interviewing, Selecting and Orienting New Employees. 4th Ed. New York: American Management Association, 2005.

17. Sherwood NE, Story M, Neumark-Sztainer D, et al. Development and implementation of a visual card-sorting technique for assessing food and activity preferences and patterns in African American girls. J Am Diet Assoc 2003:103:1473–1479.

18. Henry H, Reicks M, Smith C, et al. Identification of factors affecting purchasing and preparation of fruit and vegetables by stage of change for low-income African American mothers using the think-aloud method. J Am Diet Assoc 2003:103:1643–1646.

19. Unusan N. Effects of food and nutrition course on the self-reported knowledge and behavior of preschool teacher candidates. Early Child Educ 2007:5:323–327.

20. Mager RF. Preparing Instructional Objectives: A Critical Tool in the Development of Effective Instruction. 3rd Ed. Atlanta: CEP Press, 1997.

21. Bloom BS. Taxonomy of Educational Objectives. Handbook I: Cognitive Domain. New York: Longman, 1956. (Copyright renewed 1984 by Bloom BS, Krathwohl D.)

22. Anderson LW, Sosniak LA, eds. Bloom's Taxonomy: A Forty-Year Retrospective. Chicago: University of Chicago, 1994.

23. Anderson LW, Krathwohl D, eds. A Taxonomy for Learning, Teaching, and Assessing: A Revision of Bloom's Taxonomy of Educational Objectives. New York: Longman, 2001.

24. Krathwohl D, Bloom BS, Masia B. Taxonomy of Educational Objectives. Handbook II: Affective Domain. New York: David McKay, 1964.

25. Simpson E. The Classification of Educational Objectives in the Psychomotor Domain. Washington, DC: Gryphon House, 1972.

26. Harrow A. A taxonomy of the Psychomotor Domain. New York: David McKay, 1972.

27. O'Neil J, Marsick VJ. Understanding Adult Action Learning. New York: American Management Association, 2007.

Implementing and Evaluating Learning

"I hear and I forget, I see and I remember,
I do and I understand."

—Confucius

How does the educator or trainer successfully educate clients and employees? With clients, the practitioner seeks to promote health and reduce the risk of chronic disease. With employees, the manager seeks to enhance their ability to do their jobs. The initial three steps in planning learning, as discussed in Chapter 11, include a pre-assessment of the learner's current knowledge and competencies; the development of performance objectives in the cognitive, affective, and psychomotor domains; and the determination of educational content based on the performance objectives.

This chapter continues with the discussion of the implementation and evaluation of the learning plan. The final four steps begin with the selection of appropriate learning activities for the cognitive, affective, and psychomotor domains. These planned learning activities are implemented along with opportunities to apply theory through application and practice. An evaluation of the outcomes of learning is then completed, and if necessary, an evaluation is repeated at intervals to assure mastery of the learning plan. Finally, documentation of the educational process is completed.

SELECTING TECHNIQUES AND METHODS

Various techniques and methods of educational presentation are available to deliver the learning plan to the audience. Techniques are the ways that the instructor organizes and presents information to learners to promote the internal processes of learning.[1] They establish a relationship between the teacher and the learner and between the learner and what he or she is learning. These include activities such as lectures, discussions, simulations, and demonstrations. All are not equally effective in facilitating learning, and each has its advantages and disadvantages, its uses and limitations as summarized in **Table 12-1.**

In deciding on the method that will be most effective, the instructor may be guided by several factors. These may include the educational purpose, learner preference or style, learner needs, group size, facilities available, time available, cost, and one's previous experience or the degree of success with the techniques. One must consider what is effective for different populations, such as those from different cultural and ethnic groups, socioeconomic groups, educational and literacy levels, and age groups so that desired outcomes are reached.[2]

The domain of the performance objectives may suggest which approach is most appropriate since methods and techniques differ for cognitive, affective, and psychomotor domains. All factors being equal, the practitioner should select the technique that requires the most active participation of the learner and includes strategies for effective behavioral change. Studies show that the more actively a person is involved in the learning process, the better the retention.[3] **Figure 12-1** shows that reading and hearing information are not as productive as both seeing and hearing or, better yet, discussing information or doing something with it.

Lectures

The lecture is the presentation technique that is most familiar to people. It is a traditional passive method of informing and transferring knowledge—the lowest level in the cognitive domain—from the teacher to the learner. It is especially useful in situations with a large number of learners, a great deal of information to be communicated, and a limited amount of available time.[4] Examples are a class on sanitation for food service employees or on cholesterol and fat in relation to heart disease for work site employees or medical center clients.

In spite of the advantages of efficiency, a major drawback of lectures is that there is no guarantee that the material is learned and remembered or that food choices and eating behaviors will change. This is because the individual is a passive participant whose learning depends on listening skills. Lecture may be the least effective technique for use with adults.

Although well-educated people may respond positively to lectures because of long experience with this approach, those with less education or those from other cultures may learn better with other methods.[5-7] Their attention to lectures may wane quickly as they tune out, especially if the lecturer is not an effective speaker or if the lecture is dull. Lectures seldom meet the requirements of adult education because they lack self-directed

TABLE **12-1** | Strengths and Weaknesses of Teaching Methods

	Strengths	Weaknesses
Lecture	Easy and efficient Conveys most information Reaches large numbers Minimum threat to learner Maximum control by instructor	Learner is passive Learning by listening Formal atmosphere May be dull, boring Not suited for higher level learning in cognitive domain Not suited for manual learning

Discussion
(e.g., panel,
debate, case
study)
	More interesting, thus
	    motivating
	Active participation
	Informal atmosphere
	Broadens perspectives
	We remember what we discuss
	Good for higher level cognitive,
	    affective objectives
		Learner may be unprepared
		Shy people may not discuss
		May get side-tracked
		More time-consuming
		Size of group limited

Projects	More motivating Active participation Good for higher level cognitive objectives	Size of group limited
Laboratory experiments	Learn by experience Hands-on method Active participation Good for higher level cognitive objectives	Requires space, time Group size limited

Simulation
(e.g., scenarios,
in-basket, role-
playing, critical
incidents)
	Active participation
	Requires critical thinking
	Develops problem-solving skills
	Connects theory and practice
	More interesting
	Good for higher level cognitive
	    and affective objectives
		Time consuming
		Group size limited unless
		    on computer

Demonstration	Realistic visual image Appeals to several senses Can show a large group Good for psychomotor domain	Requires equipment Requires time Learner is passive, unless can practice

learning and problem-solving approaches. Lectures are improved by limiting the number of concepts presented, using examples and summaries frequently, and adding focused visual aids. Lectures can become more interactive by providing ample time for interactive discussion along with written handouts to reinforce what was heard.

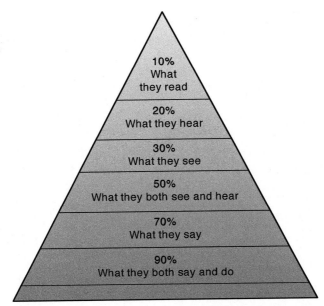

FIGURE **12-1**   What People Remember.

Discussion

Discussion tends to promote active participation by learners. This technique can be used on a one-on-one basis or in a group. Interactive discussion helps participants to examine their own thinking and internalize knowledge through the exchange of ideas and verbal responses. The instructor can guide the discussion by raising open-ended questions, posing problems, or highlighting key issues so that clients or employees make comparisons or work to draw conclusions.

Group discussion is greater when the participants are fairly well acquainted or have a common interest. With a series of classes on weight reduction, for example, clients could discuss and share what they have done to change their food choices, recipes, and shopping habits. The basis for discussion may be common experiences, written case studies, or topics that were preannounced so that the group can interact. For best results, seating should be arranged in a circle so that everyone can see and hear other participants. The instructor should facilitate but not dominate the discussion. Smaller groups of 10 to 15 people offer more opportunity for participation as learners explore their thoughts, values, and experiences, think critically, and influence others.

Facilitated discussions, such as those presented by debates and panels, may be more appropriate for a large group. In this scenario, the educator should plan content and discussion topics that attract the audience's listening interest although very few learners may actually get a chance to actively participate due to time and group size constraints.

Discussion is more time-consuming than lecture, but it can be more interesting for learners, and thus more motivating. The learning plan should include higher level cognitive and affective objectives. The key points raised in the discussion should be summarized

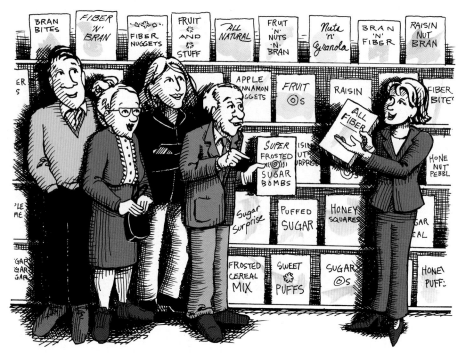

People prefer hands-on learning to lectures.

intermittently by the instructor to increase the learner's acquisition and retention of information since we remember what we say out loud.[6]

Simulation

Simulations of real-life situations are active ways to develop learner knowledge, skills, behaviors, and competencies. Several means of representation may be used such as scenarios, "in-basket" exercises, critical incidents, and role-playing. These methods involve learning by actively doing something-in other words, experiential learning rather than learning by listening or watching. Active learner involvement enhances optimum transfer of learning.[8,9]

Simulation may be based on scenarios or models of real-life problem situations. Clients on sodium-restricted diets, for example, could look at restaurant menus and determine what they should order. Learners use a process of inquiry in exploring a problem, developing decision-making and evaluative skills. Food service employees could discuss food temperatures and Hazard Analysis Critical Control Points (HACCP) procedures through preparation, holding, service, and leftovers.[10]

In-basket exercises test the person's ability to handle day-to-day challenges. The instructor can describe a critical incident by providing written memos, notes, requests, or reports to simulate a supervisor's decision-making ability in handling problems that arrive in the in-basket on the desk each day. Simulated emergencies such as fires and electrical blackouts or unusual incidents can be used. The learner has to provide a solution in handling the situation or problem.

Role-playing, in which two or more people dramatize assigned parts or roles simulating real-life situations, is another possibility. Role-playing allows learners to practice new behaviors in relatively safe environments, and it can be used to work through real problems. Role-playing is followed by a discussion of the problem, ideas, feelings, and emotional reactions such as the handling of an employee disciplinary problem or learning to say no when offered disallowed foods. Though time-consuming, simulations may be helpful in providing opportunities for individuals to make a connection between theory and practice, to engage in critical thinking as active participants, and to develop problem-solving and coping skills. Simulation may be used with cognitive, affective, and psychomotor objectives.[1,11]

Demonstration

A demonstration may be used to show how something is done or to explore processes, procedures, equipment operation, techniques, ideas, or attitudes. This technique is used to combine knowledge and skill with cognitive and psychomotor objectives. Learning to

prepare low-fat recipes and learning how to use a meat slicer are examples of instances in which demonstration is appropriate. Usually, the learner observes as the instructor makes the presentation or models the skill, although a participant volunteer may be used. The demonstration may be a dramatic learning experience if it holds the individual's attention and may be appropriate for any type of learning objective.[12,13]

If skills are demonstrated, the person will need ample opportunity to practice the task or skill soon after and evaluate the performance after passively watching

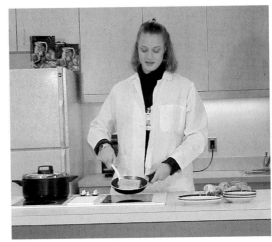

A demonstration is one approach to presentations.

the instructor. Job instruction training, discussed later in this chapter, is an example of the use of demonstration to achieve mastery.

Visual and Audio-Assisted Instruction

According to an old Chinese proverb, "one picture is worth more than 1,000 words." An effective media presentation can enhance learning by providing variety and improving memory through visual and audio stimulation. Self-directed and instructor-directed computer programs can be used with a wide variety of learners when matched to the learning situation. An audiotape can be used to hear language or dialogue. A videotape could illustrate an unfamiliar setting or piece of equipment. The newest vehicles for delivering innovative training include podcasting, cell phones, computer-interactive video-conferencing, and other electronic devices. Media is considered an adjunct to learning and should not be considered the total learning experience.[14,15] (Chapter 15 discusses media in more detail.)

TECHNIQUES FOR DIFFERENT DOMAINS OF LEARNING

For learning in the cognitive domain, most of the preceding techniques may be effective. There are additional factors to consider in fostering learning in the affective and psychomotor domains. Because learners represent different learning styles, there is an advantage to using mixed methods rather than only one method.[1,16]

In the affective domain, the educator seeks to influence the learner's interests, attitudes, beliefs, and values. This requires ongoing contacts rather than a single session. At the lowest level in the affective domain, receiving and awareness, audiovisual materials or guided discussion can begin to present the relationship between food choices and obesity. At higher levels, where the adoption of new attitudes and values is important, the individual must participate more fully in discussion of food choice options. Commitments that are made public are more likely to be adopted than those that are kept private, and attitudes are acquired through interpersonal influences.[17]

Using multiple instructional strategies that influence deeper level learning of nutrition and the modification of attitudes is more likely to promote behavior change. Promoting the active involvement of participants and interpersonal interaction in a group can help. Different types and dimensions of these techniques can address the variety of learning styles more effectively than a single teaching method.

The problem-solving process in which the instructor presents a puzzling situation or problem is an example of multiple-step learning. The learner or learner group may be asked to calculate the daily fat or sodium allowance from food labels. The steps require the learner to identify and clarify the problem, form hypotheses, gather data, analyze and interpret data, select possible solutions, test solutions, and finally draw conclusions and select the best solution to the problem. People learn how to solve problems, evaluate possible solutions, and think critically. Clients can be guided through this process so that they learn to solve their own nutrition problems.[3,12,13,17]

Modeling is also a method of influencing a person's behavior. People learn by observing others and then imitating them in unfamiliar or new situations. The teacher should behave as the learner is expected to behave, modeling the desirable attitude or behavior. People are more likely to accept new behaviors, such as healthful food choices or routine hand washing, when they meet and have discussions with people who have successfully adopted them.[18]

Skills in the psychomotor domain are learned with direct experience and practice over time. The instructor may begin with a demonstration, but then the learner needs to practice the skill under supervision. "Coaching" is a term that describes the assistance given to someone learning a new skill; it can apply to an educational experience as well as a sport. Coaching suggests a one-on-one, continuous, supportive relationship from which a person learns over time. It is perhaps the best method for on-the-job training of employees. After the demonstration, the trainer can give encouragement, promote confidence, and offer guidance as the trainee performs the task. Coaching takes into consideration different learning abilities and needs, allows actual practice, and provides people with immediate feedback regarding their performance.[16,19,20]

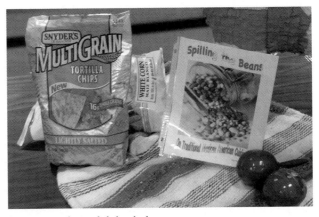

Discussion with visuals helps the learner.

TASK ANALYSIS

A task analysis is a written sequential list of the steps involved in performing any task from beginning to end and including the knowledge, skills, and abilities needed as well as the conditions under which it is performed and the proper method of performance. Usually, the major steps are numbered, and each step describes what to do. Many job-related tasks involve the psychomotor domain; thus, actions are listed in the analysis. It is often necessary, however, to have some background knowledge from the cognitive domain in performing the task. Balancing a checkbook, for example, is both a manual and an intellectual skill, as is operating a computer.

After the sequential steps are listed, each one should be examined to see whether any explanations from the cognitive domain need to be added. If step one, for example, is to plug in the meat slicer, a key point is to have dry hands to avoid the danger of electrical shock. If a final step in the wait staff's task analysis for bussing dirty dishes includes washing hands, an explanation may be added regarding the transfer of microorganisms to clean food and utensils. In food service, sanitation and safety statements are frequently needed. Other explanations of reasons why a step is necessary or notes on materials or equipment may be important to add. There are many ways to complete a task analysis.

Employees need to learn the skills related to their jobs, and clients may need to develop skills in menu planning and food preparation using a new dietary regimen, such as sodium restriction. Regardless of the kind of skill involved, the learner needs to be able to perform the skill initially and then to improve the skill through continued practice. After grasping the basics of playing tennis, driving a car, or baking a cake, for example, a person requires repeated experience to develop these skills.

If available, a job description may be used as a starting point in determining job content, but job descriptions do not give information that is specific enough for determining the content of training. All the tasks included in a job should be listed individually. If the job description is unavailable, it may be necessary to interview employees or observe their work to determine the job content. Wait staff, for example, complete a number of tasks during the day, such as greeting customers, taking their orders, placing orders in the kitchen, serving the courses of the meal, bussing dishes, setting tables, receiving payment for services, and maintaining good public relations. Each is a separate task making up the total job, and each task or set of actions can be defined in task analyses.

Once it is written, the task analysis should be used by both the trainer and the trainee. The trainer may examine the task analysis to construct learning objectives that describe the behavior expected at the end of training. In assessing the person's need for instruction, the gap representing the difference between the skill described in the task analysis and the individual's current skill must be addressed. A demonstration should show what to do and then allow the person to perform the task. The task analysis may be used as an ongoing reference since it describes what to do in sequence. Using the task analysis in coaching or in supervised on-the-job training facilitates the learning of skills.

After mastering the basic skill involved and being able to recognize the correct sequence of procedures, the individual needs repeated practice to improve the skill. With time and practice, improvements in speed and quality of work should develop.[1,21,22]

JOB INSTRUCTION TRAINING

A great deal of employee training takes place not in the classroom, but on the job. New employees require orientation and training with either an experienced worker or a supervisor. Current employees may need retraining periodically, may be assigned new tasks, or may receive promotions that require the development of new skills and abilities.

A four-step process entitled job instruction training (JIT) was delineated for rapid training of new employees. It may be used to teach skills and is based on performance rather than subject matter. The four steps are (1) preparation, (2) presentation, (3) learner performance, and (4) follow-up. This is similar to tell, show, do, and review. Before instruction, a task analysis should be completed and the work area arranged with the necessary supplies and materials that the employee is expected to maintain.[20] **Box 12-1** summarizes the main points.

Preparation

The first step prepares the employee psychologically and intellectually for learning. Since a superior may be the trainer, any tension, nervousness, or apprehension in the subordinate employee must be overcome because it may interfere with learning. A friendly, smiling trainer puts the person at ease by creating an informal atmosphere for learning in which mistakes are expected and tolerated. The trainer states the job to be learned and asks specific questions to determine what the individual already knows about it. Motivation for learning increases when employees become interested in their jobs. Finally, the trainer should be sure that the employee can physically see what is being demonstrated.

BOX **12-1**

How to Instruct

Step I.   Prepare the learner:
   1. Put the learner at ease.
   2. State the job.
   3. Find out what the individual knows about the job.
   4. Develop interest.
   5. Correct the person's position.

Step II. Present the operation:
   1. Tell, show, and illustrate.
   2. Explain one important step at a time.
   3. Stress key points.
   4. Instruct clearly, completely, and patiently, but no more than the learner can master.
   5. Summarize the operation in a second run-through.

Step III. Try out performance:
   1. Have the learner do the job.
   2. Have the learner explain key points while performing the job again.
   3. Make sure that the learner understands.
   4. Continue until you know that the learner knows the job.

Step IV. Follow-up:
   1. Put the learner on his or her own.
   2. Designate where to obtain help.
   3. Encourage questions.
   4. Taper off.
   5. Continue with normal supervision.

Presentation

The second step presents and explains the operation as the employee is expected to perform it. The trainer shows, tells, and illustrates the operation one step at a time using a prepared task analysis. Key points should be stressed. The instruction should be carried out clearly, completely, and patiently, with the trainer remembering the employee's abilities and attitudes.

Since the ability to absorb new information is limited, the trainer needs to determine how much the learner can master at a time. It may be five to 10 steps with key points, or it may be more. It may be 15 minutes or 1 hour of instruction. Overloading anyone with information is ineffectual, since the information will be forgotten. After this initial instruction, the operation or task should be summarized and performed a second time.

Performance

The third step, performance, tests how much the employee has retained as he or she tries out the operation using the written task analysis as a reference. The employee does the job while the trainer or coach stands by to assist. This is a form of behavior modeling. Accuracy, not speed, is stressed initially. As the employee completes the task a second time, the trainer should ask the employee to state the key points. To be sure of understanding, the trainer should ask such questions as "What would happen if . . .?" "What else do you do . . .?" and "What next . . .?" Employees may need to repeat the operation five times, 10 times, or however many times are needed until they know what to do. The trainer continues coaching and giving positive feedback, encouragement, and reassurance until the employee learns the operation.

Follow-up

Follow-up occurs in the fourth step as supervision tapers off. At first, the employee is left alone to complete the task. The individual should always know, however, where to obtain assistance if it is needed. Any additional questions ought to be encouraged in case problems arise. Normal supervision continues to ensure that the task is done as instructed, since fellow workers may suggest undesirable shortcuts.

Mager pointed out that when the learner's experience is followed by positive consequences, the learner will be stimulated to approach the situation, but that when adverse consequences follow, the learner will avoid the situation.[23] A positive consequence may be any pleasant event, praise, a successful experience, an increase in self-esteem, improvement in self-image, or an increase in confidence. Adverse conditions are events or emotions that cause physical or mental discomfort or that lead to loss of self-respect. They include fear, anxiety, frustration, humiliation, embarrassment, and boredom. In influencing learners in the affective domain, as well as the other domains, the dietetics professional should positively reinforce learner responses.

SEQUENCE OF INSTRUCTION

Since there is a great deal to learn, instruction requires some type of organized sequence. Sequence of instruction is characterized by the progressive development of knowledge, attitudes, and skills. Learning takes place over time, and the process should be organized into smaller units. Since the ultimate outcome is able performance or behavioral change, it is important to consider how meaningful the sequence is to the individual, not the teacher or trainer, and whether or not it promotes learning. Mager provides several recommendations for sequencing. Instruction may be arranged from the general to the specific, from the specific to the general, from the simple to the complex, or according to interest, logic, or frequency of use of the knowledge or skill.[23]

In moving from the general to the specific, an overview or large picture should be presented first, followed by the details and specifics. For example, one would present an overview of the reasons for the diabetic diet and the general principles of the diet before presenting the details. With a new employee, a general explanation of the job should precede the specifics. After the individual has digested some information, it is possible to consider a specific-to-general sequence.

Material may be organized from the simple (terms, facts, procedures) to the complex (concepts, processes, theories, analyses, applications) so that the individual handles increasingly difficult material. If the taxonomies are used in writing objectives for learning, the hierarchy of the taxonomies provides a simple-to-complex sequence.

Another possibility is sequencing according to interest, or from the familiar to the unfamiliar. One may begin instruction with whatever is of most interest or concern to the individual. Initial questions from patients, clients, employees, or other audiences suggest such interest and should be dealt with immediately so that they are free to concentrate on later information. "How long will I have to stay on this diet?" "Can I eat my favorite foods?" The information that the person desires is a good starting point for discussion.

Similarly, if the learner perceives a problem, the instructor can start with that problem rather than with a preset agenda. As learning proceeds, the individual may develop additional needs for information or goals for learning that may be addressed. Generally, people who have assisted in directing their own learning tend to feel more committed to it.

Logic may suggest the sequence. Certain things may need to be said before others. Safety precautions may need to be introduced early, for example, when discussing kitchen equipment. Sanitary utensil handling may be important to discuss with wait staff before discussing how to set a table.

Frequency of use of the knowledge or skill may also dictate sequence. The skill used most frequently should be taught first, followed by the next most frequently used skill. If training time runs out, at least the learner has learned all except the least frequently used skills. The instructor should teach first what people need to know rather than the "nice to know" information. Finally, even though learners may have been practicing individual elements of the job, they need practice on the total job. This practice may be provided in the actual job situation or through simulation.[11,20]

EVALUATION OF RESULTS

Evaluation is key to successful education. Accountability to measure effectiveness in terms of outcomes is necessary in both clinical and managerial arenas. Expected outcomes should be defined before starting the intervention rather than later. Nutrition education or employee training that does not show improvement cannot be considered effective. Evaluation is important for continuous improvement and refinement of education.

Evaluation connotes judgments about the value or worth of something compared with a standard. Everyone makes these judgments daily, both consciously and unconsciously. "The food tastes good." "The television show is worth watching." "She is not motivated." Our thoughts turn to evaluation automatically as we compare something with some standard and pass judgment.

Educational evaluation consists of a systematic appraisal of the quality, effectiveness, and worth of an educational endeavor, such as instruction, programs, or goals based on information or data. That it is systematic suggests that advance planning has taken place and that the process will provide data on the quality or worth of the educational endeavor.

Consider not only what to evaluate, but also when to evaluate and how the evaluation will be done. An evaluation plan involves several steps: defining objectives or outcomes; designing the evaluation based on objectives; choosing what to evaluate; deciding how and when to collect data to obtain timely feedback; constructing a data collection instrument or method; implementing the data collection; analyzing results; reporting them; and setting a course of action.

Although the terms "measurement" and "evaluation" are sometimes interchanged, their meanings are not equivalent. Measurement or "educational assessment" is the process of collecting and quantifying data in terms of numbers on the extent, degree, or capacity of people's learning in knowledge, attitudes, skills, performance, and behavioral change. Testing is one kind of measurement. Measurement involves determining the degree to which a person possesses a certain attribute, as when one receives a score of 85 on a test. However, such a measurement does not determine quality or worth. These systems require experimental designs, data collection, and statistical analysis of the data. The term "assessment" can also mean estimating or judging the value of the data collected, as in nutrition assessment.[24-26]

Evaluation, on the other hand, is based on the measurement of what people know, think, feel, and do. Evaluation compares the observed value or quality with a standard or criterion of comparison. Evaluation is the process of forming value judgments about the quality of programs, products, goals, and the like from the data. One may evaluate the success of an educational program, for example, by measuring the degree to which goals or objectives were achieved. Evaluation goes beyond measurement to the formation of value judgments about the data. To be effective, evaluation designs should specify not only what will be evaluated, but also when it will be evaluated, such as the score difference between a pretest and a posttest.

Purpose of Evaluation

Careful evaluation should be an integral part of all nutrition education programs and employee training programs. There are several purposes of evaluation. One cannot make judgments about effectiveness without it. Program evaluation may be used for planning, improvement, and justification. As a system of quality control, it can determine whether the process of education is effective, identify its strengths and weaknesses, and determine what changes should be made. To determine accountability, one needs to know whether people are learning, whether dietetics professionals are teaching effectively, whether programs accomplish the desired outcomes, and whether money is well spent. In times of limited financial resources, accountability requires an examination of cost–benefit ratios. Is the program useful and valuable enough to justify the cost? Is there evidence that training is changing employee behavior on the job and contributing to the bottom line? It is important to determine whether the learning objectives were accomplished and whether the individual learned what was intended or developed in desired ways.

Evaluation helps dietetics professionals make better decisions and improve education. It is helpful in making decisions concerning teaching, learning, program effectiveness, and the necessity of making modifications in current efforts or even of terminating them. Evaluation provides evidence that what you are doing is worthwhile. Plans for evaluation should be made early, in the planning stages of an educational endeavor and not after it has begun or is completed.[27]

With employees, training evaluation should show improved job performance and financial results. Another question often asked is: "Does training transfer?" One needs to determine whether the skills and knowledge taught in training are applied on the job.

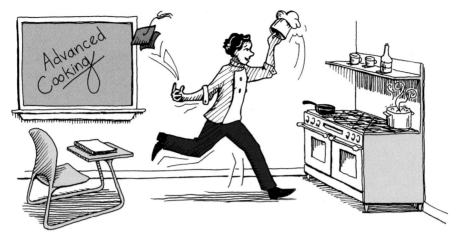

Does the training transfer from the classroom to the workplace?

If they are, this demonstrates the value of the training to the organization, and the effectiveness of the method of training. If not, change is needed.

As with other parts of his adult education model, Malcolm Knowles suggested that evaluation should be a mutual undertaking between the educator and the learner. He recommends less emphasis on the evaluation of learning and more on the rediagnosis of learning needs, which suggests immediate or future steps to be taken jointly by the dietetics professional and the client or employee. This type of feedback from evaluation becomes more constructive and acceptable to adults. Thus, evaluation may be considered something you should do with people, not to people. If problems are apparent, then solutions may be found jointly by the professional and the individual.[28]

Formative and Summative Evaluations

Formative and summative evaluations are two types of evaluations used to improve any of three processes—program planning, teaching, or learning. Formative evaluation refers to that made early or during the course of education, with the feedback of results modifying the rest of the educational endeavor. Summative evaluation refers to an endpoint assessment of quality at the conclusion of learning.

Formative Evaluation

Formative evaluation is a systematic appraisal that occurs before or during the implementation of a learning activity for the purpose of modifying or improving teaching, learning, program design, or educational materials. It is often qualitative in nature with data collection by observation, interviewing, and surveys. It can help to diagnose problems in student learning and in teaching effectiveness. It pinpoints parts mastered and parts not mastered and allows for revision of plans, methods, techniques, or materials.

Formative evaluation may be performed at frequent intervals. If the learner appears bored, unsure, anxious, quizzical, or lost, or if you are unsure of the person's abilities, for example, it is appropriate to stop teaching and start the evaluation process. Ask the person to repeat what he or she has learned. In diabetic education, if formative evaluation shows that the person does not understand the concept of carbohydrate counting, he or she will not be able to master more complex behaviors such as menu planning. Having located the problem that carbohydrate counting is not comprehended, the educator can change approaches to try to overcome the problem. Perhaps an alternative explanation that is clearer or simpler or a concrete illustration is indicated. During group learning, a collaborative member may be able to provide an explanation that an individual understands better than the explanation of the educator.

Before nutrition messages and educational materials are designed and implemented, formative evaluation or market research activities, such as focus group interviews and structured discussions with members of the target audience, are designed and implemented. This type of qualitative evaluation helps the educator to learn about individuals' thoughts, ideas, and opinions and tells whether recipients are likely to ignore, reject, or misunderstand the message or accept it and act on it.

Formative research is essential for tailoring intervention strategies. The moderator of a focus group uses open-ended interviewing strategies with groups of eight to 15 people. The focus group approach has been used to assess consumer preferences, to plan and evaluate nutrition education interventions, and to pretest print materials. It can answer questions about readability, content, and applicability.

Failure to learn may not always be related to instructional methods or materials per se, but may derive from problems that are physical, emotional, cultural, or environmental in nature. By performing an evaluation after smaller units of instruction, the educator can determine whether the pacing of instruction is appropriate for the patient, client, or employee. Frequent feedback is necessary to facilitate learning. It is especially important when a great deal of material has to be learned.

Mastery of smaller units can be a powerful positive reinforcement for the learner, and verbal praise may increase motivation to continue learning. When mistakes are made, they should be corrected quickly by giving the correct information. Avoid saying such things as: "No, that's wrong." "Can't you ever get things right?" "Won't you ever learn?" Positive, not negative, feedback should be given. Approach the problem specifically by saying, for example, "You identified some of the foods that are high in sodium, which is very good. Now let's look a second time for others."

Summative Evaluation

Summative evaluation has a different purpose and time frame from that of formative evaluation. Summative evaluation is considered final, and it is used at the end of a term, course, or learning activity. The purpose of summative evaluation is to appraise results, quality, outcomes, or worth using quantitative approaches. It may include grading, certification, or evaluation of progress, and the evaluation distinguishes those who excel from those who do not. Judgment is made about the learner, teacher, program, or curriculum with regard to the effectiveness of learning or instruction for the target population. This judgment aspect creates the anxiety and defensiveness often associated with evaluation.

Evaluation should be a continual process that is preplanned along with educational sessions. Evaluation preassessment determines the individual's abilities before the educational program, and progress should be evaluated continually during and immediately after the educational program. Follow-up evaluation at regular intervals may measure the degree to which the person has forgotten information or has fallen back to previous behaviors.[29-33]

Norm- and Criterion-Referenced Methods

Besides formative and summative evaluation, there are norm- and criterion-referenced interpretations. In norm-referenced results, the group that has taken a test provides the norms for determining the meaning of each person's score. A norm is like the typical performance of a group. One can then see how the individual compares with the results of the group, whether above or below the norm. In criterion-referenced results, a standard is used as a basis for the level of proficiency required. Instead of comparing learners with each other, the instructor compares each individual with a predefined, objective standard of performance of what the learner is expected to know or to be able to do after instruction is complete. A criterion-referenced measurement ascertains the person's status in respect to a defined objective or standard, and test items, if tests are used, correspond to the objectives. If the learner can perform what is called for in the objective, he or she has been successful. If not, criterion-referenced testing, which tends to be more diagnostic, indicates what the learner can and cannot do, and more learning can be planned.

Some instructors may believe that a test should not be too easy, but the degree of difficulty of a test may not be as important as whether a person can perform. The instructor may believe that some of the questions have to be difficult so that a spread of scores is produced to separate the brightest from the rest, the A's from the B's and C's. Some tests are developed with the intent that not everyone will be successful and variation in individual scores is expected. Students are graded in a norm-referenced manner by comparison with other individuals on the same measuring device or with the norm of the group. A norm-referenced instrument indicates, for example, whether the individual's performance falls into the 50th percentile or the 90th percentile in relation to the group norm. This method is not as appropriate for affective and psychomotor objectives.

With criterion-referenced evaluation, everyone can do well by attaining a minimum standard. Instruction has been successful when learners reach a defined level of expertise. The Registration Examinations for Dietitians and for Dietetic Technicians are examples of criterion-referenced tests.

Formative evaluation is almost always criterion-referenced. The instructor wants to know who is having trouble learning, not where they rank compared with others. Summative evaluation may be either norm- or criterion-referenced.[34,35]

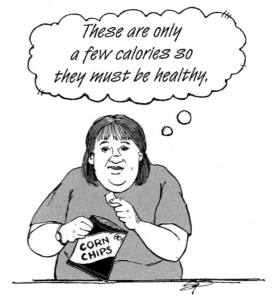

These are only a few calories so they must be healthy.

We need to evaluate what people learn.

TYPES OF EVALUATION AND OUTCOMES

After considering the purpose (why) and timing (when) of evaluation, the educator should resolve the question of what to evaluate. Several types of evaluation can be used in measuring effectiveness. These are (1) measurement of participant (client, employee) reactions to programs; (2) measurement of behavioral change; (3) measurement of results in an organization; (4) evaluation of learning in the cognitive, affective, and psychomotor domains; and (5) evaluation of other outcomes.[34] The evaluation of health education is usually focused on one or more types: knowledge, attitudes or beliefs, change in behavior, and other measures.

Participant Reaction to Programs

The first type of evaluation deals with participant (employee, client) reactions to educational programs and whether or not they are favorable. Preferences may vary by age of the participants, cultural or ethnic group, gender, socioeconomic status, and other variables. You need to decide what should be evaluated. Were participants pleased and satisfied with the program, subject matter, content, materials, speakers, room arrangements, physical facilities, and learning activities? When a program, meeting, or class is evaluated, the purpose is to improve decisions concerning its various aspects, to see how the parts fit the whole, or to make program changes.

The quality of learning elements, such as objectives, techniques, materials, and learning outcomes also may be included. Hedonistic scales or happiness indexes, such as smiley faces or numerical scales, have been used to determine the degree to which participants "liked" various aspects. Although these judgments are subjective, they are not useless, since learners who dislike elements of a program may not be learning.

Behavioral Change

A second type of evaluation is the measurement of change in behavior. Did employee or client behavior or habits change based on the learning? In measuring behavior, the focus is on what the person does. In employee training, for example, you may assess changes in job behaviors to see whether transfer of training to the job has occurred. Continual quality improvement has influenced the need for this type of evaluation. It is necessary to know what the job performance was before training and to decide who will observe or assess changed performance—the supervisor, peers, or the individual. This type of assessment is more difficult to measure and can be done selectively.

The ultimate criterion for effectiveness of nutrition education is not merely the improvement in knowledge of what to eat, but also changes in dietary behaviors and practices as the individual develops better food habits, Is the person consuming more fruits and vegetables, for example? These changes are difficult to confirm and often depend on direct observation, which is time-consuming; on self-reports; and on indirect outcome measures, such as weight gained or lost in a person on a weight reduction diet, reduction in blood pressure in hypertensive persons, or better control of blood sugars in diabetes mellitus.[17,34]

Organizational Results

Professionals involved with employee training gather a third type of evaluative data to justify the time and expense to the organization. Management may want to know how training will positively benefit the organization in relation to the cost. Results in terms of the following aspects may be attributed, at least in part, to training: improved morale, improved efficiency or productivity, improved quality of work, better customer satisfaction, less employee turnover, fewer accidents or worker's compensation claims, better attendance, dollar savings, number of employee errors, number of grievances, amount of overtime, and the like. Did changing employees' behavior on the job improve business results? If not, it is not useful.

Learning

Whether learning has taken place is a separate question, even if the program rated highly on entertainment value. The learning of principles, facts, attitudes, values, and skills should be evaluated on an objective basis, and this task is more complex. If the learning objectives are written in terms of measurable performance, they serve as the source of the evaluation. To what degree were the objectives achieved by the learner?

Whether a person has succeeded in learning can be determined by developing situations, or test items, based on the objectives of instruction. A program is ineffective if it has not achieved its objectives. It is important for the test items to match the objectives in performance and conditions discussed in Chapter 11. If they do not match the objectives, it is not possible to assess whether instruction was successful, that is, whether the learner learned what was intended.

Mager pointed out that several obstacles must be overcome to assess the results of instruction successfully. Some obstacles are caused by poorly written objectives, whereas others result from attitudes and beliefs on the part of instructors who use inappropriate test items.[23]

One of the problems in evaluation results from inadequately written objectives. If the performance is not stated, if conditions are omitted, and if the criterion is missing, it will be difficult to create a test situation. If these deficiencies are discovered, the first step is to rewrite the objective.

Mager suggested a series of steps to select appropriate test items:[34]

1. Note the performance (what the person will be able to say or do) stated in the objective. Match the performance and conditions of the test item to those of the objective.
2. Check whether the performance is a main intent or an indicator. If the performance is the main intent, note whether it is covert (invisible) or overt (visible, audible).
3. If the performance is covert, such as solving a problem, check for an indicator behavior, a visible or audible activity by which the performance can be inferred.
4. Test for the overt indicator in objectives containing one rather than the main performance.

The first step is to see whether the performance specified in the test item is the same as that specified in the objective. If they do not match, the test item must be revised, since it will not indicate whether the objective has been accomplished. If the objective states that the performance is "to plan low-fat menus," or "to operate the dish machine," for example, the test should involve planning menus or operating the dish machine. It would be inappropriate to ask the learner to discuss the principles of writing menus or to label the parts of the dish machine on a diagram.

In addition to matching performance, the test should use the same specific circumstances or conditions that are specified in the objective.

EXAMPLE: (Given the disassembled parts of the meat slicer) is able to reassemble the parts in correct sequence.

The conditions are "given the disassembled parts of the meat slicer." The practitioner should provide a disassembled machine and ask the employee to reassemble it. An inappropriate test would be to ask the learner to list the steps in reassembling the meat slicer or to discuss the safety precautions to be taken.

If the learner must perform under a range of conditions, you may need to test performance using the entire range. If a client eats at home and in restaurants, the dietetics professional must determine whether the person is capable of following the dietary changes in both environments. If students are learning to take a diet history, they should be taught to handle the range of conditions, including people of different ages, socioeconomic levels, and cultural groups. Not every condition will be taught and tested, but the common conditions that the individual will encounter should be included in the objectives and in testing.

The main intent of an objective may be stated clearly, or it may be implied. The main intent is the performance, whereas an indicator is an activity (visible, audible) through which the main intent is inferred:

EXAMPLE: (Given a copy of a sodium-restricted diet) is able to plan a menu for a complete day.

In this example, the main intent is to discriminate between foods permitted and omitted on the diet, and the indicator is the ability to plan menus. You can infer that the client knows what is permitted and what is not if accurate sodium-restricted menus are planned. Test for the indicator in objectives that contain one. This, of course, does not prove that the person will change eating behaviors.

Covert actions are not visible, but are internal or mental activities, such as solving problems or identifying. If the performance is covert, an indicator should have been added to the objective, as explained in Chapter 11, and the indicator should be tested.

EXAMPLE: Is able to identify the parts of the slicer (on a diagram or verbally).

For this example, the employee should be provided with the indicator, a diagram of a meat slicer, and asked to identify the parts.

Although some performances are covert, others are overt. Overt actions are visible or audible, such as writing, verbally describing, and assembling. If the performance is overt, determine whether the test item matches the objective.

EXAMPLE: Is able to reassemble the parts of the meat slicer.

The employee should be provided with the parts of the meat slicer and asked to reassemble them. Performance tests are appropriate when skills are taught. If the employee is being taught to use equipment, the evaluation should be to have him or her demonstrate its operation. If a student is learning interviewing skills, an interview session is indicated as the evaluation.

The discussion so far has used examples of objectives in the cognitive and psychomotor domains. Affective objectives describe values, interests, and attitudes that are thought to predispose dietary changes. While the cognitive and psychomotor domains are concerned with what individuals can do, the affective domain deals with what they are willing to do. These changes are covert or internal and develop more slowly over a period of time. Evaluation of their achievement is more difficult and needs to take different forms.

Attitudes are inferred based on the evidence of what people say or do. To assess whether the individual has been influenced by education, the professional may conduct a discussion and listen to what the individual says or observe what he or she does, since both saying and doing are overt behaviors. In measuring attitudes and values, the person needs the opportunity to express agreement rather than deciding on right or wrong answers. A self-reported attitude survey may be used, for example. Statements can be given to which the person responds on a 5-point scale, from "strongly agree" to "strongly disagree." To evaluate change in the learner's behavior, the practitioner attempts to secure data that permit an inference to be made regarding the person's future disposition in similar situations. In the affective domain, this is a more difficult task.

It is conceivable that the individual may display a desirable overt behavior only in the presence of the practitioner. The attitude toward following a diabetic diet or an employee work procedure may differ depending on the dietetics professional's presence or absence. Since time is required for change in attitudes and values, evaluation may have to be repeated at designated intervals. To determine realistically how the person is disposed to act, the measurement approach needs to evaluate volitional rather than coerced responses.

Other Outcomes

An outcome is a result and can be defined as what does or does not happen after an intervention. The criterion of nutrition education program effectiveness has generally been improvement in knowledge, awareness, and in dietary behaviors or physiologic parameters, or both. This criterion can be measured in many ways depending on the application and outcome data available. For professional education programs, the use of hard copy and electronic portfolios representing evidence of skills and competency is one way to assess outcome measures.[36–38]

Outcomes should have clear interpretations related to the dietitian's intervention in improving nutrition and health status. They may be of several types: (1) physiological or biological measures, (2) behavioral change based on self-report, (3) diet-related psychosocial measures, and (4) environmental or other measures of dietary behavior.

SELF-ASSESSMENT

You have just discussed sodium restriction with a man with hypertension. How can you assess what he has learned?

Biological indicators are changes in clinical or biochemical indices, such as serum lipid levels in cardiovascular disease, hemoglobin or serum albumen level in pregnancy, and glycosylated hemoglobin level in diabetes. Eating behavior changes such as decreasing fat intake or increasing fiber intake are based on self-reports, which can be subject to bias. Psychosocial outcomes include increased nutrition knowledge, attitude change, or self-efficacy for behavior but do not prove the change in food choices. Other changes are in body mass index or weight, increases in the level of physical activity, decreased blood pressure, or reduction in risk factors for disease and improved health (both long-term goals). Care must be taken in interpreting some of these results, since they may reflect variables other than education. Stress, for example, can affect a person's blood sugar even when the diabetic diet is followed. In nutrition education interventions, behavior has been measured in different ways ranging from observable food choices to dietary intakes. These may include reports by teachers or parents of children's food preferences, such as refusing a food, willingness to taste a new food, and selecting a more nutritious food when other choices were available. Actual food choices and consumption, plate waste, and self-reported intake can be used to evaluate dietary intake. Other measures include 24-hour dietary recall, food records and food frequency questionnaires, and changing food preparation practices and recipes, or percentage of participation after an intervention.

Physical measures can include laboratory values, blood pressure, weight indices, urinary output, and physical activity status. Mean maternal weight gain, infant's birth weight, and Apgar scores at birth can be used to evaluate pregnancy outcomes and the health of newborn infants.[24]

Organizational changes included changes in school lunch menus, such as to lower fat and sodium, or food choices and nutrition information offered at the worksite. Data can be collected on the number of work-related injuries or food sanitation incidents after safety training.

DATA COLLECTION TECHNIQUES

There are many techniques for collecting evaluation data: paper-and-pencil tests, questionnaires, interviews, visual observation, job sample or performance tests, simulation, rating forms or checklists, individual and group performance measures, individual and group behavior measures, and self-reports. As measurement devices that will be analyzed statistically, they require the use of specific experimental designs. Regardless of the particular instrument or technique used, it should be pretested with a smaller group before actual use. Since comparisons are desired, it is usually necessary to collect preliminary data on current performance or behaviors.[31,32]

Tests

Tests, especially written tests, are probably the most common devices for measuring learning. Tests sample what one knows, and schools depend heavily on them. Multiple-choice, true-false, short answer, completion, matching, and essay questions are used to measure learning in the cognitive domain. These tests are appropriate when several people are expected to learn the same content or material. Sometimes, both a pretest and a posttest are used to measure learning. This method assists in controlling variables, but be careful not to attribute all the changes noted on the posttest to the learning experiences since other factors may have been involved.

Although tests are appropriate with school-aged children, adults may respond less favorably. The dietetics practitioner should avoid evoking childhood memories associated with the authoritarian teacher, the dependent child, or the assigned degree of success and failure based on right or wrong answers. In one-on-one situations, the practitioner could ask the individual to state verbally what he or she learned as though telling it to a spouse or friend. Or, a self-assessment instrument may be used.

Questionnaires

Questionnaires may be preplanned and are often used to assess attitudes and values that do not involve correct answers. Questions may be open-ended, multiple-choice, ranking, checklist, or alternate response, such as yes/no or agree/disagree. In evaluating behavioral change on the job, trainees and supervisors can both complete a questionnaire.

Interviews

Interviews conducted on a one-to-one basis are another form of evaluation. They are the oral equivalent to written questionnaires used to measure cognitive and affective objectives. Before the interview, the instructor should preplan and draw up a list of questions that will indicate whether learning has taken place. After instruction, evaluation may consist of asking the learner to repeat important facts. An advantage of an interview is that the evaluator can put the person at ease and immediately correct any errors. Another advantage is that the interviewer can probe for additional information. Although this method is time-consuming, it is appropriate for people with low literacy or those less educated. Focus group interviews, mentioned earlier, are an example of a qualitative, formative evaluation.

Observation

In many cases, visual observation is an appropriate method of evaluating learning. The behaviors to be observed should be defined, and an observation checklist may be helpful. When employees are under direct supervision, systematic ongoing observation over a period of time is a basis for evaluating learning. The supervisor can observe and report whether the employee is operating equipment correctly or following established procedures properly. If the employee has been taught sanitary procedures, for example, the professional can see whether or not they are incorporated into the employee's work. Evaluate the performance, using what was taught as a standard. If discrepancies are found, further learning may be indicated.

Performance Tests

When direct observation is not possible or would be too time-consuming and costly, a simulated situation or performance test can be observed. Performance tests are appropriate in the cognitive and psychomotor domains. You can ask a wait staff member to set a table, a cook to demonstrate the meat slicer, or a client to indicate what to select from a restaurant menu. The client could be given a list of foods and asked to differentiate those appropriate for his or her diet. With permission from the learner, audiotape or videotape may be used to record the teaching session. The instructor and learner may discuss the results together and plan further learning to correct any deficiencies. The observer needs to delineate which behaviors are being observed and what is to be acceptable behavior.

Rating Scales and Checklists

Rating scales and checklists have been used to evaluate learner performance and teacher effectiveness. Categories or attributes such as knowledge level or dependability are listed and should be defined in detail to avoid ambiguity. Emphasis should be placed on attributes that can be confirmed objectively rather than judged subjectively. A 5- or 7-point scale is used, allowing a midpoint, and the ratings should be defined, for example, from "excellent" to "poor" or from "extremely acceptable" to "very unacceptable." The list should include as a possible response, "No opportunity to observe."

Rating scales are subject to several errors. Two evaluators may judge the same individual differently. To avoid error, definition of the terms and training of evaluators are essential. The ratings may suffer from personal biases. In addition, some raters have the tendency to be too lenient. Error may result if the rater is a perfectionist. Some evaluators tend to rate most people as average, believing that few people rank at the highest levels. Another possible error is the "halo" error, in which an evaluator is so positively or negatively impressed with one aspect of a person that he or she judges all other qualities according to this one impressive aspect.

Performance Measures

In employee training programs, individual and group performance measures may be assessed. These may include work quality and quantity, number of errors, days of absenteeism, number of grievances, and other types of problems that affect work performance.[20]

Self-Reports

Self-reports, self-evaluation, and self-monitoring are another approach to evaluation. In the affective domain, written questions or statements are presented and the individual supplies responses. "What changes, if any, have you made in your food choices?" "What are you doing differently?" Self-reports, such as a 3-day food record, have been used to measure behavioral change. Responses may be distorted or biased if the individual can ascertain the acceptable answer.

All methods of evaluation have advantages and limitations, which need to be considered. Although evaluation may not provide proof that an intervention and education worked, it does produce a great deal of evidence.

RELIABILITY AND VALIDITY

The concepts of reliability and validity are essential to the measurement of the effectiveness of nutrition education outcomes and employee learning. Validity indicates whether we are measuring what we intend to measure. There are different types of validity, such as content-related, construct-related, and criterion-related (concurrent and predictive) validity, all of which help to "defend" the validity of the instrument. Content-related validity, which is the simplest and perhaps the most important, refers to whether the test items or questions correspond to the subject matter or purpose of instruction or to the knowledge, skills, or objectives they are supposed to measure for a specific audience by culture, age, literacy level, and the like. If one is interested in determining knowledge of dietary fiber, for example, are the questions appropriate in content?

Reliability refers to the consistency and accuracy with which a test or device measures something in the same way in each situation or over time. For example, if a test is given twice to the same students to sample the same abilities, the students should place in the same relative position to others each time if the test is reliable. Methods for determining the reliability and validity of tests may be found in the educational literature.

In all cases, keep in mind that the measuring device should assess whether the learner has attained the requisite knowledge, skill, or competence needed and whether behavior has changed. Pretesting evaluation instruments with the intended audience is essential. If the learner has not attained the intended knowledge or skill, additional learning may be indicated.

After the data from evaluation are collected, they should be compiled and analyzed. The statistical analysis of data is a lengthy subject of its own beyond the scope of this book. Future plans or programs may be modified based on the results of the evaluation. Results should be communicated through evaluation reports to others such as participants, management staff, decision makers, and future learners.[29,31,34]

LESSON PLANS AND PROGRAM PLANS

A lesson plan is a written summary of information about a unit of instruction. It is prepared and used by the instructor. Various formats for lesson plans are available, but the content is essentially the same. A lesson plan is a blueprint that describes all aspects of instruction. It includes the following:[13,23]

- Preassessment of the participants or needs assessment
- The performance objectives identified
- The content outline (introduction, body, conclusions)
- How the content will be sequenced
- A description of the activities participants will engage in to reach the objectives
- Instructional procedures (techniques and methods)
- Educational materials, visual aids, media, handouts, and equipment
- Amount of time allotted or scheduled
- Facilities to be used
- Method of evaluating whether the learner reached the objectives, outcomes, or other results
- References

Once written, a lesson plan is a flexible guide to instruction that can be used with many different individuals or groups. A series of lesson plans or activities may be grouped into a larger unit of instruction covering a longer time frame, such as a whole

---

B O X 12-2

Sample Lesson Plan on Sanitary Dish Handling

- I. Target audience: New wait staff
- II. Objective: When setting tables, wait staff will be able to handle dishes and utensils in a sanitary manner.
- III. Time allotted: 15 minutes
- IV. Preassessment: Question new employees to determine what they already know about sanitary dish and utensil handling.
- V. Content and sequence:
  1. Wash hands. Handling of flatware by the handles.
  2. Handling of cups by the base or handle and glassware by the base.
  3. Handling plates and bowls on the edge without touching the food.
  4. Use a tray.
  5. The hands and skin as major sources of disease-causing bacteria and their transmission to food and utensils.
  6. Proper bussing of dishes to avoid contamination of the hands.
  7. Hand washing.
- VI. Learning activities:
  1. Demonstration and discussion of proper handling of dishes and utensils when setting tables, serving food, and bussing tables.
  2. Discussion of hand washing.
  3. Actual practice by new wait staff.
- VII. Materials: Dishes, utensils, tray, handout of important points to remember.
- VIII. Evaluation: Whether or not dishes and utensils were handled properly during the actual practice; continued observation of the employee's performance on the job.

---

day or several days. The term "program planning" is also used. A plan for a longer program would include essentially the same components as a lesson plan with the addition of the names of speakers or others responsible, and cost considerations. Sample lesson plans are found in **Boxes 12-2** and **12-3**.

DOCUMENTATION

Dietetics professionals are accountable for the nutrition care they provide in all settings, including in consulting and private practice and at the work site. Accepted standards of practice for quality control and accreditation agencies, such as the Joint Commission on Accreditation of Healthcare Organizations (JCAHO), mandate that dietetics services be documented and communicated to other health professionals providing care.[39] Patient records also provide evidence in malpractice suits and are important to the denial of legal liability. This is increasingly important when transferring information to others over the Internet.[40]

BOX **12-3**

Sample Lesson Plan on Calcium in Pregnancy

I.   Target audience: Pregnant women

II. Objective: To be able to identify foods and quantities of foods that will meet the daily calcium needs for pregnancy and plan menus using these foods.

III. Time Allotted: 30 minutes

IV. Preassessment: Question audience about which foods contain calcium and how much of these foods should be eaten daily during pregnancy. Determine any previous pregnancies and what was eaten.

V.   Content and sequence:

1. Total daily calcium needs, with the important functions of calcium during pregnancy.

2. Dairy foods as a source of calcium, with quantities of calcium in each.

3. Other foods as good sources of calcium, with quantities of calcium.

4. Calcium sources for lactose-intolerant individuals.

5. Have audience suggest a breakfast, lunch, dinner, and snacks that meet the need for calcium.

6. Questions from the audience.

7. Have each person plan her own menu for tomorrow.

VI. Learning activities: Group discussion of food sources of calcium. Show actual foods and food models for portion sizes. Group planning of a day's menu followed by each individual planning something appropriate for herself for the next day's menu.

VII. Materials: Actual food samples, food models, paper and pencils for menu planning, chalkboard or flip chart for writing menus, handout with good sources of calcium and the amount of calcium in each, including the daily recommended intake (DRI) for pregnancy, and a sample menu.

VIII. Evaluation: The menu planned by each individual. Discussion with individuals during their follow-up prenatal visits.

Documentation provides a developmental history of nutrition services to clients. Measurement and documentation of desired outcomes—medical, clinical, educational, and psychosocial—are essential. The information communicated demonstrates what services have been delivered that contribute to health care delivery and that these services provide the patient or client with a specific benefit that will offset the cost of the service.

The usual place for documentation is in the medical or client's record. Although several formats are available, traditionally the professional makes notes on the patient's medical record using the SOAP procedure.[39] The acronym SOAP stands for Subjective, Objective, Assessment, and Planning. The American Dietetic Association has recently implemented a nutrition diagnosis and intervention three-step process using Problem, Etiology, and Signs or Symptoms (PES) that endeavors to standardize language used in the nutrition care process.[41] Chapters 4 and 5 cover these systems in more depth. Documentation of employee education and training programs is also essential. Records should be kept of all information included in employee orientation. The use of an orientation checklist is helpful in ensuring that everything the employee needs to know has been communicated to him or her. Records should be kept on file showing the date and content of ongoing training sessions, such as inservice programs, and off-the-job experiences, such as continuing education.[1]

This chapter has examined the selection and implementation of learning activities in the cognitive, affective, and psychomotor domains. Task analysis and job instruction training were described. Finally, the evaluation process in which data is collected and analyzed to determine the success of educational endeavors was outlined.

CASE STUDY 1

Susan Grey, RD, has decided that there is a need for prenatal nutrition classes in the outpatient clinic. Many of the patients are teenagers with limited incomes who are on suboptimum diets. The clinic nurse is also interested in cooperating to reduce the time she spends in individual counseling with patients.

1. Develop a lesson plan for a prenatal nutrition class.
2. What audiovisual materials would you suggest?
3. What handout materials would you recommend?
4. How long should the presentation be?

CASE STUDY 2

Sally Parker manages the kitchen at a major medical center with 600 beds. In the past month, there has been some employee turnover, and three new employees are involved in the preparation of hot foods. Susan is unsure of their knowledge of sanitation and knows that it is past time to be sure that they know the standards and the HACCP procedures.

Sally decides to get the three employees together to assess their knowledge and discuss standards for personal hygiene and time-temperature standards for cooking and holding hot foods.

1. What are some ways to determine what the new employees know already, that is, their current level of knowledge?
2. What are possible ways to approach and fill any gaps in their knowledge?
3. How can Sally follow up and evaluate the results of her discussions?

REVIEW AND DISCUSSION QUESTIONS

1. What are the advantages and disadvantages of the educational methods and techniques?
2. What methods and techniques are appropriate for objectives in the cognitive domain? The affective domain? The psychomotor domain?
3. Explain how a task analysis would be used with Job Instruction Training.

4. In what ways may educational instruction be organized or sequenced?
5. What are the purposes of evaluation?
6. Differentiate the following: formative and summative evaluation; reliability and validity; criterion-referenced and norm-referenced evaluation.
7. What are the major types or levels of evaluation? If you had to describe each to someone desiring to evaluate employee training, what major elements of each would you emphasize?
8. If you had to evaluate a diabetes education program, what would you do? How would you go about it?
9. What are the parts of a lesson plan or program plan?
10. What should be documented in the medical record?

SUGGESTED ACTIVITIES

1. Complete a task analysis for using a procedure or a piece of equipment (coffee urn, meat slicer, dish machine, mixer, oven, grille, broiler, etc.), listing the sequential steps and key points.
2. Using the job instruction training sequence and a task analysis, teach someone to use an unfamiliar piece of equipment.
3. Plan learning using one of the techniques in the chapter (other than lecture), such as discussion, simulation, or a demonstration. Carry out the plan.
4. Develop one or two performance objectives on a topic of interest for a target audience defined by age, sex, socioeconomic status, and educational level. The audience may be pregnant women, mothers, schoolchildren, adolescents, adult men or women, elderly, employees, executives, sports figures, or a person with a chronic disease. Plan the pre-assessment, content, techniques for presentation, teaching aids and handouts, and evaluation methods. Carry out the educational plan.
5. Develop one or two visual aids to use in teaching.
6. Give a pretest of knowledge on a subject. Instruct the learner on the subject. Follow up with a posttest to examine results.
7. List three ways in which you might evaluate whether an employee learned from a training program. List three ways in which you might evaluate whether a patient comprehended instruction regarding a diabetic diet.

WEB SITES

http://www.aicr.org   American Institute for Cancer Research
http://www.amanet.org   American Management Association
http://www.americanheart.org   American Heart Association
http://www.astd.org   American Society of Training and Development
http://www.cancer.org   American Cancer Society
http://www.cnpp.usda.gov   U.S. Department of Agriculture (USDA) Center for Nutrition Policy and Promotion
http://www.diabetes.org   American Diabetes Association

http://www.eatright.org   American Dietetic Association

http://www.foodsafety.gov   Food safety information

http://www.healthanswers.com   Streaming video

http://www.healthfinder.gov   Fact sheets, games, Spanish site

http://www.healthtouch.com   Patient educational materials

http://www.hrsa.gov   Health Resources and Services Administration (HRSA)

http://www.ific.org   International Food Information Council

http://www.ifst.org   Institute of Food Science and Technology

http://www.igpe.edu   Institute for General Practice Education

http://www.nal.usda.gov/fnic   USDA Food Nutrition Information Center

http://nccam.nih.gov   National Center for Complementary and Alternative Medicine

http://www.niddk.nih.gov/health/health.htm   National Institutes of Health (NIH)

http://www.nraef.org   National Restaurant Association Education Foundation

http://www.usda.org   USDA

http://www.nutrition.gov   Links to government resources

http://www.vrg.org   Vegetarian Resource Group

http://www.wheatfoods.org   Wheat Foods Council

REFERENCES

1. Lucas RW. People Strategies for Trainers. New York: American Management Association, 2005.
2. Arthurs JB. A juggling act in the classroom: managing different learning styles. Teaching Learning Nurs 2007:2:2–7.
3. Gravani MN, Hadjileontiadou SJ, Nikolaidou GN, et al. Professional learning: a fuzzy logic-based modeling approach. Learning Instruction 2007:17:235–252.
4. Ernst H, Colthorpe K. The efficacy of interactive lecturing for students with diverse science backgrounds. Adv Physiol Educ 2007:31:41–44.
5. Allen ML, Elliott MN, Morales LS, et al. Adolescent participation in preventive health behaviors, physical activity, and nutrition: differences across immigrant generations for Asians and Latinos Compared with Whites. Am J Public Health 2007:97:337–343.
6. Henry H, Reicks M, Smith C, et al. Identification of factors affecting purchasing and preparation of fruit and vegetables by stage of change for low-income African American mothers using the think-aloud method. J Am Diet Assoc 2003:103:1643–1646.
7. Sherwood NE, Story M, Neumark-Sztainer D, et al. Development and implementation of a visual card-sorting technique for assessing food and activity preferences and patterns in African American girls. J Am Diet Assoc 2003:103:1473–1479.
8. Sweet M, Michaelsen LK. How group dynamics research can inform the theory and practice of postsecondary small group learning. Educ Psych Rev 2007:19:31–47.
9. Johnson DW, Johnson RT, Smith K. The state of cooperative learning in postsecondary and professional settings. Educ Psych Rev 2007:19:15–29.
10. Gibbons JR, McLymont VE, Wiprovinick J, et al. Effect of a multidisciplinary team approach to implementing HACCP guidelines for enteral feeding. J Am Diet Assoc 2006:106:A54.
11. Sasson JR, Alvero AM, Austin J. Effects of process and human performance improvement strategies. J Organ Behav Manage 2006:26:43–78.
12. Scheuer O, Muhlenbrock M, Melis E. Results from action analysis in an interactive learning environment. J Interactive Learning Res 2007:18:185–205.

13. Everett DR. Lesson planning made elegant. Bus Educ Forum 2006:61:48–52.

14. Williams DD, Hricko M, Howell SL, eds. Online Assessment, Measurement, and Evaluation: Emerging Practices. Hershey, PA: Information Science Publications, 2006.

15. Islam KA. Podcasting 101 for Training and Development: Challenges, Opportunities, and Solutions. San Francisco: Wiley-Pfeiffer, 2007.

16. O'Neil J, Marsick VJ. Understanding Adult Action Learning. New York: American Management Association, 2007.

17. West DS, DiLillo V, Bursac Z, et al. Motivational interviewing improves weight loss in women with type 2 diabetes. Diabetes Care 2007:30:1081–1087.

18. Bassi M, Steca P, Delle Fave A, et al. Academic self-efficacy beliefs and quality of experience in learning. J Youth Adolesc 2007:36:301–312.

19. Arthur D. Recruiting, Interviewing, Selecting and Orienting New Employees. 4th Ed. New York: American Management Association, 2005.

20. Kirkpatrick DL. Improving Employee Performance Through Appraisal and Coaching. 2nd Ed. New York: American Management Association, 2005.

21. Mager RF, Beach KM. Developing Vocational Instruction. Belmont, CA: Fearon Publishers, 1967.

22. Stolovitch HD, Keeps EJ. Telling Ain't Training. Alexandria, VA: American Society of Training and Development, 2002.

23. Mager RF. Analyzing Performance Problems, Or, You Really Oughta Wanna. Belmont, CA: Pitman Management and Training, 1984

24. Haessig CJ, LaPotin AS. Outcomes Assessment for Dietetics Education. Chicago: American Dietetic Association, 2002.

25. Medeiros LC, Hillers VN, Chen G, et al. Design and development of food safety knowledge and attitude scales for consumer food safety education. J Am Diet Assoc 2004:104:1671–1677.

26. Chima CS, Farmer-Dziak N, Cardwell P, et al. Use of technology to track program outcomes in diabetes self-management program. J Am Diet Assoc 2005:105:1933–1938.

27. Maillet JO, Skates J, Pritchett E. American Dietetic Association: scope of dietetics practice framework. Appendix: standards of practice in nutrition care for the registered dietitians, standards of practice in nutrition care for the dietetic technician, registered, and standards of professional performance for dietetics professionals. J Am Diet Assoc 2005:634–645, 645e1–645e10.

28. Knowles MS. The Adult Learner: A Neglected Species. 4th Ed. Houston: Gulf Publishing, 1990.

29. Mertens DM. Research and Evaluation in Education and Psychology: Integrating Diversity with Quantitative, Qualitative, and Mixed Methods. 2nd Ed. Thousand Oaks, CA: Sage, 2005.

30. Norcini JJ, McKinley DW. Assessment methods in medical education. Teaching Teacher Educ 2007:23:239–250.

31. Eggen PD, Kauchak DP. Strategies and Models for Teachers: Teaching Content and Thinking Skills. Boston: Pearson Allyn Bacon, 2006.

32. De Champlain AF. Ensuring that the competent are truly competent: An overview of common methods and procedures used to set standards on high-stakes examinations. J Vet Med Educ 2004:31:61–65.

33. Foshay WR, Tinkey PT. Evaluating the effectiveness of training strategies: performance goals and testing. Ilar J 2007:48:156–162.

34. Mager RF. C.R.I.: Criterion-Referenced Instruction: Analysis, Design, and Implementation. Los Altos Hills, CA: Mager Associates, 1976.

35. Byrd-Bredbenner C, Mauer J, Wheatley V, et al. Food safety hazards lurk in the kitchens of young adults. J Food Protect 2007:70:991–996.

36. Passerini K. Performance and behavioral outcomes in technology-supported learning: The role of interactive media. J Educ Multimedia Hypermedia 2007:16:183–211.

37. Hicks T, Russo A, Autrey T, et al. Rethinking purpose and processes for designing digital portfolios. J Adolesc Adult Literacy 2007:50:450–458.

38. Fahey K, Lawrence J, Paratore J. Using electronic portfolios to make learning public. J Adolesc Adult Literacy 2007:50:460–471.

39. Joint Commission on Accreditation of Health Care Organizations. 2007 Comprehensive Accreditation Manual for Hospitals: The Official Handbook. Oak Brook, IL: Joint Commission Resources, 2007.

40. Ashley RC. Telemedicine: legal, ethical, and liability considerations. J Am Diet Assoc 2002;102:267.

41. American Dietetic Association. Nutrition Diagnosis and Intervention: Standardized Language for the Nutrition Care Process. Chicago: American Dietetic Association, 2007.

CHAPTER 13

Group Facilitation and Dynamics

OBJECTIVES

- List the factors increasing group cohesiveness.
- Discuss the suggestions for promoting group change.
- Explain the informal work group.
- Identify the group facilitation skills.
- List and explain facilitator and participant functions in groups.
- Differentiate between formal and informal groups.
- Develop skill by leading a small group discussion.
- Identify the benefits and limitations of cohesive groups.
- List the strengths and weaknesses of group decision making.

Never doubt that a small group of thoughtful, committed citizens can change the world. Indeed, it is the only thing that ever has.
—MARGARET MEADE

Dietitians and other health care professionals manage employee groups in addition to interacting with client groups, community groups, colleagues, and other health care professionals. Employee training and patient or client education are often accomplished in a group setting.

Besides interpersonal communication skills, practitioners need to demonstrate the ability to "work effectively as a team member." Knowledge of both "concepts of human and group dynamics" and "human resource management" is required by the Commission on Accreditation for Dietetics Education.[1]

As you peruse the list of objectives for this chapter, you may be surprised at the range of communication behaviors related to groups that health care professionals are expected to develop. Activities such as conducting performance appraisals, counseling, disciplining staff, facilitating group meetings, team building, enhancing morale through the building of group cohesiveness among staff, initiating change, and managing the resulting resistance all

291

require well-honed communication skills. This chapter focuses on providing readers information on teams; groups; cohesiveness in groups, and its relationship to change; group facilitation skills; and facilitator–participant functions.

A group may be defined as a collection of individuals interacting with one another as members who share a common goal or identity. The chapter attempts to parse the deceivingly simple definition, explaining each of its components. Although much of the chapter is devoted to exploring skills required of the group facilitator and participants, the reader is cautioned that one cannot develop these skills simply from reading a chapter, or even from reading it again and again. To develop these skills, you must make a personal commitment to risk feeling unsure and awkward as you attempt to practice. In fact, the time to develop group skills is while you are still a student or staff member. You can practice these skills with friends, with family, and in the community. In this way, when you advance to a position of authority, you will have refined your skills from the earlier practice and experience.

Although interpersonal and group interaction skills can be taught, the most effective way for people to learn them is through experiencing, observing, and modeling others whom they admire and view as effective communicators. Communication skills often are more effectively "caught" than taught, and professionals need to be conscious of their opportunities to develop these skills among staff and clients through their own modeling of appropriate behaviors. Whether or not you intend it and whether your behavior is optimal or not, the professional is a role model for staff and clients. By learning interpersonal and group skills and then consciously applying them, health care professionals constructively and proactively enhance the development of these skills among staff and clients.[2]

> *A committee is a group that keeps minutes*
> *and loses hours.*
> —MILTON BERLE

CHARACTERISTICS OF AN EFFECTIVE TEAM

Political, economic, and social change is pressuring health care organizations to reinvent themselves. Staff and directors alike live with the anxiety arising from the question of whether or not the belt-tightening efforts, combined with structural changes and strategic alliances, will achieve the necessary improvements in efficiency and help to secure the viability of an organization.

A spate of studies in health care are examining the value of the team approach toward achieving that goal. Furthermore, the studies are being done not only within separate disciplines but also across disciplines and among the multiple disciplines that are included in health care. Topics such as team building, using communication strategically to improve health, group-think, essential group communication facilitation and competencies, and the effects of the group skills of the health care provider on patient or client satisfaction continue to be investigated.[3–10]

By and large the studies confirm the superiority of the team approach, albeit directed by an enlightened director or facilitator, over the traditional authoritative style. Twenty-first century team members are more likely to cooperate when they sense that their opinions are both sought and respected. They are more likely to resist when they sense disinterest or disregard, accompanied by an expectation of compliance. The studies cited confirm that the team approach is more cost-effective and efficient and promotes more harmony and less resistance among staff and between the team leader and the work team. The contemporary health care professional, therefore, needs to be skilled in the practices of team leadership and development. The most critical of these skills is the operational knowledge of how to create the appropriate atmosphere among the team members—a climate that is comfortable, informal, and relaxed and yet encourages the team to perform optimally, free from obvious tensions, and to work together while involved and interested.

The contemporary team leader recognizes that his or her role is not to dominate or unduly defer to the group. The leader understands that leadership often shifts, depending on the circumstances. Different members, because of their special knowledge or experience, may be in positions at various times to act as resources for the group. The leader of a health care team, therefore, needs to know the specific skills of the employees, so that on an ad hoc basis appropriate people can be summoned to lead. In such teams, there is generally little evidence of a struggle for power; the issue is not who controls but how to get the job done.[11,12]

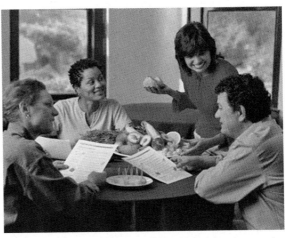

The team leader also has the responsibility for motivating team members to stay focused on the team's goals and objectives. For example, if two team members are not getting along, the team leader is responsible for bringing the discussion back to the team's goals and off individual personalities.

Groups should be seated in a circle so all members can see everyone else.
Source: United States Department of Agriculture.

The team leader reinforces member behavior that promotes healthy team dynamics. One of the key functions is to teach team members to monitor themselves and their work-related responsibilities. A well-functioning team processes their progress and attempts to discern what may be interfering with the operation. Whether the problem is that of an individual whose behavior is interfering with the accomplishment of the group's objectives or whether it is a matter of procedure, the preferred method of resolution for today's workforce is open discussion until a solution is found.[11]

Another of the team leader's responsibilities is to stimulate a climate in which the members communicate openly and frankly. Although they are cohesive, they are not afraid to disagree or be rejected by teammates for sharing a contrary view. Conflict is regarded as healthy, and members understand that "managed" disagreement often leads to synergetic solutions. Members expect to voice their alternative opinions so that mutually satisfying solutions may be found. Criticism is frequent and frank and given with a minimum of anxiety. When members feel invested in one another, they feel freer to express their feelings authentically. When all members of the team participate in the problem-solving and decision-making processes, team members feel responsible and committed to the successful implementation of the team's decisions and objectives.[12]

STIMULATING CHANGE IN TEAMS AND GROUPS

Groups and teams are similar but not the same. All teams are groups, but not all groups are teams. A group is a collection of people who are together because of a common cause, goal, or purpose; it is not just a collection of people. The word "team" implies all of what constitutes a group, plus more. Teams ordinarily have structure imposed to facilitate the accomplishment of their agenda, and a team has a director, a coach, and a facilitator whose task it is to act as their catalyst. To be such a catalyst, team leaders or facilitators require group skills to manage change with both staff teams and client groups.[13]

Ongoing change in organizations is inevitable. When changes are minor, the administrator can simply announce the changes and expect others to follow without resistance; however, other changes may be perceived as threatening by the staff. When changes arouse a sense of fear, ambiguity, and uncertainty, they are resisted. One of the first steps in overcoming this resistance is to facilitate the overt expression of concerns, even when such disclosures may provoke conflict. The professional needs to learn how to process the conflict that arises in the group so that it can be managed constructively.

A direct correlation exists among the amount of time, consideration, and participation in the proposed change allotted to those affected by the change and the amount of resistance likely to occur. When people are given consideration and an opportunity to voice their anxieties and questions, with their recommendations being incorporated whenever possible, they are less likely to resist the changes and more likely to assist in upholding them among others who may resist. When an entire work group is involved in discussion of problems and potential changes, with their supervisor acting as facilitator, collaborative agreement can be reached to use new methods, procedures, or solutions. The members of the group who later object are reminded by the others that they had adequate opportunity to make suggestions and express their concerns and that objecting now is inappropriate.[11]

Communication among work groups is affected by a constellation of variables, each of which is related to every other. Currently, no theoretical model takes into account all the elaborate networks of sender, receiver, and message variables in small groups. In this section the two most salient variables, "change" and "cohesiveness," are explored. It is to the practitioner's advantage not only to understand the power and influence of the two phenomena on organizational life, but also to understand and apply appropriate strategies to use the change and cohesiveness variables for the good of the organization, department, and staff.

COHESIVENESS IN GROUPS

Cohesiveness is an elusive concept that cannot be described by a single definition. An eclectic definition is perhaps the best way to discuss the concept. A cohesive group has strong feelings of "we-ness," that is, members talk more in terms of "we" than "I;" display

---

BOX **13-1**

Factors Increasing Group Cohesiveness

1. All members perform worthwhile tasks and feel they are appreciated by the group.
2. Members clearly perceive the group's goals and consider them to be realistic.
3. Members perceive the group as an entity in its own right and refer to it as such, calling it "the group" or "our group."
4. The group develops a history and tradition. All cohesive groups (church, state family, work, etc.) perform traditional rites and rituals, passing on to new members the "secrets" of the past and strengthening the existing ties among the group's veterans.
5. The group has prestige.
6. Members possess knowledge or material needed by the group.
7. Member participation in the determination of the group's standards is full and direct.
8. Members perceive the issues at hand to be of importance.
9. Personal interaction among members is based on equality, with no one exercising much authority over anyone else.
10. Members share ideals and interests, a common enemy outside the group, or a common satisfaction of individual needs for protection, security, and affection.
11. Members are not jealous of or competitive with one another.
12. Group size is small rather than large.
13. The group is more homogeneous than heterogeneous.

---

loyalty and congeniality to fellow members; work together for a common goal, with everyone ready to take responsibility for group tasks; and possibly endure pain and frustration for the group and defend it against criticism and attack. A summary of factors influencing group cohesiveness is found in **Box 13-1**.

Facilitating Cohesiveness

Because employee turnover is constant in most organizations, intense cohesiveness in work groups is rare; however, a knowledgeable manager can enhance the group's level of attraction and support toward one another through an understanding and application of what behavioral scientists have determined regarding group cohesiveness.

The specific reasons why cohesion thrives in some groups, dissipates in others, and fails to emerge at all in still others are as elusive as its definition. The most fundamental reason for groups tending to gravitate toward cohesive units stems from a basic tenet of human nature: people like to be liked. This desire to be accepted and liked leads people to engage in actions that will maintain or increase the esteem they receive from those around them. There is, therefore, a tendency to go along with the group. After a group feels cohesive, it attempts to preserve the state. Cohesiveness, however, is not static. Even highly cohesive organizations change employees, altering the nature of the internal structure and the interaction patterns of members. Over a period of time, therefore, a group may lose its cohesiveness.[14] Not all teams are cohesive, and those that are may not remain so indefinitely. Cohesiveness relates to the feelings of belonging and acceptance that each member feels in the group. Unless the norms of authenticity, openness, and nonjudgmental acceptance of differences are regularly reinforced among the members, the level of cohesiveness will diminish.

Benefits of Participation in a Cohesive Group

In addition to the increase in self-esteem that generally accompanies members' participation in a cohesive group, other benefits emerge as well: members or individuals can be honest in their dialogue with other members, and they can relax and not be continually on their guard. Because members feel a stake in the group, they are more likely to disagree and argue about decisions affecting it. When a decision is made, each member feels committed to it and takes responsibility for it. Even if meetings are uninhibited and less structured, the topic is more likely to be fully explored; errors are more likely to be pointed out, and poor reasoning or attempts at manipulation on the part of various individuals are more likely to be exposed in the cohesive group than in the more self-conscious and cautious noncohesive group. Maintaining high cohesiveness provides a highly desirable work climate, especially when the manager uses participative decision-making and group problem-solving strategies.

Noncohesive Groups

People in noncohesive groups are likely to argue less, to be more polite, and to be more easily bored. When members disagree, they feel less secure in expressing themselves and often give no overt signs; instead, they may frown, look away, or plead ignorance. Members who are worried about their own security hesitate to challenge others; therefore, noncohesive groups frequently stick to irrelevancies or safe topics or procedures rather than becoming involved in discussing the real issues. Unlike members of cohesive groups, members of noncohesive groups generally do not fully explore the topic, expose manipulation or poor reasoning, argue for what they believe, or take full responsibility for the group's decision. Agreement may be only for the sake of apparent cohesion (external), in which case the individual does not feel bound to the group's goals or decisions. Clearly, the quality of any group decisions or solutions to work-related problems made in these groups is poorer than those made in more cohesive work groups. It is the manager's responsibility to create a climate in which individuals dare to differ from the group without fear of expulsion. If, for example, someone challenges the majority opinion, and others respond defensively to the challenge, it becomes the manager's responsibility to remind the group of values inherent in group debate. The norm reinforced by the manager is the right of each member to challenge without fear, with the result often being group synergy, decisions and solutions superior to those that emerge without challenge.

Generally, the newer members of a group are the most easily intimidated because they are more likely to feel inferior to the established members of the work group. The individual's sense of acceptance in the work group is a highly prized possession, and anything that produces disharmony or conflict of views is likely to disturb it. New members are the most likely to accept and adopt the group's norms because of the pressures of being in a group in which everyone else is acting, talking, or thinking in a certain way. This can occur even without any overt or conscious pressure by group veterans.[15]

Communication and Group Dynamics

The major advantage of the cohesive group is its tendency toward a greater quality of communication, with the interaction more equally distributed than in the noncohesive group. Members feel freer to disagree and challenge one another, provided that they do not perceive the message as a threat to their own status or security. Messages are usually more fully explored in the cohesive group, and the communicator has a better chance of achieving a shared understanding of the message, which could lead to a favorable attitude change in the entire group. If, however, the group interprets a message as a threat to its cohesiveness, it will reject it more hastily than the noncohesive group will.

Conforming to norms may stifle a person's identity and creativity and may restrict, inhibit, and change the values of individual members. It is paradoxical that cohesive teams or groups also provide individuals with opportunities for need fulfillment and personal growth through work satisfaction and camaraderie and are the most likely to achieve synergy. Developing cohesiveness within the team and then using it to produce superior problem solving and decision making can only be achieved consistently through the enlightened facilitator's careful monitoring and "fine-tuning" of the group's dynamics. The manager needs to solicit and reinforce authentic reactions from individuals within the group while at the same time safeguarding the sense of unconditional acceptance among the other team members.

Facilitating Group Change

Various theories of change and organizational development have been emerging since the middle of the 20th century.[16–18] Group change can be fostered through coercion and intimidation, but permanent change promoted in this way is rare. Group change is most easily and optimally developed in meetings and workshops, where trust, team building, and open communication are facilitated among members. Change has the best chance for acceptance and permanence when the need for and value of the change arise from within the group. Change occurring under these conditions receives mutual support and reinforcement from the entire group. After all channels of communication are opened and the needs for change explored, the members may experience a short-lived increase in hostility, but eventually after all have shared perceptions and arrived at mutual agreement or compromise, the new norms are enforced.

Although some group members may disagree with the change and revert to the old behavior, frequently group pressures and individuals' perceptions of their own dissonance cause them to abide by the group-accepted behavior. Suggestions for promoting group change are summarized in **Box 13-2.**

Box **13-2**

Suggestions for Promoting Group Change

- If attitude change is desired, small open-ended, off-the-record discussion groups in which the person feels secure are most effective.
- When people need to change behaviors, participation in group discussions is 2 to 10 times more effective than a lecture that presents the reasons for and pleas for change.
- Active discussion by a small group to determine its goals, methods, work, and new operations, or to solve other problems is more effective in changing group practices than separate instructions, supervisor's requests, or the imposition of new practices by an authority. Group involvement brings about better motivation and support for the change and better implementation and productivity of the new practice.
- Group change is easier to bring about and more permanent than change in the individual members of the group. The supposed greater permanence stems from the individual's assumed desire to live up to group norms. It follows that the stronger the group bonds, the more deeply based are the individual's attitudes. Another explanation suggests that the public commitment to carry through the behavior decided on by group members creates an awareness of the expectations that members have for each other, thus creating forces on each member to comply.
- The best way for a manager to initiate change is to create an atmosphere that leads to a shared perception by the entire group of the need for change. Then the members will call for the change themselves and enforce it. After all facts have been shared with all members and all channels of communication have been opened, there is frequently a sudden but short-lived increase in hostility; however, without this complete sharing among all group members, there can be no real change, only mistrust and subtle hostility.
- High-status persons have more freedom from group control than do other members. The greater the prestige of individual group members, the greater the influence for change they can exert on the others.
- The "buddy system" of change, in which the change is suggested by a peer, is better than having it demanded by an authority figure.

Modified from Galanes G, Adams K, Brilhart J. Effective Group Discussion. Dubuque, IA: McGraw-Hill, 2003.

People's attitudes, beliefs, and values all are rooted in the various groups to which they belong. The more genuinely attached people are to their groups and the more attractive these groups become in fulfilling the various needs of group members, the more likely these members are to be in close and constant contact with their group. Under these conditions group-anchored behaviors and beliefs are extremely resistant to change, with the group being able to exercise firm control over its members. The more attractive a group is to its members, the greater its power to change them. For the group itself to be used most effectively as an agent of change, it must first be cohesive with a strong sense of oneness existing between those who are to be changed and those who desire change. Attempts at changing group members must be aimed at either countering the influence of the group or encompassing it in the

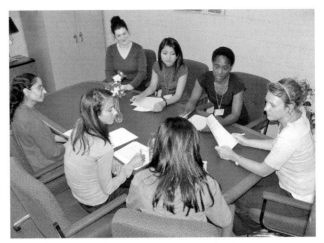

Groups can provide solutions superior to those of one individual.

change. Either way, all attempts at changing individuals must also consider the dynamics of their groups.[19-22]

INFORMAL WORK GROUPS

Health care professionals need to be aware of the inherent power and influence of the informal work group. Since the 1920s, when the Hawthorne studies were carried out at the Western Electric plant near Chicago, social scientists have been studying the Hawthorne Effect. The Hawthorne Effect refers to the theory and its corollaries that employees perform more efficiently when they believe that they are being given special attention. The theory suggests that the major influences affecting efficiency and production are group social structures, group norms, and group pressures.

Professionals need to be sensitive to the dynamics and influences of the informal work group. They must learn ways to provide a forum in which social, task-related, and organizational concerns can be expressed, responses can be offered, and any resistance to change can be overcome. To become conscious of the influence inherent in the informal work group and to tap into the grapevine of informal communication, the manager needs to be aware of the networks of communication that exist within the department as well as the networks within the organization.

Communication networks are the patterns of message flow or linkages of who actually speaks to whom. In all organizations, there are distinctions between the "permissible" structured or organizational channels and the actual channels of communication and network linkages. The permissible channels are the linkages dictated by the organization's structure, which determines the hierarchy of power and influence; the actual channels are the patterns that do, in fact, occur. Often, administrative assistants are ultimately more influential, because of their connections within the network, than others who are considerably higher on the organization chart.

MANAGING GROUPS

The United States in the 21st century continues to be more multicultural than any other country in the world. Among both the workforce supervised and client groups served by health care professionals, no single style will suffice. When managing groups, therefore, the professional's style needs to be appropriate for the persons he or she is attempting to influence. Although they constitute a minority, some people, for example, perform best when under the direction of an authoritarian leader, one who objects to being challenged or questioned and does not want consultation with subordinate members. When persons come from backgrounds in which they have not been encouraged to think and have been punished for initiating ideas, predictably in a work situation they will lack the self-confidence to offer suggestions within a group. If treated with patience, however, and given continued positive reinforcement each time they risk contributing an idea, they may gradually gain the confidence to become valuable group members. In general, however, members of today's workforce have grown up with a preference for egalitarian treatment—overt acknowledgment of each person's value, dignity, and worthiness of respect—and perform best in groups with a leader who can act as a facilitator, involving employees rather than prescribing to them.

In other words, to be successful as leaders, contemporary managers must understand and utilize group facilitation skills. Facilitators are those who understand the value of group decision making and see their function as helping the group to get started, to establish a climate of work, to give support to others, to guide the group, and to keep the group on track so that its objectives are achieved. The group's activities and the facilitator's attitude toward the group are based on respect for what can be accomplished through group discussion and on the fostering of a group climate in which people feel comfortable and secure enough to contribute their ideas.[11,13–15]

Facilitator Preparation

Facilitators' responsibilities begin even before the discussion, in their preparation of the appropriate meeting environment. They must make sure that the room itself is comfortable, with adequate ventilation and lighting and with a consciously arranged seating pattern. Sitting in a circle, for example, allows group members to see one another's faces, which tends to increase interaction among them. When people are arranged at long rectangular tables, they tend to interact most with those in direct view and little with those on either side of them.

When meetings involve persons who do not know one another, the facilitator should supply nametags or cards for everyone in the group. A sense of group spirit develops more quickly when people use one another's names as they interact. Allowing members time to introduce themselves is time well spent toward developing a comfortable climate. "Small talk" in groups is not a small matter. Just hearing one another allows the members to make some assumptions that help them to reduce anxiety. An individual's tone of voice, dress, diction, and manner provide valuable clues to his or her character. Often, negative inferences disappear after the other's voice is heard and some information regarding the person's background is gathered.

> *Facilitating is like driving—you've got to pay*
> *attention a lot.*
> —KEVIN ELKENBERRY

Group Facilitation Skills

Nutrition counselors and managers need to assist in group problem solving by developing their roles as expert information disseminators, diagnosticians, team members, empathizers, and group facilitators. Most practitioners eventually need to direct in groups and facilitate interaction among them. Effective facilitation requires training and discipline to stay in the role of guide, monitoring unobtrusively and adding interjections only as needed to maintain group process and functioning, while not actually becoming a participant. Described in the following paragraphs are specific skills that need to be practiced as you train to develop group facilitation skills.[7,22]

Relieving Social Concerns

A tenet of group dynamics suggests that social concerns take precedence over task-related or work-related concerns. In other words, a person's first concern is with being accepted and acknowledged as worthy. If people feel anxiety about being with unknown others or others who may bear them ill will, they generally do not participate. One way in which a facilitator can attend to social concerns is to spend a few minutes at the beginning of each meeting allowing people to interact socially, providing "open-time" to establish or reestablish positive regard for one another. If ill will does exist among some of the participants and the facilitator is aware of it, he or she can attempt to have the members resolve their conflict before the meeting, or, if they are willing, the conflict can be resolved at the meeting. Only after the members have had their social concerns met can they wholeheartedly participate in task concerns.

Tolerating Silence

After facilitators have made opening remarks, have made sure that everyone knows everyone else, have articulated the desire for everyone's participation, and have stated the reasons or purpose for the meeting, they might rephrase the topic in the form of a question and then invite someone to comment. Because members frequently hesitate to express opinions with which their superior might disagree, they often wait to hear the supervisor's opinion first. At times no one may want to initiate discussion and reduce the tension. Silence is likely to occur most during the early stages of an ongoing group. After the group comes to understand that the facilitator, the group's guide or monitor, truly does not intend to dominate, lead, or force opinions, members begin to use the meeting time to interact with one another. For those first few meetings, however, the facilitator should repeat the intention not to participate, should encourage others to participate, and then should just sit patiently. Ordinarily, if the silence is tolerated long enough, someone eventually takes the responsibility for directing the discussion.

Guiding Unobtrusively and Encouraging Interaction

The facilitator guides indirectly, helping the members to relate better to one another and to complete the task. Facilitators ought not to allow themselves to become the focus. The facilitator can encourage interaction among the group members by looking away from speakers in the group as they attempt to harness his or her eyes. Although this behavior may seem rude, the speaker quickly gets the idea and looks to the other group members for feedback and response as the talk continues. The facilitator should resist the temptation to make a reply after others talk, but should instead wait for someone else to reply. If no one else makes a comment, however, the facilitator can ask for reactions. A question such as "What are your reactions to that?" is preferable to a statement such as "My reaction is. . . ."

Because facilitators wish to keep the focus on the group, they should remind group members during the first few minutes of the meeting that their purpose primarily is to get things started and then simply to serve as a guide. This assertion will eventually be tested. Most people have heard the same sentiment expressed by teachers and others and have learned that while some do mean it, the majority are paying it lip service only, want things done their way, and expect ultimately to be followed.

Knowing When and How to Resume Control

Just as a facilitator who rules and dominates in an authoritarian manner can stifle the group's creativity, facilitators who are too timid, uncertain, or frightened and who let the group wander can hinder the group's potential for synergy, that is, for finding superior solutions. Facilitators need to determine whether the group is capable of facilitating for itself. When it is, the facilitator's function is to remain on the sidelines. Only when no competent participant is available to perform the necessary functions does the facilitator become an active member of the group.

Reinforcing the Multisided Nature of Discussion

The facilitator can reinforce the nondogmatic, multisided nature of discussion by phrasing questions so that they are open-ended. Examples are: "How do you feel about that?" "Who in your opinion . . . ?" and "What would be some way to . . . ?" Facilitators need to think before asking questions to avoid closed and leading questions, questions that can be answered by only one or two words, and questions that suggest a limited number of alternative responses.

Exercising Control Over Loquacious Participants

The most common problem that facilitators have is knowing what to say to someone who is overly talkative. There are many appropriate ways of handling this type of participant, and individual facilitators need to decide which techniques they feel most comfortable using, keeping in mind that when they interact with any single member of the group, all other participants experience the interaction vicariously. If the facilitator treats individual participants without respect or humiliates or embarrasses them, all members are affected by the experience.

Several techniques may be effective in dealing with the loquacious participant. The facilitator may interrupt the participant, commenting that the point has been understood, and begin immediately to paraphrase concisely so that the participant knows that he or she has been understood. Although some group members talk excessively because they enjoy talking and because they believe that they are raising their status within the group through the quantity of their interaction, other talkative members often repeat themselves because of insecurity. They are not convinced that they have been understood. Usually, this kind of participant stops talking after being paraphrased. Of course, this process may need to be repeated several times during the course of the discussion.

A second problem arises with the participants who simply enjoy talking and perceive increased status from it. These people do not stop talking after being paraphrased. They may need to be told that short concise statements are easier to follow, that they need to limit the length and number of comments, or that the group is losing the point from their extensive commentary. If that does not work, the facilitator may need to talk with the participant privately. Often, talkative group members are unaware that others are offended by their domination. The facilitator can point out to them that he or she has noticed others stirring and wanting to enter the discussion. It needs to be stressed to these participants that their practicing and learning to be concise allows additional time for others to contribute to the discussion. Establishing additional meeting guidelines on an ad hoc basis can also control "time-wasters." The facilitator, for example, may say, "Because of the brief time remaining, we will no longer be able to permit interruptions."

Encouraging Silent Members

For various reasons, including boredom, indifference, felt superiority, timidity, and insecurity, there are usually some members who refuse to participate. In addition, as mentioned earlier in this section, group members, either client or staff, are almost always multicultural in their background. In some cultures silence from subordinates or people younger than the group's leader is viewed as "respectful." The facilitator's action toward them depends on what is causing them to be silent. The facilitator can arouse interest by asking for their opinions of what a colleague has said. If the silence stems from insecurity, the best method is to reinforce positively each attempt at interjection. A smile, a nod, or a comment of appreciation for any expressed opinion is sufficient. Sometimes silent

Agenda

- ☐ Review / Approve Minutes
- ☐ District Reports
- ☐ Project Updates
  - • Legislative Actions
  - • Community Outreach
  - • Labeling Changes
  - • New RDAs
- ☐ New Business
- ☐ Adjournment

Meetings should have an agenda.

members "shout out" nonverbal signals. An overt frown, nod, and pounding fingers all are signals that should be interpreted as the silent member's willingness to be called on to elaborate; however, if silent members have their heads down and blank facial expressions, it would be a mistake to force them into the discussion.

If the facilitator is confident that the silent members are reserving their comments because of a cultural belief that by doing so they are showing respect, then the topic needs to be handled directly, with the facilitator's reminding them that the reason groups meet, rather than having an individual make the decisions or solve the problems alone, is based on the belief in collaboration as a superior problem-solving technique. For collaboration to occur, everyone's opinions and insights need to be expressed.

Halting Side Conversation

Generally, the facilitator should not embarrass members who are engaged in private conversations by drawing attention to them in the presence of the group. If the side conversation becomes distracting to other members of the group, those engaged in the conversation might be called by name and asked an easy question. For example, one might say, "John, I would be interested in your perspective on this issue," or "John, do you agree?"

Discouraging Wisecracks

If someone in the group disrupts with too much humor or too many wisecracks, the facilitator needs to determine at what point the humor stops being a device to relieve tension in the group and starts to interfere with the group's interests. When facilitators believe that the humor is taking the focus off group issues and onto the joker, they need to interrupt, preferably smiling, with a comment such as "Now let's get back to business." If the comment needs to be made a second time, intense eye contact with the joker and no smile as the same remark is repeated usually halts the disruption.

Helping the Group Stay on Topic

When the group itself seems unable to stick to the agenda and wanders, a device underused by facilitators is a flip chart to jot down points that have been agreed on as a way to chart the group's progress. With a minimum of interaction, the facilitator can prod the group on by simply summarizing and writing down the points. Generally, the group's reaction is to go on to the next item on the agenda.

Avoiding Acknowledgment of the Facilitator's Preferences

Facilitators hinder the group when they praise the ideas they like and belittle those they dislike. It is particularly important that they avoid making comments that may be taken as disapproval, condescension, sarcasm, personal cross-examination, or self-approval. Once the group members know the facilitator's preferences, they will tend to incorporate these preferences in their own comments. Because facilitators are in a position to reward or punish attendees, the group members quickly learn that if what supervisors want is to be followed and not disagreed with, that is how they will behave toward them.

Facilitator and Participant Functions

In addition to the specific skills required of facilitators, there are numerous group skills that both participants and facilitators should possess. There is a mistaken notion that it is the facilitator's responsibility alone to see that the group's tasks are accomplished and that a healthy group spirit is maintained. In reality, these responsibilities belong to anyone who has the training and insight to diagnose the group's weaknesses and who has the skills to correct them. Because most people are used to being "led" in groups, the facilitator may need to reinforce verbally the functions that all participants are expected to perform. The following paragraphs describe some of these skills and functions that both facilitators and participants have a mutual obligation to develop in themselves.

Initiating

Groups need members to propose new ideas, goals, and procedures. Individual members are expected to accept the responsibility of initiating. Any member who has an insight into what should be initiated and waits for someone else to do it is ignoring an obligation. The facilitator might also remind participants of the spate of behavioral literature that verifies the correlations between employee–participant involvement and superior decisions.

Information and Opinion Seeking

Everyone shares the responsibility of seeking information and opinions. You do not need to have vast knowledge of the topic being discussed to be a valuable member. Asking the right questions and seeking information from others in the group who have knowledge are valuable functions.

Clarifying

Clarifying what others have said by adding examples, illustrations, or explanations is a major contribution. People are not all on the same wavelength. Because of background, cultural group, life experiences, education, natural intelligence, and environment, some people tend to understand one another more easily than do others. Two people who have grown up under similar conditions, for example, have an easier time communicating than two people from different backgrounds. People who understand what someone else in the group is struggling to make clear and add examples and explanations to clarify the thoughts for the others have made significant contributions. Simply nodding in agreement and saying nothing is a disservice to the others.

Coordinating

Another function related to clarifying is coordinating relationships among facts, ideas, and suggestions. If one member has the insight to understand how the ideas and activities of two or more group members are related and how they can be coordinated, that member serves a valuable function in expressing this relationship to the others.

Orienting

"Orienting" is a term given to the function of processing for the group the pattern of its interaction and progress. The orienter clarifies the group's purpose or goal, defines the position of the group, and summarizes or suggests the direction of the discussion. Orienting by providing frequent internal summaries, for example, allows the group an opportunity to verify whether everyone is understanding the direction in which the group is going and provides those who disagree or who have misunderstood with the opportunity to speak.

Supporting

Perhaps the least understood and most valuable function a person can perform for a group is being a supporter. Supporters are those who praise, agree, indicate warmth and solidarity, and verbally indicate to the others that they are in agreement with what is being proposed. It is a valuable function because without verbal support from others, good ideas and suggestions are often disregarded. If one person expresses an idea that the majority dislikes and that no one supports, the idea is quickly dismissed. Generally, if only one person supports the idea, the group will seriously consider the proposal. Frequently, a minority opinion can gain majority support because a single supporter agrees, causing the group to consider seriously the possible merits of the proposal. Support can be given by briefly remarking, "I agree," "Well said," "I wish I had said that," or "Those are my sentiments, too." Generally, one person alone cannot influence a group: one person with a supporter, however, has an excellent chance of doing so.[21]

Harmonizing

Harmonizing is also a valuable contribution to the group. It includes mediating differences between others, reconciling disagreement, and bringing about collaboration from conflict. It is common for group members to sit silently as they hear the valid arguments on both sides of an issue. One of the ways in which discussion differs from debate, however, is that discussion assumes that most issues are multisided, whereas debate tends to lend itself to two-sided issues only. The group member who verbally reinforces the positive aspects of the various factions and helps to suggest new and alternative solutions that include the best points of all sides is harmonizing.

Tension Relieving

Conflict, stress, and tension in groups are inevitable. When the stress or the tension mounts, it can enhance the conflict and the disagreement. People who can find humor in the situation, reduce the formality or status differences among group members, and relax the others are called tension relievers. A problem can occur when the tension reliever seeks recognition for himself or herself and continues to joke, drawing the attention away from the issues. Relieving tension is valuable up to a point, after which it can be disruptive.

Gatekeeping

The final function in this discussion is gatekeeping. In gatekeeping, facilitators or participants notice which members have been sending out signals that they want to speak but have not had the courage or opportunity to enter the discussion. Gatekeeping ensures that all have an equal chance to be heard. As pointed out in the discussion of the facilitator's functions, there is a difference between people who are nonverbally signaling that they have strong feelings—by raising their eyebrows, tapping loudly, or grunting—and people who are silent. Group members become uncomfortable when they sense that other members might force them to talk. All members share the responsibility to protect others from being coerced into sharing opinions. Gatekeepers tend to say things such as "You look like you have strong feelings," or "I can tell by your face that you disapprove." Such comments are generally all the prodding the silent participant needs to enter the discussion.

Too often individuals believe that in the ideal group, a single leader is responsible for each of the functions just discussed. In fact, all members—participants as well as facilitators—are responsible, and they need to be alert to perform as many of the functions as they see a need for. Some people may be natural harmonizers or natural orienters or may be able to effortlessly perform some other valuable function. However, if the group needs a gate-keeper and none is present, the natural harmonizer who sees the need must exercise the gatekeeping function. One of the ways in which people familiar with group dynamics and with the skills needed to enhance the working of groups can detect members who have had training in the same area is by their willingness to act on their insight to correct a weakness in the group. The mind operates several times faster than the speed of human speech. While members of the group are talking, other sophisticated group members need to be reflecting on the dynamics of the group and on the needs at the moment. This process leads to an understanding of which functions need to be performed to help the group accomplish its task and maintain its healthy spirit.[22–25]

PARADOX OF GROUP DYNAMICS

There is a paradox inherent in groups. They possess the potential, on the one hand, to stimulate creative thinking and to promote a decision or solution that is superior to what any individual working alone could accomplish. On the other hand, groups possess the potential to stifle creative thinking and thus promote a quality of outcome inferior to what individuals working alone might accomplish. Ordinarily, no one person is solely respon-sible for what happens in any given session; however, whether a group becomes a force to promote creative thinking and problem solving or a force that inhibits these functions depends primarily on the skills of its leader and, to a lesser degree, on the skills of the par-ticipants. Specific behavior patterns help a group to function effectively; others hinder the progress. Knowing how to facilitate positive behavior in groups and how to inhibit the negative behavior is an asset to dietetics practitioners.

SYNERGY

Professionals need to appreciate "group process" and to discover what can be done to stimulate their staff or client groups so that they become a creative force that promotes synergy. Synergy refers to the phenomenon in which the group's product (i.e., conclu-sion, solution, or decision) is qualitatively or quantitatively superior to what the most resourceful individual within the group could have produced by working alone.[22] Today, much is understood about the phenomenon; however, it has not yet filtered into manage-ment practice. Although greatly influenced by the style of their facilitators, all groups pos-sess the potential to be either a force for creative, innovative thinking or a force that works to preserve the status quo and stifle new ideas.[22] The purpose of this section is to offer suggestions on how to promote the former. The major variables that affect the group's potential for synergy are the availability of a single expert within the group, the hetero-geneity or homogeneity of the group, and the existence of training of the group and its facilitator in the consensus-seeking process.

Facilitators should begin each meeting by stating their desire to promote a climate of acceptance and freedom of expression. Hearing the facilitator express this desire helps to set a group "norm" whereby everyone has a responsibility to participate. A norm is an unwritten rule to which the group adheres. Members pick up the code of appropriate behavior by noticing what the facilitator reinforces positively, ignores, tolerates, or rejects. Eventually, the facilitator's expressions of his or her desire for everyone to participate and the rights of each member to express subjective opinions without being abused by others will be tested. It is not enough to articulate norms; they must be enforced. If people are abused by others, told to be silent, embarrassed, humiliated, or insulted, for example, and the facilitator does not intervene to protect them, his or her articulated norm will be discounted and the actual behavior that has been tolerated will be considered the "real" norm. For that reason, it is critical that group facilitators realize the importance of their function to stimulate group interaction while protecting group members from being verbally abused or stifled. Realizing that synergy is most likely to occur in groups in which people can react authentically and are free to challenge the facilitator and the other participants, the health care professional needs to convince the group members that they need to listen and respond honestly to one another's ideas.

As a rule, if a single expert is available and the rest of the group members are relatively ignorant of the matter being discussed, the expert should make the decision. In practice, however, there is usually no single expert available, and some group members are more informed than others, with a wide range of opinions being represented in the group. Under these conditions, the potential for synergy exists.

The variable of a heterogeneous versus homogeneous group of participants is more complicated. When group members are untrained in the *consensus-seeking process* and form a homogeneous group, they have less conflict and generally produce superior decisions to those produced by an untrained heterogeneous group. It is understandable that people who are similar in age, background, culture, life experiences, values, and the like have an easier time agreeing than with those with whom they have little in common.[26]

The heterogeneous group that is untrained is likely to respond in one of the following ways. If the members of the group do not know one another, they will probably remain silent. Most people become anxious in the presence of strangers, whose response to them is unpredictable. Rather than risk sharing a contrary opinion and being insulted, humiliated, or embarrassed, they tend to go along with the opinions expressed by other members of the group. Decisions in such groups may appear to be produced by consensus, because there is no apparent disagreement, but in fact consensus may not be present. Because there is no group commitment and cohesion, conflict presents a threat to the group's interpersonal structure. Members try to smooth conflicts rather than resolve them. When disagreement arises, the members make quick compromises to get along. They resort to conflict-reducing techniques, such as majority rule and trade-offs. The quality of decisions made in these groups tends to be low.

The other possibility is that a great deal of verbal conflict will occur among the untrained members in a heterogeneous group, with each member insisting on his or her own point of view, so that the group never arrives at a decision with which everyone can be satisfied. This tends to occur most often in ad hoc groups with high-power personalities.

The variable of training in the consensus-seeking process is the most critical of all for producing synergy. In studies conducted by Dr. Jay Hall, a social scientist, trained and untrained groups were measured; both types of groups produced synergy. In the trained groups, however, synergy occurred 75% of the time, whereas in the untrained groups, synergy occurred only 25% of the time.[26] The implications are obvious: group leaders, facilitators, managers, supervisors, and all those who try to work with others in a participative manner need to understand the principles of training and instruct their groups in the process. A second conclusion was that under conditions of training, heterogeneous groups performed better than homogeneous groups. In fact, the broader the range of opinions presented, the better are the group's chances of arriving at superior decisions. The implication here is that a group of "lemons," group members who fight and cannot agree, can be turned into lemonade, if the facilitator trains them in the consensus-seeking process.

Guidelines for Seeking Consensus

The training required to move a group from 25% to 75% efficiency in achieving consensus is based on a set of guidelines for group behavior; it is simple and not time-consuming. Professionals who decide to use this method with staff need to understand, however, that it may take several weeks of regularly reminding the group of the guidelines and interrupting each time the guidelines are not followed, before the process becomes natural to the group. The following are guidelines for achieving consensus in groups:

1. All group members have the responsibility and obligation to share opinions.
2. After group members have expressed opinions on a particular issue, they have the right to ask others to paraphrase these comments to their satisfaction.
3. After being paraphrased, they may not bring up their perspective again unless asked to do so by another group member. Insisting on one's own point of view or blocking discussion is not acceptable.
4. Everyone has the responsibility to understand the arguments and opinions of the other members and may ask questions for clarification.
5. After all perspectives are understood, the group needs to arrive at a solution or decision that can satisfy everyone. In accomplishing this task, the group may not immediately resort to the stress-reducing techniques of majority rule, trade-offs, averaging, coin-flipping, and bargaining.
6. Differences of opinion should be viewed as natural and expected.

Members need to be encouraged to seek out the perspectives of others so that everyone is involved in the decision process. Disagreements can help the group's decision because with a wider range of information and opinions, there is a greater chance that the group will develop superior solutions. Frequently, when the group members suspend their own judgment, new solutions emerge that no single individual would have been able to develop alone. These solutions tend to incorporate the best points of all views—of both the majority and the minority. Such solutions tend to be synergistic. At times, however, after considerable discussion, no new solution emerges. In these instances, alternative problem-solving techniques can be applied.[22,26]

Alternative Problem-Solving Techniques

When a group is unable to agree on a solution, several other methods—each with its advantages and disadvantages—can be used. One method is for the leader to make the decision. The advantage is that the decision is arrived at quickly; the disadvantage is that those who dislike it may not support it. Leaders may feel that they have "won," but others who feel that they have "lost" may attempt to subvert the decision or solution. Another possibility is for some members to accommodate others by no longer insisting on their preferred solution. This method immediately relieves the group of conflict, but those who accommodated may later resent having done so and may not feel obliged to uphold the solution. Perhaps the most common method is compromise, each side giving in a little until both can agree. The problem with compromise is that often what is given up is sought back eventually. Compromise solutions tend to be short-lived. Other conflict-reducing techniques such as majority rule, trade-offs, and coin-flipping also tend to be short-lived because the members who gave up something to satisfy the immediate need for a solution feel no obligation to support the solution.

GROUP PARTICIPATION IN DECISION MAKING

There are both advantages and disadvantages to participative decision making. The practitioner needs to be aware of them to decide, on a contingency basis, when this method is appropriate.

Advantages

1. When managers meet their team members one at a time, problems of communication and perceptual distortion may occur. Each time the manager discusses the issues on a one-to-one basis, the superior's manner and language vary, with each subordinate asking questions from a different perspective. Meeting together to discuss such matters as operational activities and politics provides an opportunity for everyone to hear the same descriptions at the same time and to ask questions, which may clarify perceptions, so that everyone shares a common understanding.
2. Interpersonal relationship problems can be resolved, particularly when the staff is aware of the need for teamwork.
3. Motivation can be enhanced, since the individuals involved in the decision may become more committed to it and may better understand how it is to be carried out. Resistance to change is reduced when individuals consider the alternative actions together and decide together on the goals and objectives for achieving change. They experience a greater commitment to changes that they themselves have either initiated or participated in developing.
4. The synergy of problem solving can occur, allowing the group to arrive at solutions that are qualitatively superior to any that a single individual could arrive at alone.

Disadvantages

1. Group participation in decision making can be time consuming; however, the time spent in goal setting, problem definition, and planning can result in more rapid implementation of the solution and less resistance to change.
2. Cohesive groups can become autonomous and work against management's preferences.
3. Groups can sometimes become a way for everyone to escape the responsibility for taking action, since each person may assume that someone else is ultimately responsible.

4. The goals and interests of employees and those of management may not be compatible.

5. Employees may not be qualified to participate. Participation requires not only a desire to be involved, but also knowledge or experience in the problem area, as well as an ability to communicate insights, reactions, and desires. Not everyone possesses these qualities and skills to the same degree, and some who have the desire, but not the ability, may need to be trained.

6. People whose ideas are continuously rejected can become alienated.

7. Managers may use groups as a way to manipulate employees into making the decision that they, the managers, have already decided on.

8. Work group involvement may raise expectations among employees that cannot always be met or that the manager did not intend; once started, employees may want to be included in all decision making, whether or not their participation is appropriate.

9. The hazards of "group-think" refer to the phenomenon of a group stifling individual creativity to preserve the status quo. It is the mode of thinking that persons engage in when seeking concurrences becomes more important in a cohesive group than a realistic appraisal of the alternative courses of action. The symptoms of group-think arise when group members avoid being too harsh in their judgments of their leaders' or their colleagues' ideas for the sake of preserving harmony. All members are amiable and seek complete concurrence on every important issue to avoid conflict that might spoil the cozy, group atmosphere.[22,26]

Dr. Irving Janis, social psychologist and pioneer researcher in this area, is the leading expert on the group-think phenomenon. Below are some of the remedies he suggests to prevent its occurrence. Health care professionals need to consider ways of adapting these practices to their own style of group facilitation with staff.[27]

1. At each meeting, the facilitator should verbalize the desire that all participants assume the role of "critical evaluator." Members need to be encouraged to look for the weaknesses in one another's arguments. The facilitator's acceptance of criticism from others is critical if the others are to continue the practice with them and with one another.

2. The facilitator should adopt from the start an impartial stance rather than stating preferences and expectations. Such a stance encourages open inquiry and impartial probing of a wide range of policy alternatives.

3. The organization should routinely or periodically set up several alternative policy planning and evaluation groups to work on the same policy question, with each group deliberating under a different leader. This practice can prevent the insulation of an in-group.

4. Before reaching a final consensus, the group members should discuss the issues with qualified associates who are not part of the decision-making group and should then report back to the others the results of their informal surveys.

5. The group should invite one or more outside experts to some meetings on a staggered basis and encourage the experts to challenge the views of the dominant group members.

6. At every meeting of the group, whenever the agenda calls for an evaluation of policy alternatives, at least one member should be assigned to play the "devil's advocate," challenging the testimony of those who advocate the majority position.

7. After reaching a preliminary consensus about what seems to be the best policy, the group should hold a "second-chance" meeting, during which members express all their residual doubts as vividly as they can. This meeting gives everyone a last opportunity to rethink the entire issue before making a definitive choice.[28–31]

This chapter has stressed the necessity for practitioners to study group process and internalize the behaviors needed to participate in, facilitate, and model group interaction skills. With proper facilitation, groups can stimulate solutions and insights the individual might not experience otherwise. Once health care professionals develop the skills needed to diagnose group needs and the ability to correct them by focusing on the group's resources, they can function as change agents and as communication models for the other group members, while at the same time becoming more effective when placed in a management position.

CASE STUDY

Betty Smith, RD, CDE, is planning a series of group meetings for her clients who are parents of children who have been recently diagnosed with type 1 diabetes mellitus. Her concern today is planning for optimum group participation in the first session, which will be 1 hour long. She also wants to be sure to meet the needs of the group so that they will return for future sessions.

1. What suggestions do you have for the first session?
2. State a common education goal applicable to this group.
3. Document the method of outcome assessment for the effectiveness of the education session.
4. How should Betty set up the meeting room?
5. What can she do to introduce group members?
6. What should Betty do to indicate her desire for group participation?
7. How may she implement "group facilitation skills?"

CASE STUDY

Doris Johnson, RD, has worked for the past 5 years in a school lunch program at an elementary school. In the past year, there has been 35% turnover of employees. Although all new employees have received training, Doris has noticed that sanitation has slipped considerably. It is not as high a level as in the past.

Doris has decided to bring together a group of employees at the end of the lunch service for a discussion of the problem. About 10 employees will be present.

1. How should Doris introduce the problem?
2. What role should Doris take in the discussion?
3. What should she do to facilitate discussion?
4. How would Doris go about promoting a synergistic solution?
5. How should Doris set up the meeting room?

REVIEW AND DISCUSSION QUESTIONS

1. What is the role of the team leader?
2. What distinguishes autocratic from participative leadership?
3. Why is a team approach superior?
4. How should a facilitator halt a side conversation?
5. Discuss the significance of the informal work group.
6. What is synergy and how can it be stimulated in groups?
7. Discuss several of the participant functions and how they generally either aid in promoting the group's effectiveness or assist in accomplishing the group's task.
8. Discuss two suggestions for promoting group change.

SUGGESTED ACTIVITIES

1. In groups of three, discuss the best small group experiences you have ever had. What occurred that qualifies them as superior? Describe specific behaviors of both the group's leader or facilitator and the participants that seem to have made a difference. Time should be allotted for each group to share its insights with the others.
2. In groups of three, plan to meet in three different settings over the next 2 days, with different seating, room size, lighting, and the like. Report your observations on the effects of the environment to the entire class. Notice whether different groups had simpler reactions and were influenced by the same factors. A simpler variation on this activity would be to hold a discussion for 10 minutes with the group arranged in a circle and then to continue the discussion with the group sitting in a straight row.
3. Make a list of at least three small groups in which you have been active, and describe the functions you performed in each. Compare your perceptions of yourself as a contributing group member with the perceptions that your friends or classmates had of you. Do you notice that you performed different functions in different groups? Do some functions overlap from group to group? Are your classmates in agreement with you regarding your functions within their group?
4. Thinking back to some recent experiences in group discussions, complete each of the following statements:
   A. "My strengths as a group participant are. . . ."
   B. "My strengths as a group facilitator are. . . ."
   C. "What is keeping me from being more effective both as a participant and facilitator is. . . ."
   D. "My plans for improvement are. . . ."
5. How do you determine whether needed leadership and facilitative services are being provided during a discussion? Compare your observations with those of your classmates.
6. Write a question or description of a food or nutrition problem or issue, preferably from your own personal or professional experience, for which you do not have a solution. Present it to a small group and facilitate their discussion. Possible questions might include "What populations need to take vitamin supplements?" "What are the best food

choices when eating at a fast food outlet?" and "What recommendations should one give to someone who desires to reduce calories or exercise more?"

7. Group together four to five people who have a common problem such as wanting (1) to lose weight, (2) to start eating breakfast, (3) to control excess consumption of snacks, (4) to select nutritious meals, (5) to increase the fiber content of their diets, or (6) to exercise more often. State the problem, and have the group attempt to solve it.

WEB SITES

CHANGE IN TEAMS AND GROUPS

http://www.managaementhelp.org/grp_skll/teams/teams.htm
http://www.richmond.edu/~dforsyth/gd

COHESIVENESS IN GROUPS

http://www.accel-team.com/work_groups/informal_grps_04.html
http://www.brookes.ac.uk/services/ocsd/2_learntch/small-group/sgt1.7.html
http://interzone.com/~cheung/SUM.dir/humcohesive.html
http://www.mapnp.org/library/grp_skll/theory/theory.htm
http://sgr.sagepub.com/cgi/content/abstract/21/2/234

TEAM MANAGEMENT

http://www.leadingteams.org/use/consultants.htm
http://www.tms.com.au/

SELF-MANAGEMENT IN TEAMS

http://www.russellconsultinginc.com/docs/white/tdosmwt.html

DEVELOPING GROUP LEADERSHIP SKILLS

http://adrenaline.ucsd.edu/onr/disaster/summary.htm/   Consensus in groups
http://www.adv-leadership-grp.com/articles/motivate.htm
http://crs.uvm.edu/gopher/nerl/group/a/h.html/   Developing group facilitator skills
http://www.healthcaredynamics.com/hcd-pas.html/   Group dynamics in healthcare
http://www.powerful2lead.com

REFERENCES

1. Commission on Accreditation for Dietetics Education. Eligibility Requirements and Accreditation Standards. Chicago: American Dietetic Association, 2006.
2. Walker W, Brokaw L. Becoming Aware. Dubuque, IA: Kendall/Hunt, 2004.
3. U.S. Department of Health and Human Services. Healthy People 2010. McLean, VA, International Medical Publishing, 2001:2801.
4. Townsend M, Johns M, Shilts M, et al. Evaluation of a USDA education program for low-income youth. J Nutr Educ Behav 2006;38:30–41.

5. Dutta-Bergman M. The relation between health-orientation, provider-patient communication, and satisfaction. Health Commun 2005;18:291–303.

6. Dysart-Gale D. Communication models, professionalization, and the work of medical interpreters. Health Commun 2005;17:91–103.

7. Goldman, M. Facile facilitation. Leadership Excellence 2006;6:17–18.

8. Goldsmith M, Morgan H. Team building or time wasting. Leadership Excellence 2006;4:3–5.

9. Rider E, Keefer C. Communication skills competencies: definitions and a teaching toolbox. Med Educ 2006;40:624–629.

10. Bones C. Group-think doesn't unite, it divides. Hum Resources 2005;6:24–26.

11. Robbins S, Judge T. Organizational Behavior. 12th Ed. Upper Saddle River, NJ: Prentice-Hall, 2007.

12. Robbins S, Coulter M. Management. Upper Saddle River, NJ: Prentice-Hall, 2007.

13. Burtis J, Turman P. Group Communication Pitfalls. Thousand Oaks, CA: Sage, 2006.

14. Poole M, Hollingshead A. Theories of Small Groups, Thousand Oaks, CA: Sage, 2005.

15. Keyton J. Communicating in Groups. New York, NY: Oxford University Press, 2005.

16. Kewin K. Field Theory in Social Science. New York: Harper and Row, 1994.

17. Kotter J. Leading changes: why transformation efforts fail. Harv Bus Rev 1995;59–67.

18. Farias G, Johnson H. Organizational development and change management. Joint Appl Behav Sci 2000;376–379.

19. Weber V, Joshi M. Effecting and leading change in health care organizations. Joint Comm J Qual Improv 2000;26:388–399.

20. Horak B. Dealing with human factors and managing change in knowledge management. Top Health Manage 2001;21:8–18.

21. Wilson G. Groups in Context. Dubuque, IA: McGraw-Hill, 2005.

22. Adams K, Galanes G. Communicating in Groups. Dubuque, IA: McGraw-Hill, 2006.

23. Fujishin R. Creating Effective Groups. San Francisco: Acada Books, 2001.

24. Galanes G, Adams K, Brilhart J. Effective Group Discussion. Dubuque, IA: McGraw-Hill, 2003.

25. Young K, Wood J, Phillips G, et al. Group Discussion. Prospect Heights, IL: Waveland Press, 2001.

26. Hall J. Decisions, decisions, decisions. Psychol Today 1971;6:61.

27. Janis I. Groupthink. Psychol Today 1971;6:43.

28. Druskat V, Wolff S. Building the emotional intelligence of groups. Harv Bus Rev 2001;79: 80–98.

29. Hinojosa J, Bedell G. Team collaboration. Q Health Res 2001;11:206–211.

30. Soloman C. Team spirit. Health Facil Manage 2001;14;41–59.

31. Bliese P, Britt T. Social support, group consensus and stressor-strain relationships. J Organ Behav Special Issue 2001;22:425–437.

Creating and Delivering Effective Oral Presentations and Workshops

OBJECTIVES

- Describe the process of presentation preparation.
- List the three components of a presentation and their content.
- Discuss effective speaker delivery techniques.
- Identify challenges and postulate ideas to overcome barriers.
- Outline special issues when presentations involve media professionals.
- Deliver a presentation to others and complete a postpresentation critique.

"When you have nothing to say, say nothing ..."

—CHARLES CALEB COLTON

Food and nutrition experts need to be good communicators. The Commission on Accreditation for Dietetics Education of the American Dietetic Association includes oral communication as a knowledge, skill, and competency requirement for professional practice.[1] Most practitioners will be required to give an oral presentation to share their expertise during their careers.[2–5] The presentation skills discussed in this chapter apply to a wide variety of professional venues involving students, clients, peers, and employees in both small and large group settings. As is true for so many of the other skills discussed in this book, the confidence needed to deliver a message orally and articulately cannot be achieved by reading alone. Prepare to digest the information and then have the courage to try by applying the techniques in real situations. Mastering the ability to communicate a message to an audience is an acquired skill. The goal of an effective message is to produce a desired outcome such as changing behavior, understanding new information, appreciating new trends, or developing new skills.

There is a large body of literature on the general subject of oral communication, presentation planning, and public speaking.[6–9] The purpose of this chapter is to provide information on how to create and deliver effective focused oral presentations and workshops. This process includes preparation, organization, delivery, and evaluation. Other chapters in this book cover planning the learning process (Chapters 11 and 12) and creating audiovisuals (Chapter 15), which are necessary complementary skills for effective oral communication.

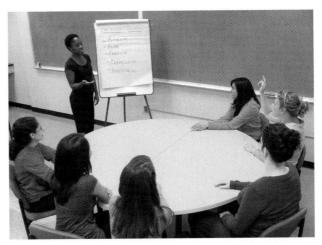

In discussing emotional eating, the professional enhances her presentation with visuals.

PREPARATION OF AN EFFECTIVE PRESENTATION

The key to an effective oral presentation is preparation. The speaker must assess the needs of the planned presentation through a series of audience, program, and content analysis activities. This philosophy incorporates both an inside and an outside viewpoint of audience and speaker goals. The program planner can often provide input supplemented by the presenter's own preparation analysis.[6,8]

Audience Analysis

The first step is an audience analysis. This step is necessary if the speaker is to maintain the delicate balance between what the audience expects to learn and what the presenter wants them to learn. Many experts use the acronym WIIFM, or "What's in it for me?" Collect basic information about the planned audience, such as age, gender, educational level or occupation, years of experience, and knowledge of the topic. What is the audience's goal in attending the presentation? Are individuals volunteering to attend or is this a mandatory training session? What is their perceived value of the sessions? Did they pay to come and listen or is this a free event? The presentation will be more successful and focused if many of the audience's goals and expectations are incorporated in the program.[7,10]

Program Analysis

The second step is program analysis. The speaker needs to know the setting and overall structure of the program. Will there be only one presenter or multiple speakers? If one is the sole presenter, there may be more flexibility regarding content and delivery style. If the presentation is part of a larger program, find out which topics and speakers both precede and follow your presentation. Ask for the learning objectives and planned content of the entire program as well as other speakers' presentations to ensure that you complement, rather than duplicate, that information.

For either program situation, consider the position of the presentation in relationship to scheduled meal and refreshment breaks. Assess what instructional media are available for use. Ask if handouts are expected and, if they are, obtain submission deadlines and quantity required, and find out who is responsible for providing them to the audience. Some programs require that handouts be provided in advance so they can be incorporated into a packet given at the time of registration. Others may assume they will be distributed on the day of the presentation. Determine time constraints. Evaluate the allotment of presentation time in relation to the time required for audience questions. Collect information on the physical layout and location of the venue. Will there be a podium and microphone? Where do the presenters sit while other speakers present? How will the room be set up? Will the audience be seated in chairs or at tables? What will be the potential distractions? Can audience members enter and leave the room? Will they be eating lunch or drinking beverages after a refreshment break? Discuss the expectations of the sponsoring organization and the presenter's role in the overall program. The goal is to anticipate all program setting issues that may be present as part of your preparation so you can be ready to address their effect.[8,11]

Content Analysis

The third step is content analysis. The key to holding the attention of an audience, particularly an audience with limited time to absorb the speaker's ideas, is to be coherent and to communicate simply. Otherwise, listeners' minds will wander. The secret to brevity and simplicity is to know one's objectives before planning the talk. The content of the presentation needs to match the learning objectives. What does the speaker want to accomplish? What changes are intended in the knowledge, attitude, or behavior of the audience? Will they perform a task or recall some information? A common mistake made among untrained presenters is to attempt to cover too much in the time allotted. Inexperienced speakers often feel the need to parade their expertise and overload the audience with information. For example, the content of a presentation on food safety should vary depending on whether it is given to seasoned employees, or new employees, or a combination of the two groups.

In contrast to reading, which allows a person to go back to reconsider an idea, listening requires ongoing concentration. When the brain begins to feel overloaded and saturation sets in, it protects itself by shutting down or wandering elsewhere. You have probably had the experience of pretending to be listening to an overly meticulous speaker while your mind was elsewhere, having lost interest in the speaker's message. The content of oral presentations needs to be limited to a few major points, generally formatted as three to five learning objectives. The listener can absorb focused content particularly when it is reinforced through details, examples, and a variety of media. Too much information and too many different points defeat the purpose. When listeners know where the presentation is going and are able to follow the presenter's reasoning, they are much more likely to give their full attention. They are more likely to grasp examples and internalize them with greater ease.[12–14]

COMPONENTS OF AN EFFECTIVE PRESENTATION

The three main organizational components of a presentation are the introduction, body, and summary. Most people are not aware that the organization of a presentation is critical to the response of the audience. Although an audiences might retain about the same amount of information after hearing an organized or a disorganized presentation, only attendees at the organized presentation would consider its message seriously or possibly change their attitude toward the subject matter. An audience that hears an organized speaker who gives the audience a sense that he or she knows exactly where the talk is going by structuring the talk with a defined beginning, middle, and end, is more likely to infer that the speaker is competent in the area. Many brilliant and qualified professionals are not taken seriously when giving presentations because they sound too "loose," too unprepared, or too disorganized.[15–17]

Title and Speaker Introduction

Two important pieces precede the presentation itself: the creation of the presentation title and format of the speaker introduction. The title, as the initial impression, sets the stage by providing an interest level to the audience of the presentation. The title should be engaging but informative. It should prompt a degree of curiosity without deterring from the actual purpose of the presentation. The program organizer may suggest a title early in the process. The presenter should strive to have input into the final decision as a method of ensuring an initial energy level of audience expectation. For example, compare the following title options: "Diabetic Management" and "Innovative Methods to Improve Diabetic Management." The audience anticipates the active learning setting that the second option suggests.[11]

The introduction of the speaker should provide the information necessary for the audience to establish his or her credibility with the subject matter in a concise manner. The goal is to highlight only the pertinent information relevant to the audience rather than share the speaker's entire life history. The speaker introduction is most effective when it weaves professional information with a personal touch to connect the audience with the speaker. The speaker should provide a brief written introduction to the presenter to help guide his or her comments and link the content to the audience's recognition of the speaker's professional expertise. For example, the introduction could begin with pertinent educational and work experience. The introduction could continue with a suggested phrase such as ". . . You may have read Mary's current article on this subject in the June issue of the *Journal of the American Dietetic Association* . . ." or ". . . You will be interested to know Mary engages in the physical activity philosophy she will share today by being an avid walker herself. . . ."

SELF-ASSESSMENT

How would you be introduced if you were asked to give a talk on nutrition? Write out an introduction for yourself.

Each of the three main organizational components of the actual presentation serves a specific function. The introduction begins the presentation by providing basic information to create interest. The body presents the actual data, details, and substance of the topic. The summary concludes the presentation and provides a take-home message for the audience. Generally, the introduction and summary sections should each take about 5 to 10 minutes of presentation time. The body should comprise the remainder of allotted time to cover the material while allowing for audience questions after the summary.[8,11,13] A detailed discussion of each component follows.

Introduction

The introduction serves as a transition to the body of the talk. The introduction content describes to audience members how the topic relates specifically to their needs. Start with an opening sentence or two that will set the stage for the general purpose of the presentation and gain listeners' attention. Follow with additional information to maintain the audience's interest, providing data to support the topic or briefly describing the scope of the problem. This information heightens listeners' perception of the value of the presentation to them personally. Finally, the introduction outlines the specific learning objectives.

The objectives direct the listeners to the body of information that will follow. The speaker should engage the audience by "promising" a specific outcome (i.e., what listeners will know) at the end of the presentation. This may include ways to better control their health, provide more nutritious meals to their families, be more secure, be in a position in which others think better of them or respect them more, think more of themselves, or feel they have the knowledge to develop and apply new skills in their job. The learning objectives prepare the audience to be attentive to the forthcoming message. Not every human need can

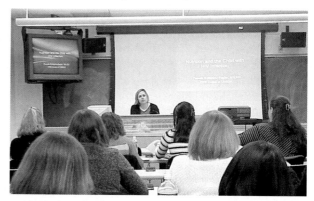

A presenter should be familiar with the site and equipment.

be related to every topic, but as many as possible and as appropriate should be incorporated during the introduction.

An opening statement to consumers who come for a free presentation on the topic of heart disease might be: "You are here today to learn more about heart disease and how to make changes in your eating lifestyle to reduce your risk." This statement will start the connection. Brief statistics could then follow, showing the number of heart disease deaths that occurred within the last year that were diet-related. The learning objectives continue the introduction by previewing the information in the body of the presentation. "Today I intend to discuss three specific points. First, we will examine the relationship of diet to heart disease. Second, I will discuss how to read food labels for the fat and cholesterol content of foods, and finally, I will provide guidelines on how to apply your new nutrition heart-savvy knowledge when eating out."

Not only does the introduction help the audience to listen to the talk with an expectation of what is to come, but the organization itself adds to the "halo effect" and increases the audience's perceptions of the speaker's credibility. The speaker should return to the learning objectives within the body of the presentation, if possible, to remind audience members of how the listening process is fulfilling their own needs.

Body

The body of the presentation expands the points mentioned in the introduction by providing the actual information and data. Presenters need to have a rationale for the way they decide to organize this major section to achieve the learning objectives. The body of the presentation also should ensure that audience members fully understand the content message, believe the speaker, and are comfortable enough with the speaker to share their objections in the event that they are confused or wish to challenge the presenter. Audience members expect to be able to do something differently after a presentation. Examples are to start reading food labels, to try a new recipe, to purchase a different food at the store, to eat breakfast, or to change the way they train other employees.

The speaker needs to construct the message clearly and concisely by presenting the information in a logical order. The content level is critical. It is necessary to direct the level of information from the baseline knowledge of the audience to a higher level that can be accomplished within the time allotted. This can be challenging when the audience has various levels of knowledge and expertise. The audience's understanding is enhanced by designing and incorporating any or all of the following: visual aids, handouts, and participative experiences that may cover a wider scope of content than is covered in the presentation time. For example, a reference or simple handout of the principles of a heart-healthy diet that will not be discussed in depth during the talk may be given in addition to a specific handout focusing on the heart-healthy fats covered in depth during the body of the talk. In this way, the speaker meets the needs of both the audience members who need more information on the basic concept and those with advanced knowledge.

The presenter increases validity of the content and speaker credibility when he or she provides references, documentation, and sources along with the information presented. Finally, the speaker needs to develop a rapport with the audience during the body of the presentation by pacing the information through the presentation. Audience members should feel confident about the information presented and ask questions at the end of the presentation. If the speaker moves too quickly from one point to another, audience confusion and frustration may result. The breadth and depth of the content should match the time allowed. It is the responsibility of the speaker to end the presentation at the specified time with enough time for questions. It is unfair to both the audience and the next speaker to take more time than planned due to poor organization or preparation.[8,11,13]

Summary

The summary and conclusion signal the audience that the presentation is "winding down" and about to end. This transition needs to be gradual and smooth. When possible, review the initial learning objectives to remind the audience they have participated in the achieving the overall goals of the presentation.

Concluding remarks such as "That's all folks," "Thank you for your attention," or "Any questions?" are unprofessional and sound haphazard. Remember that the speaker's credibility is influenced by the audience's perceptions of how well he or she has organized the presentation. Verbal clues such as "In conclusion . . . ," "To summarize . . . ," or "Before concluding, I want to leave you with one more thought . . ." are helpful in letting the audience know that the presentation is about to terminate. Many speakers use a final quote or anecdote to reinforce an important point one last time, display their contact information if not already provided on the handout, or use a standard slide with a question mark to set the stage for audience questions.

Be proactive in asking whether your listeners have any questions. Of course, people are often hesitant to ask questions. The speaker should prepare a few for the audience, and then ask for a reaction from a participant who has been paying attention. You might say, "I noticed that you smiled when I was discussing the list of foods to avoid. Can you share what food will be most difficult for you to give up and some ideas you may have for an acceptable alternative?" After responding to the first question, which was generated by the presenter, it is often simpler to get others to respond when the question is asked, "What *other* questions or comments do you have?"

Remember to bring business cards and to remain after the presentation to speak with people who may want to share comments or ask questions. Speakers who have maintained good eye contact and have prompted the inference of warmth through smiling almost always find themselves interacting with audience members who wish to engage them after the presentation. This is frequently a chance to develop contacts for additional speaking engagements, and it is therefore an opportunity for the best kind of face-to-face public relations. When a long line of people is waiting to talk and time is limited, encourage the

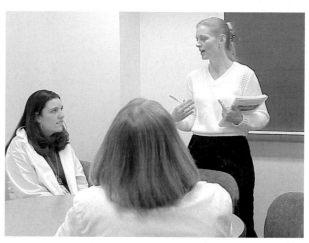

Barriers between the presenter and audience should be omitted.

remaining people to use your business card information to contact you. Be sure to follow up as promised.[18]

IMPLEMENTATION OF AN EFFECTIVE PRESENTATION

Using some basic techniques, described next, speakers can create and deliver an effective presentation.

Audience Connection

Audiences identify with speakers who appear worthy and knowledgeable. Speakers, therefore, should subtly let listeners know during their presentation that they are qualified. For example, one might say, ". . . in an article I wrote last year for the *Journal of the American Dietetic Association* . . .," or "of the several hundred patients I have worked with in the past. . . ." Audiences tend to be more attentive when they believe that the person speaking to them is able to relate to their circumstances or demonstrate any connection they may have with a particular group. For example, you might say, "I have lived in this community for 15 years . . . ," or "I was once 25 pounds overweight myself . . . ." If one gives it some thought, almost all audiences have some traits with which the speaker can identify.[11,14]

Presenters are evaluated by the audience, and the audience's perceptions add to the ambiance from the moment they enter the room. Whenever possible, presenters should arrive early and make an effort to meet people. Their own self-confidence, whether real or feigned, will relax the audience and increase attendees' perceptions of the speaker's desire to share information. Presenters should never volunteer negative information regarding their own stress or fear of speaking. The audience wants to learn and enjoy, and when they are aware of the speaker's fragility or stage fright, they tend to become nervous themselves in sympathy.[19,20]

If the presenters are waiting to be introduced and are seated among the audience or on a stage, they should be aware that audience members who know they are the guest speakers will be watching their every move. That means that even before beginning the presentation, speakers must be careful to smile, look confident, and extend themselves to others. After the speaker is introduced, the way he or she walks up to the podium is critical. During those first moments, an initial impression is being created. The speaker should walk confidently, looking and smiling toward the audience. Before uttering the first words to the audience, a good technique is to spend a long 3 seconds just looking out at the audience, smiling and establishing eye contact with several people. This allows them to infer poise, confidence, and the speaker's desire to connect with them.

Trained speakers see almost everything from their position in front of the room. If they are alert, they may see people who are beginning to fidget, and they can interpret and act on this feedback. Speakers might decide consequently to give the audience a brief interaction, such as responding to a question by asking audience members to raise their hands; they might heighten their own movements to regain attention; or they might engage in a new activity, perhaps one that involves audience participation. They might see some people coming in late, looking awkwardly for a seat. This gives them the opportunity to publicly welcome them and ask others to move over to provide seating. The audience will begin to send signals and participate when they realize the speaker is sensitive to them.[6]

Although individual situations may make it difficult to adhere to this structure, a general rule, when speaking for an hour or less, is to plan on at least 10 minutes for audience interaction. When speaking for more than an hour, audience participation activities are essential to keep the audience engaged and invested in your presentation.

> *If you refuse to accept anything but the best,*
> *you very often get it.*
> —W. CLEMENT STONE

Use of Visuals

Media are a direct extension of the speaker and consequently reflect directly on the speaker's credibility. Media may include computer slides, handouts, blackboard, flip chart, and even actual foods. Media that are prepared, designed, and implemented with high professional standards set the stage for a superior presentation. For example, a speaker who uses PowerPoint slides in large print with attractive clip art, rather than a black-and-white transparency with small print, allows the audience to infer that he or she is an experienced and considerate presenter. Even the quality and color of the paper used in handouts can add or detract from the overall impression.[21,22] More information on creating effective media is found in Chapter 15.

Delivery Techniques

The written text and the oral presentation are entirely different. There is no objection to a presenter writing out the entire talk, carefully organizing it according to topics, causes and effects, chronology, or whatever else seems appropriate. However, once the talk is written, the speaker needs to recognize that the written manuscript represents the "science" of a presentation; the actual delivery represents the "art." Each time it is delivered, the presentation should be somewhat different, with different words, examples, anecdotes, and so forth, to suit particular audiences and situations. The choice of words in spoken language also tends to differ from that in written language. Sentences in oral speech tend to be simpler, shorter, and more conversational, including common words and contractions, whereas a written manuscript may be more erudite and academic. The only way for speakers to develop this art is to rehearse from a simple outline and not a manuscript and to rehearse in front of real people who will react and comment, rather than in front of mirrors, walls, or car windshields.

Never read or memorize! There are other good reasons for not rehearsing from a manuscript. The speech tends eventually to become memorized and that can be deadly. Once a speech is memorized, speakers tend to become more speech-centered than audience-centered, which means that they tend to become more concerned about whether they can remember each line exactly as it is written on the manuscript and less concerned about whether the audience is enjoying, learning, listening, and understanding. Another problem that arises from manuscript speaking is that it is *dull!* Because the speaker's facial expressions and vocal intonations are not spontaneous, the monologue tends to sound memorized and can easily become boring to listeners.[23–25]

One of the worst things that presenters can do is to admit to an audience that they are scared, ill prepared, missing material, sick with a cold, or have done the presentation

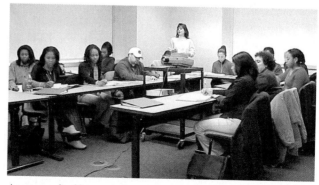

A presenter should arrange the seating area in advance.

better in the past for other groups. The audience does not know what it may be missing and is generally much less critical of speakers than speakers are of themselves. The speaker must act confident, even when he or she does not feel it internally. Speakers experience themselves in the situation from the inside out; the audience experiences them from the outside in. This means that if asked whether they are nervous or anxious, speakers should always answer "No!" Audience members see only the tip of the iceberg when they observe the speaker; they do not feel the intensity of the speaker's anxiety and are probably totally unaware of it unless it is brought to their attention through the speaker's own confession.

The feelings commonly referred to as "stage fright" may date back to the dawn of the human race, when our prehistoric ancestors had to survive by living in caves and sharing the food supply with other beasts. Faced by a predator, our ancestors had a genuine use for a sudden jolt of energy, which gave them the power to do battle or run (i.e., fight-or-flight response). The vestiges of this power, stemming from the secretions of the adrenal gland, still manifest themselves today when people sense danger. Who hasn't felt that ice block in the stomach while being reprimanded by the boss or experienced sweaty palms and racing heart while walking into a room full of strangers? Occasionally, one still reads newspaper accounts of a person exhibiting superhuman strength under conditions of fear or danger, as in the father who lifts a car off his child who has been pinned under the wheels. This is an example of the power that comes with the adrenaline jolt; however, when a person is unable to fight, run, or in some other way utilize this surge, he or she may become overwhelmed by the internal feelings themselves. This feeling before and during a presentation is commonly labeled "stage fright."

The best safeguard against stage fright is adequate preparation and rehearsal. The more one practices in front of *live people,* the less nervousness one exhibits. Other ways of dealing with these feelings include being active during the presentation and "acting" calm and confident. If presenters know they are going to be full of extra energy because of their excess adrenaline secretions, they could plan to include demonstrations during the presentation such as passing out materials, using a pointer, or any other activity that involves motion. Motion is a release for tension and anxiety and allows the audience to infer enthusiasm from the speaker's movement rather than fright, nervousness, or tension. It may not work for everyone, but many people can learn to control their public behavior if they visualize themselves as acting.[19,20,25]

All movement should be meaningful. Do not pace. Presenters ought to look for opportunities to break the invisible barrier between themselves and their audience. Walking toward the audience, walking around the audience, walking in and out of the audience, and walking among the audience all are acceptable ways of delivering a presentation. What is not acceptable is pacing back and forth, particularly with eyes down, as the speaker pulls his or her thoughts together before uttering them. Movement into an audience is a communication vehicle in itself. When presenters penetrate that invisible barrier between themselves and the audience, they are nonverbally indicating their desire to connect, to be close, to better sense what it is the audience is feeling about the speaker and the content. In fact, as speakers walk among the audience, the audience can begin to be seen from a different perspective. The speaker may gain new insights into how better to clarify particular points and issues from this experience.

Environmental Control

Take control of seating the listeners before everyone settles down. It may be their boardroom, gymnasium, or meeting hall, but it is the presenter's "show." Make conscious decisions about whether or not to pull the group into a circle, half-circle, rows; sitting around tables; and so forth. When it is possible to know beforehand which persons are the most influential, their seats should be reserved and placed in the best position to see, hear, and appreciate visual aids as well as the speaker. **Box 14-1** provides a final checklist for presentations.

Presenters do best when they omit all barriers between themselves and their audience. Avoid using a podium or lectern, if possible. Sometimes, due to the room setup or requirements of other speakers, this cannot be avoided. Even in this situation, however, use of a table, which can feature handouts and other materials, is preferred. A podium or lectern should be used only when the speaker does not intend to move about but intends to lecture and needs a stand to rest against and place notes on. Adults generally do not learn optimally through the lecture method. Unless the speaker is extraordinarily good, a straight lecture presented from behind a podium should be avoided. When delivering a message while standing in front of a group without a barrier, the speaker is more disposed to stop the talk to respond to the verbal or nonverbal feedback of listeners. Gestures and movement, too, can be expansive and visible without the lectern barrier.[6,8]

B O X 14-1

Checklist for Oral Presentations

Customizing and completing this checklist before presentations will help avoid last-minute problems.

✓ Do I have my presentation notes?
✓ Do I have all my supporting materials?
✓ Are there enough handouts for each of the attendees?
✓ Will the facility be unlocked and open?
✓ Are the tables and chairs arranged to suit my design?
✓ Do I understand how to operate the lighting system?
✓ Do I understand how to operate the ventilation system?
✓ Do I know the location and operating condition of the electrical circuits?
✓ Do I know how to operate the media?
✓ Do I have backup accessories? (i.e., extra bulb, extension cord, marker, laser pointer)
✓ Will the projection screen be in place and adequate for this size group?
✓ Do I have the type of sound system I require? Is it working?
✓ Have arrangements been made to handle messages during the presentation?
✓ Will there be a sign to announce the presentation location?
✓ Will someone be introducing me, and have I given all the information I want shared with the group?

Practice the use of the media in relationship to the speaking location. Evaluate the use of media with the available lighting and determine if a change in the lighting settings is necessary or possible. Check the arrangements for distribution of the handouts, if applicable. Identify the person who is responsible for introductions and verify the information as necessary.

Determine the options in microphone use. Whenever possible, try to use a clip-on or wireless system, which allows more movement than a positioned microphone at a podium. Ask for a glass of water to be provided during the presentation. Drinking from a bottle of water is distracting.

Be rigorous about time constraints. Bring a small travel clock with large numbers or a timer to help monitor time available or locate a clock if present. Calculate prior to the presentation actual transition times between the introduction, body, and summary of the presentation. The presenter can also designate a member of the program committee or a colleague in the audience to signal when to begin stating the conclusion.

Voice and Diction

Vocal inflection and variation add interest and the impression of speaker enthusiasm. For some people, controlling this variation is simple and natural; for others, it is a challenge. Nevertheless, the presenter needs to attend to voice modulation. The goal when speaking in front of a group is to sound natural and conversational. However, what sounds natural and conversational when standing in front of a large group is not the same as what sounds conversational in a small face-to-face group. "Natural and conversational" from the presenter's point of view is exaggerated. The highs need to be a bit higher and the lows need to be a bit lower. What may sound to the presenter's ear as phony and theatrical generally sounds far less so to the listener. The good news is that this trait can be fairly easily and quickly developed, even in those who recognize a problem in this area. It requires risking sounding foolish and exaggerated in front of trusting others, until adequate reinforcement has convinced the presenter that the increase in vocal variation is really an advantage. In any case, a delivery that is of narrow range or monotone is difficult to respond to for more than a few minutes.

When talking in front of a group, the speaker should generally attempt to speak more slowly than in ordinary conversation. What is an appropriate rate during a small face-to-face discussion is probably too fast for a group presentation. For some reason, there seems to be a correlation between the speech rate of the speaker and the size of the audience. What might be easily grasped at a more rapid rate in face-to-face conversation is not understood as quickly in large groups. Speaking at a slower rate also allows the presenter to scan the audience while speaking to see if he or she is being understood, to see if some people need an opportunity to disagree, to see if he or she needs to talk louder, or to increase the variation because some listeners look bored.

Professional speakers attend to their diction, particularly when pronouncing words such as "for," "can," "with," "picture," "going to," and "want to." In ordinary conversation one is not likely to judge negatively a speaker who mispronounces common words and engages in sloppy diction, saying, for example, "fer," "ken," "wit," "pitcher," "gunna," and "wanna," for the words listed above. However, when that speaker is in front of an audience, these mispronounced words often stand out and lead to negative inferences regarding the speaker.

Professionals who present themselves in front of groups must attend to their diction because they risk losing credibility if it is poor.

Once speakers have become conscious of their diction and have decided to improve it, several steps are required. First, speakers can ask trusted others who are often around them to listen critically and to stop them each time a diction error occurs. Second, after they learn of the common diction problems, speakers need to train themselves to hear the errors. Because the human mind operates generally at five times the rate of human speech, it is possible to listen critically to ourselves during speech. Like learning to ride a bicycle or use a computer, this learning and training task is uncomfortable at first, but improvement comes quickly. Third, speakers need to recognize that working on diction is an ongoing task. Professional speakers never stop listening to the way their words are coming out and continually plan ahead to pronounce them correctly. When necessary, phonetically clarify difficult words or phrases on small cards, and guard against stumbling or mispronunciation by practicing these challenges over and over until they flow easily.

Gestures and Body Language

It is good practice to keep your hands away from your body and from one another. Allow them to be free to gesture. Avoid holding anything in them while talking unless it is a useful prop like a laser pointer or a visual aid. A laser pointer should selectively illustrate important points. Audiences are distracted when laser points move in a wild or circular manner repeatedly on the screen. Presenters often feel awkward with their hands hanging loosely at their sides. Perhaps if they could see themselves on videotape in this posture, they would realize that it is natural looking, but even more important, they would probably see that one tends not to stay in that position. If hands hang loosely at the presenter's sides, eventually the hands begin to rise and gesture spontaneously to emphasize important points.

It is dangerous to begin a presentation holding a pen, paperclip, rubber band, or other instrument not directly related to the presentation. Unconsciously, the fingers begin to play with the instrument, and the audience becomes fascinated with watching to see what the speaker will do. Presenters need to train themselves to keep their faces animated, using a variety of facial expressions. For many of the same reasons expressed earlier, it is important that speakers use all the communication vehicles available to them to maintain the audience's attention. Facial expression is itself a communication vehicle. When it is lively, animated, expressive, and changing regularly while the speaker reacts to the feedback coming toward him or her from the audience, it enhances the verbal message and allows the audience to go on unconsciously inferring the speaker's audience-centeredness. This is easier for some people to do than for others; however, everyone can improve. Because it is not easy for a speaker to "act" expressive does not mean that this person cannot grow considerably in the ability to look expressive.

Eye contact is a vehicle of communication. Use eye contact to see everyone and respond to the nonverbal feedback. When speakers have the opportunity to present themselves and their ideas to an audience, they want the audience to understand them, to believe them, and to follow their recommendations. A speaker has the best chance of being successful in achieving these goals when able to interpret the audience's ongoing reactions. Presentation speaking is often considered a one-way form of communication in which the speaker talks at the audience as they listen. Effective speaking is actually a two-way situation in which audience and speaker communicate with one another constantly and simultaneously.[7]

Facial expressions are important. Presenters must remember to smile and look as if they are enjoying the experience of sharing information. Smiling can be rehearsed and may feel phony, but it needs to be built into the design of the presentation. Speakers do not need to be constantly grinning, but they do need to maintain an expression of gentleness, approachableness, and nondefensiveness. The easiest way to convey these impressions is by smiling often. Unfortunately, it is not easy to smile when one is unsure of the material. All the preceding techniques can be implemented only after the speaker has sufficiently mastered the content and has consciously, through rehearsal, developed skills.

Professional Appearance

Professional dress suggests to the audience one's status as a speaker by providing a sense of confidence. Ironically, this means selecting appropriate clothing that does not attract attention and that the audience will not remember! A well-tailored business suit for men paired with a neutral color shirt (off-white or light colors for camera work) and a tie that complements in a similar color tone are good choices. Women can choose skirt or pant suits and neutral or pastel business blouses. Comfortable, polished shoes are important. Heels should be flat to prevent loss of balance with movement. The audience may view the shoes more easily in a raised stage environment. Bright colors, large patterns, unusual designs, light-reflecting jewelry, and dangling earrings all may distract from the speaker's message by drawing too much of the audience's focus away from the oral message.[6,8]

EVALUATION METHODS

Effective speakers use feedback from every presentation they give to fine-tune their skills. Standard program evaluations often rate the speaker on the planned learning objectives. More in-depth program evaluations may add information on effectiveness and presentation traits. Ask the program planner to provide a copy of the audience evaluation of the presentation, when available. Obtain an audiotape or videotape, if available. Some speakers tape their presentations or ask a trusted audience member to do so on their behalf.

ADAPTATIONS

Although workshops and media interviews rely on many of the general presentation guidelines outlined, each of these situations warrants specific adaptations to be successful and effective in its own arena.

Workshop Format

There are significant differences between a presentation and a workshop format. The differences are in the amount of time needed, the amount of audience participation recommended, and the goals of the leader. Presentations generally run no more than 90 minutes, whereas workshops may run from 90 minutes to several days. Audience participation is an integral part of workshop design. The goals of workshops are generally to teach and train participants to become proficient in a group of skills or knowledge competencies. This is contrasted with a presentation's goal to persuade the audience to accept a specific proposal or behavior change. The following suggestions are particularly appropriate when designing workshops.

Workshop leaders should plan on using techniques that involve all participants. Open communication should occur between the leader and the participants as well as among the participants themselves. Strategies to encourage participation include dividing the larger group into smaller groups, giving smaller groups time to get to know one another, and then assigning each small group sets of activities related to the workshop topic. These small group activities may include such things as case studies, role-playing, questionnaire completion, brainstorming, or discussion. Occasionally, participants may be asked to complete preworkshop assignments, such as filling out a questionnaire, reading material related to the workshop, or performing some other task. Reactions to these tasks can be processed among the participants in small groups.[26]

Frequently, the most important point in determining the climate and direction of the workshop occurs during the first 20 minutes. Some suggestions for using the opening minutes to establish an open climate include using a group introductory activity to promote a relaxed and open atmosphere. When the group is small enough, generally 20 or fewer people, spending time allowing participants to express themselves by identifying their major concerns and questions tends to promote involvement. Workshop leaders can relieve participant anxiety by introducing themselves, sharing both personal and professional information, and giving a brief overview of their objectives for the workshop, the main topics to be covered, their sequence, and the approximate time span. They should also reinforce that they have expectations in terms of participants' cooperation and involvement. Even when such introductory activities take as long as an hour, they are justifiable because of their importance in establishing a common frame of reference with shared goals in a relaxed and receptive setting.

The workshop leader should be aware of signals of fatigue or boredom from participants and have strategies to deal with this possibility. Strategies to maintain the group's attention and interest include identifying two or three participants, whose behavior provides some type of clue to group climate; providing a variety of activities to break up the routine; and providing a change of pace. Most successful workshops are a blend of information-presenting activities and hands-on experiential-type of activities. Another way to safeguard understanding and attention is regularly to summarize what has occurred, especially before moving on to a new topic. Continuity of training is promoted through purposeful and periodic reviews and summaries during the workshop. Leaders should note that it is not essential to do the summarizing; in fact, having the participants do it provides feedback about the group's grasp of the important points.

Just as the introductory period of the workshop should not be rushed, the closure, too, should be carefully planned. In a full day's workshop of 6 to 8 hours, allowing a full hour at the end for closure is appropriate. Of course, it depends on how much time is available for the entire workshop. During the closure, loose ends are tied and the presenter has a final opportunity to verify whether the group's original expectations have been met. Requiring the group to complete an evaluation of the workshop during the allotted time is the method most likely to yield the largest return. These evaluations are most helpful to leaders who want to continue improving their skills, by enabling them to make changes in subsequent workshops based on the responses. The emphasis in a workshop is always on quality, not quantity. It is not how much the audience has heard; it is how much they have learned, will remember, and will use in the future that is the final measure of the workshop's success.[10,24]

Media Interview Format

Increasingly, public health and dietetics interventions depend on effective health communication. The influence of media politics, the accuracy of media reporting, the use of media for health education and advocacy, the availability of training in media relations for staff members, and questions about whether media interaction facilitated or impeded achievement of public health objectives have shown that an organization's image and credibility are clearly influenced by both the manner and content of its media spokespersons. This portion of the chapter on presentation skills deals specifically with tips for presenting oneself or one's organization in the media.

When given the opportunity to present information through the mass media, one needs to understand the power of the media to influence and the inferences that listeners or viewers make based not only on the speaker's presentation and speaking skills but also on the speaker's manner. After grasping the enormous persuasive power of mass media, a presenter can train to use it to his or her advantage. However, if the presenter is unaware and makes no special adaptations for the media, the presentation will be unsuccessful—even though the content is excellent.[27]

Presenter's Style

When communicating through the mass media, speakers need to remember that in more than 50% of listeners, interpretation of the message is influenced not by the content, but by the form—the speaker's manner, energy, and level of enthusiasm, and the vehicles and media used for transmission. It is best to present the information directly in a conversational manner with only a brief outline as a guide. Speakers who paraphrase, quote, or read directly from a manuscript ordinarily will not convey the same tone of confidence, integrity, passion, and sincerity that a person, who is speaking for himself or herself will be able to demonstrate. To demonstrate passion, for example, the speaker needs to know the material thoroughly, have strong feelings about it, and allow himself or herself to emulate the message and not read just empty words.[5,8,14]

Airtime is expensive and interviewers may interrupt or give signals to wind up the comments. When invited to be interviewed or share information through the mass media, speakers need to verify how much time they will be allotted and plan accordingly. When time is limited, the speaker needs to decide ahead of time what points are most essential, have these points highlighted, and express them first. If additional time is provided he or she can then elaborate or add additional information.[5,13]

Chances of being selected for a media presentation increase if one or more videotaped clips or focused content outlines are submitted. Once something is taped, the performance becomes a permanent record that can appear anywhere or anytime in the future, so preparation and focus are key components of success.

Often radio and television interviewers do not have time to become well informed regarding the specifics of their guests' causes. Always maintain a professional manner. Being short with an interviewer may well be interpreted as arrogance and reflect negatively on the speaker's cause. Keep the message simple. It would be wise to rehearse and tape answers and then listen carefully. Use commercial breaks to clarify the direction of the conversation.

Humor is a powerful communication vehicle, but not all people have the gift. Interviewees should be particularly careful about trying to be funny. It may make them look foolish unless they are confident they have the special gift. When, however, the material itself is genuinely funny and has been tried successfully in other audiences, the humor should be brought out.[28]

Often television and radio programs conduct preinterviews to determine whether the guest is articulate and interesting enough to hold the audience. This is the time to do your best. Just because the host is being kind and polite does not mean that he or she won't decide to omit the least interesting or articulate guests.

After presenting in the mass media several times, one becomes adept at processing the experience while it is happening. Presenters need to develop a third eye to monitor themselves in the media and send back messages to themselves about how they are doing during the presentation or interview. Because the human mind whirls several times faster than speech speed, it is possible to see and hear yourself while talking and to modify accordingly. The rule generally is that for the mass media, one's natural behavior should be exaggerated somewhat larger than life, but without being outrageous. Speakers need to behave in a way that generates inferences of self-confidence, sincerity, and even charisma.

Hand gestures on television should be carefully controlled; they tend to be distracting on the screen. Speakers need to sustain interest through their dynamic voice, cadence, inflections, pauses, tone, and facial expression. Although large expansive gestures generally don't work well, variety and variation do work.

Handling Questions and Problems

Very few nonprofessional presenters are able to improvise and come off looking professional. Answers to questions that the interviewee expects to be asked should be rehearsed and not read from notes. If asked a question you can't answer, the smartest thing to do is admit it and offer to locate the answer and forward it to the appropriate people or say, "While I can't exactly answer that, I can tell you that. . . ." This brings the discussion back to the presenter's main message. Part of the self-monitoring process should include the interviewee judging the length of his or her own answers. Avoid long-winded answers or monologues. They tend to bore listeners and irritate the interviewer. Dress is a communication vehicle itself. The best advice is to dress conservatively and in good taste and to avoid being flashy or drawing attention through clothes.

When one is representing an organization, often the same questions will be asked over and over, day after day. Remember, this is the first time many in the audience may be hearing this message; presentations need to sound fresh each time, even though it may be the speaker's 20th time in 2 days answering the same questions.

Bored listeners and viewers change channels. Guest interviewees and presenters need to prepare themselves with interesting anecdotes and aphorisms. Personal experiences tend to hold attention. The deadliest mistake is to become too intellectual or abstract.

When several guests are on the same panel or are involved in a simultaneous interview, someone may attempt to dominate or interrupt. Be prepared to assert yourself if this occurs. Push back into the conversation and say something like, "Let me finish my point," or "Hold that thought while I finish one point." This should be done with a smile and kind voice, but it should, by all means, be done. Listeners and viewers respect the person who stands up for himself or herself—politely. Never get defensive to a member of the audience or another panelist who takes the offensive angrily. The speaker should simply look to the moderator to move the program on.

If you feel offended publicly, grin and bear it rather than reacting emotionally. You can say "I don't agree" or "let's look at this from another perspective," but do not snap back a retort because it may come off as being weak or overly sensitive.

Because so much of what is produced for the media eventually is repeated, speakers should avoid mentioning the time, place, or date of the live broadcast. If a piece isn't "dated," it has a better chance of being used at a later date by other affiliates who may need material.

There may be times when the speaker thinks he or she has been invited to talk about a specific cause, but once there the interviewer steers to other topics. When this happens, it is speaker's responsibility to get his or her original message across even if the host isn't considerate enough to afford the right opportunities. If questions become inappropriate or are about topics that you would rather not discuss, simply say, "I would rather not discuss that." Don't waffle or use "double-talk." Credibility is destroyed when listeners infer deception.

Final impressions count, especially in the media. The speaker should use the final public moments to leave a positive impression of a composed, assertive, and controlled person. Privately, before leaving, the speaker should look for the producer and director and thank them personally as well. A firm handshake and looking people in the eye while talking adds a separate nonverbal message itself, apart from the verbal one being expressed.[19,25]

The suggestions provided in this chapter need to be practiced rather than memorized. Presenters need to involve participants in their presentations. Straight lecture without interaction among participants is less effective in bringing about change than lecture with discussion.

Developing presentation skills and handling the myriad of problems that can occur with media or interviewers constitute a process that occurs over time. Presenters get better and better with each subsequent opportunity or practice.

CASE STUDY 1

Joan Stivers, RD, works in a corporate wellness program. She has noticed that some employees who eat in the employee cafeteria make less than optimum food choices for lunch. Others go out to a nearby fast-food restaurant. She is asked by management to give a 30-minute presentation on healthy, nutritious lunches.

1. Write a brief abstract summarizing the presentation.
2. What should Joan do in the introduction?
3. What are the objectives of the body of the presentation?

(continued)

CASE STUDY 1

(continued from previous page)
4. What approaches would you recommend with this audience?
5. How should she handle the conclusion?
6. Outline several methods to evaluate the effectiveness of the presentation.

CASE STUDY 2

The state university campus wellness center has assessed the need for nutrition education programs. One finding was that some of the athletes on campus do not seem to understand the importance of maintaining fluid intake and balance before, during, and after sports events. Coaches have asked the dietetics professional on campus to give a presentation on fluid balance to reinforce what they have told players. John Little, RD, has agreed to give the presentation and to be available for individual counseling sessions on nutrition as well.

1. What additional information should John gather before planning his presentation?
2. What are five to six major points he should cover in his presentation?
3. How can John evaluate the outcome or success of his presentation?
4. What could John mention in his introduction to secure the audience's motivation to listen to him?

REVIEW AND DISCUSSION QUESTIONS

1. What are the three analysis processes used when preparing a presentation?
2. What are the major components of an effective presentation?
3. Describe and analyze several experiences you have had as an audience member.
4. Why is it important for a presenter to proofread all materials used in the presentation?
5. What does it mean to be audience-centered?
6. How can presenters overcome challenges such as nervousness, fear, and stage fright?
7. Why are a presenter's verbal and nonverbal expressions important?
8. What is the difference between a presentation and a workshop?

SUGGESTED ACTIVITIES

1. Design and deliver a 10-minute presentation on some issue related to foods, nutrition, or dietetics, such as safety of the food supply, a new food product, fiber in foods, reduced fat or calories in foods, snacks, restaurant meals, or sodium.
2. Design and deliver a presentation intended for a group of parents of obese children. A minimum of two visual aids should be used. Included with the 20-minute presentation should be 5 full minutes of audience–speaker interaction.
3. Design and deliver a 30-minute presentation intended for a group of people who have recently learned they have diabetes. A minimum of three visual aids are required, including flip chart and handout material. Plan on at least 8 minutes of interaction

with the audience; this should be prompted by the speaker's perceptions of the non-verbal feedback emanating from the audience.

4. Design and deliver a 60-minute presentation intended for a group of people who have paid to be taught or trained by you in an area related to your specialty in the area of dietetics. Develop whatever aids seem appropriate.

Note: If possible all presentations should be videotaped. Presenters should provide reaction sheets to the audience and later write a critique of the taped presentation responding to their own subjective reactions, the critique sheets of the audience, and the instructor's comments.

WEB SITES

PUBLIC SPEAKING TIPS

http://www.mindtools.com

http://www.speaking-tips.com

http://thecreativemindz.com

http://www.toastmasters.org

REFERENCES

1. Commission on Accreditation for Dietetics Education. Foundation Knowledge and Skills and Competency Requirements for Entry-Level Dietitians. Chicago: American Dietetic Association, 2002.
2. Short JE, Chittooran MM. Nutrition education: a survey of practices and perceptions in undergraduate dietetics education. J Am Diet Assoc 2004:104:1601–1604.
3. Peregrin T. A place at the table: marketing dietetics professionals' expertise to other health care providers in a clinical setting. J Am Diet Assoc 2004:104:1781–1783.
4. Goldberg JP, Hellwig JP. Nutrition communication: exciting opportunities for dietitians. J Am Diet Assoc 2003:103:25–26.
5. McManamom B, Pazder N. Pitching your ideas to the media. J Am Diet Assoc 2000:100:1451–1453.
6. Macinnis JL. The Elements of Great Public Speaking: How to Be Calm, Confident, and Compelling. Berkeley, CA: Ten Speed Press, 2006.
7. Beebe SA, Beebe SJ. Public Speaking: An Audience-Centered Approach. 6th Ed. Boston: Allyn & Bacon, 2005.
8. Gilman AD, Berg KE. Get to the Point: How to Say What You Mean and Get What You Want. Dubuque IA: Kendall/Hunt Publishing, 1995
9. Hadfield-Law L. Effective Presentations for Healthcare Professionals. Oxford: Butterworth Heinemann, 1999.
10. Gibson J. The breakfast of champions: teaching audience analysis using cereal boxes. Texas Speech Commun J 2007:31:49–50.
11. Anholt RR. Dazzle'em with Style: The Art of Oral Scientific Presentation. St. Louis: Academic Press, 2005.
12. Canter DD, Nettles MF. Dietitians as multidepartment managers in healthcare settings. J Am Diet Assoc 2003:103:127–240.
13. Hoff R. Say It in Six. Kansas City, MO: Andrews and McMeel, 1996.

14. Khodarahmi S. I hear what you are saying. Commun World 2007:7:11–12.

15. Pearson JC, Child JT, Kahl DH. Preparation meeting opportunity: how do college students prepare for public speeches? Commun Q 2006:54:351–366.

16. Gutgold ND. Successful paper presentations. Tex Speech Commun J 2007:31:45–48.

17. Charlesworth D. Thinking critically, speaking famously, and writing effortlessly: an alternative performative public speaking assignment. Commun Teacher 2005:19:1–4.

18. Baxter B. Activities for Oral Communication and Presentations. Westminster, CA: Teacher Created Resources, 2004.

19. McCullough SC, Russell SG, Behnke RR, et al. Anticipatory public speaking state anxiety as a function of body sensations and state of mind. Commun Q 2006:54:101–109.

20. McKenzie L, Saunders J. Facing the fear: methods for addressing speech anxiety in public speaking class. Texas Speech Commun J 2007:31:53–54.

21. Kosslyn SM. Clear and to the PowerPoint: How to Use 8 Psychological Principles to Produce Brilliant PowerPoint Presentations. New York: Oxford University Press, 2007.

22. Howell DD, Howell DK, Childness M. Using PowerPoint in the Classroom. Thousand Oaks, CA: Corwin Press, 2006.

23. Smith TE, Frymier AB. Get "real": does practicing speeches before an audience improve performance? Commun Q 2006:54:111–125.

24. Fredricks SM. Teaching impromptu speaking: a pictorial approach. Commun Teacher 2005:19:75–79.

25. Madden SJ, Fellows KL. Persuasive speaking: it's just a game! Commun Teacher 2006:20:49–52.

26. White JV, Pitman S, Denny SC. Tool kits for teachable moments. J Am Diet Assoc 2003:103:1454–1456.

27. Leff D. How to write for the public. J Am Diet Assoc 2004:104:730–732.

28. McRoberts DA, Larson-Casselton C. Humor in public address, health care and the workplace: summarizing humor's use using meta-analysis. N Dakota J Speech Theater 2006:19:26–33.

CHAPTER 15

Planning, Selecting, and Using Instructional Media

OBJECTIVES

- Describe the key points for making visual materials.
- Identify when to best use various instructional media.
- Measure literacy level of educational materials.
- Explain the potential uses of asynchronous and synchronous education.
- Plan, use, and evaluate instructional media used in a presentation.
- Identify several ways in which technology is changing education.

> *"The truth isn't the truth until people believe you, and they can't believe you if they don't know what you are saying, and they can't know what you are saying if they won't listen to you, and they won't listen to you if you're not interesting, and you won't be interesting unless you say things imaginatively, originally, freshly."*
> —WILLIAM BERNBACH

Instructional media are the teaching tools that enhance teaching through the use of various technologies. Using media correctly and effectively enhances your delivery of a message.[1] Whether making a presentation or working one on one with an individual, visual displays such as food models or attractive bulleted points, charts, and graphs make your message more understandable, more professional, and more interesting. This chapter examines the types of instructional media most commonly available, offers suggestions for use, and discusses the advantages, limitations, and evaluation of various forms of media. In whatever aspect of dietetics you work, communication is a part of the business and media can help enhance communication. In the 21st century, the challenges are to choose among the increasing variety of formats and methods available and to learn how to think differently to teach differently.

BENEFITS OF VISUAL MEDIA

"A picture is worth a thousand words." How true. Four pictures, therefore, are worth 4,000 words. The more you want to get across, the more visual assistance is needed. When people can see materials rather than merely hear them or read about them, they remember more. Visual media are especially helpful to groups with limited reading ability and people who speak little English.

According to Albert Mehrabian, during presentations learners absorb 7% of text, 38% of verbal information, and 55% of visual information.[2] Another estimate holds that people learn 10% from reading, 20% from listening, and 80% from what they see.[3] Although the estimates vary, the trend is clear. What happens when learners try to recall information 2 weeks later? They remember 20% of what they hear, but 50% of what they both see and hear and 90% of what they say and do.[4] Giving the audience visuals helps enhance learning and remembering; lecturing, alone, whether it be about healthy eating or about sanitation, only gets limited results. Visual methods help. But active participation is the key to learning.[4]

Visual media are part of the instructional input. Visuals enhance written and oral communication methods and make them more interesting. Pictures and sounds have the power to compel attention, to enhance understanding, and to promote learning in a shorter time frame than by using solely verbal explanations. But a strong presentation does not overly rely on visual aids. The presenter should be able to do without any visuals if necessary.[5]

PLANNING VISUAL MEDIA

Planning what instructional media to use is part of the overall program planning for any learning situation. Answers to the following seven questions will help your thinking:

1. What are the objectives or aims of the session? What should audience members learn or be able to do?

2. What methods or activities (lecture, discussion, individual counseling, simulation and the like) will facilitate accomplishing the objectives? Where can media fit into these plans?

3. Who is the audience? What is the size of the

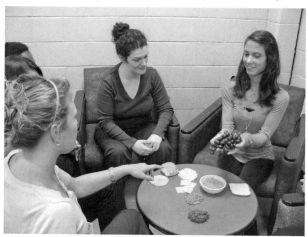

A picture is worth a thousand words.

audience? What are the characteristics of the learner, such as age, gender, educational and literacy level, and cultural or ethnic group?

4. What is the learner's current level of knowledge of the topic? A presentation to a lay group, for example, would need different visuals than a presentation to a group of professionals; and new employee training may need a different approach from that for long-term employees.
5. What purpose(s) do the visuals serve? Is it to generate interest in the subject; to affect attitudes, emotions, or motivation; to entertain; to present information; to attract and hold attention; to involve the learner in mental activity promoting learning; or some combination of purposes?
6. How can you concisely organize and sequence the points to be made and emphasize them with visuals? How are the key messages being reinforced? Can you break down the learning into key steps and assess knowledge at each step?
7. How will you evaluate the effectiveness of the total presentation, including visuals?[3,6]

The instructional media selected depend on the goals, the size of the audience, the physical facilities, equipment and time available, and the learning style of the audience. Before discussing types of visuals, let's identify key principles for all visuals.

ART AND DESIGN PRINCIPLES

The quality and effectiveness of media may depend to a great extent on art and design principles. A dietetics practitioner does not have to be a great artist, but some understanding of simple principles improves results. First and foremost, the visual must be large enough for all participants to see. Know the size of the facility and the type of presentation before creating the visuals.

Simplicity and Unity

The presenter should try to convey only one idea at a time, since too many ideas confuse the audience. Decide what should be at the center of attention or interest and then build around it. Focus on it immediately and reinforce the message. The inclusion of three main messages is enough for most presentations.

Wording and Lettering

Be concise and use the fewest words possible. Use an image when you can. Working on conciseness of wording should help to organize the thoughts that the presenter wants to get across. Titles and labels are placed at various locations. Headings or headlines need to clarify the emphasis and should be in larger print.

Standardizing the size of the lettering (type size) and the kind of lettering (fonts) conveys a more professional appearance. Times Roman and Gothic are more readable than some stylized script fonts. See **Box 15-1** for examples of fonts. The size must be large enough to be read by the reader who is sitting the farthest away. Limit the number of fonts to one or two. Type size also needs to be considered in handouts. For handouts, a minimum of 12-point type is recommended.[6] For the elderly, a 14- or 18-point type size and dark colors on light background work better.

Box **15-1**

Type Styles, Fonts, and Print Sizes

10 point type

12 point type

14 point type

18 point type

24 point type

36 point type

48 point type

Times New Roman
Century
Courier New
Freestyle Script
Arial
Copperplate Gothic Bold
Rockwell
Lucida Handwriting

For slides, the number of words should be limited to 20 to 36. The "rule of six," is to use not more than six lines and not more than six words per line with type size of 24 point or higher.[5] Capital letters are appropriate for short titles of five to six words or less, but a combination of capital and lower case is preferable for longer titles, allowing space for readability. A Combination of Upper and Lower Case Letters Is Preferable. ALL CAPS ARE MORE DIFFICULT TO READ. You may wish to number lists or use bullets (•), underline words for emphasis, or add stars to key points.[7]

Color

Color can enhance visuals and demand attention. You may combine colors that are pleasing aesthetically and do not clash. It is best to decide on the focus of the visual and select the color for that element first. Colors have meanings for people. In most Western countries, red and orange are considered "hot," whereas green, blue, and violet are considered "cool" colors.[3] Cool colors are most pleasing to many. The presenter should start by considering the background color. If it is light, any bright colors may be used. With a dark background, lighter shades are needed, and print must be larger to be readable. Use a color or theme and only change it for major reasons.

Images

Visuals can illustrate difficult concepts well. This includes proportions, relationships, similarities, and differences. An illustration evokes a visual picture of a procedure or technique. A cartoon can add fun to the presentation and increase the viewer's memory of a concept. As with the other principles, the dietetics professional should consider the layout of the illustration and its effect on the audience's understanding. Is it too crowded? Confusing? Is it serving its purpose? A complex table or chart may be better as a handout than as a slide or in a simplified format. Select relevant images, not useless or distracting ones. If inserting audio or visual elements, try to limit them to 2 minutes or less.

Balance and Emphasis

There are two kinds of balance, formal and informal. Informal balance is asymmetrical and more attention-getting and interesting than symmetrical balance. Formal balance occurs when one half is the mirror image of the other half. Bear in mind that our society reads from left to right and top to bottom, so that is the way your audience will view any visual.[6] **Figure 15-1** illustrates balance.

Backups

Have a plan to deal with media and equipment that do not work or are too small for the space. Ask about backup projectors and bulbs, have a backup copy of a presentation, and have a printed copy. Be ready to do the presentation without the assistance of media.

Copyright and Permission

Obtain permissions before using web-based images and reference materials.[2,7]

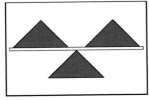

Formal balance

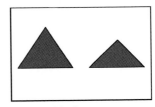

Informal balance

FIGURE **15-1**   Formal and Informal Balance.

ASYNCHRONOUS OR SYNCHRONOUS LEARNING

Instructional information may be given in a synchronous or asynchronous manner. In synchronous learning, all the participants are learning at the same time. This may be one on one, as a small group, or as a large group. Traditionally, synchronous learning was done in one location in an office, classroom, or conference room. Today, synchronous learning can occur at two or more sites via videoconferencing and cable or telephone connections, compressed video connections, telephone or computer conference calls with materials distributed over the Internet, or live chats on the Internet, called "Webinars." Asynchronous learning is "anytime learning." Reading a journal article or watching a DVD or CD-ROM or participating in an e-mail discussion based on your schedule are examples of asynchronous learning. Asynchronous learning gives learners much more freedom over their approach to learning. They can read, listen, or watch the material until they are comfortable with it. Both types of education should be designed so the student must actively participate in the learning whether by participating with others or by completing tutorials and quizzes.

Computer-based learning modules are common in many work sites. Computer-based instruction can be used in various ways. It provides time flexibility and a consistent message.[8] Learners read or listen and do practice or comprehensive tests. This method is particularly good for learning facts, such as medical terminology, or calculations, such as designing a parenteral nutrition solution. The clients or employees are given rapid feedback on how well they comprehend the material. Tutorials, games, and simulations may augment the learning.

Today, the technology and teaching methods have advanced to the point that very interactive facilitated learning between teacher and student can occur via the computer. The addition of interaction between teacher and student, and student and student via the Internet has allowed computer-based distance education to grow rapidly across the world. A computer-based distance education class generally has all the components of a traditional class: textbooks, readings, assignments, and tests. The class discussion is replaced by a web-based discussion facilitated by the teacher. The lecture is replaced by readings, websites, written lectures, and audio or video streaming or compact discs (CDs). The students and faculty generally need high-speed Internet connections.

For "just-in-time" patient, client, or employee education, many institutions are using stand-alone computer kiosks (terminals). This touch-screen approach allows access to information from convenient locations with visual and audio components. Clients can get information when they need it. It does not replace, but rather augments, the dietetics professional's message. Many community education projects use kiosks. One such project at the University of Georgia tested the use of a multiple-person screen setup versus a sit-at-the-screen solo setup in English and Spanish. The kiosks were designed to share information on the multiple facets of diabetes. Many of the participants were elderly.[9] They found the eating and exercise information most useful. The sit-down model was preferred.

A recent study comparing web-based versus classroom learning on diet and physical activity showed that both worked to change behavior in the short term.[10] Another study demonstrated that telemedicine and in-person diabetes education both improved glycemic control and were well accepted by the patients.[11]

KINDS OF VISUAL MEDIA

After considering what needs to be communicated and thinking about the audience, the dietetics professional selects the appropriate media for the purpose. Any one or several may be applicable. **Box 15-2** outlines the possibilities. This section discusses the types of media to consider—from real objects to multimedia presentations.

Real Objects

Nothing is more realistic than showing actual foods or food packages. A lesson on food labeling, for example, may include a variety of food packages so that the audience can participate hands-on with actual products in learning to read and understand the labels. To avoid audience distraction, keep items covered or out of sight when they are not being used. Passing items around may be a major distraction.

A tour to the grocery store is another possibility. When an actual tour is not possible a video tour or a virtual tour can be used. Supermarket tours are common across the country. Food demonstrations are also common.

B O X 15-2

Types of Media

Real Objects and Presentations
Foods
Food demonstrations
Food packages and labels
Food models
Food service equipment

Audio Formats
Audiotapes
Compact discs
DVDs
iPODS
Cell phones

Display Media
Chalkboard or whiteboard
Flip chart
Bulletin or display boards
Photographs
Pictures
Magnets and pens
Instant messaging

Graphics
Diagrams
Charts
Cartoons
Clip art
Menus

Projected Visuals
Overhead transparencies
Slides and computer-based
    presentations
VHS tapes
CD-ROMs
Webcams

Moving Images
Videos
CD-ROMs and DVDs
Screencasts

Print Media
Handouts
Brochures and newsletters

Making recipes to be tasted in group sessions when teaching about nutrition or modified diets increases familiarity with foods and cooking techniques. A person with heart disease, for example, who has seen the dietetics professional prepare a tasty recipe, sampled it, and received the recipe is more likely to try it at home because she or he is familiar with it. In a series of classes, audience members may assist and provide recipes. A study on preschoolers showed that tasting foods was a valuable way of educating them to eat healthier.[12]

In training employees, it is preferable to train them using the real object, such as a meat slicer, dish machine, cash register, or other equipment. Actual hands-on experience is preferable. Breaking the learning into small segments is also preferable to facilitate learning.

Advantages

- Realistic.
- Hands-on learning and audience participation enhance motivation and retention.

Limitations

- Some foods are perishable.
- Cooking facilities may not be available.
- Not suitable for large groups.
- More preparation time often is needed

Pictures, Packages, and Menus

Pictures from magazines or catalogs or clip art may be displayed on posters or on computer screens. Sample packages and containers of recommended foods may be displayed. To discuss a "Nutrition Facts" label or ingredients labeling with a client, it is helpful and realistic to have actual labels available. Labels may be removed from packages and mounted on cardboard or into a book for display or as photocopies. You may want to have different collections, for example, when teaching about healthy snacks, low-fat food choices, sodium-controlled, low-calorie foods, and the like. Photocopies of labels work well and reduce storage space or the amount of material that needs to be carried to an alternate site.

One method of teaching about the values on the label and the ingredients is to have clients guess the product by the nutrient composition and ingredient list. Menus from local eating establishments are excellent for learning about eating out. Scanning the items into a computer will allow for presentation to a larger group.

Advantages

- May be colorful and eye catching.
- Generally inexpensive.
- Packages and pictures are portable.

Limitations

- Lack motion.
- Can be overdone unless the message is focused.

Food Models and Measurements

Food models are representations of the real objects. Many professionals maintain an inventory of three-dimensional plastic food models. They are helpful in estimating client portion sizes, for example, during an assessment of food intake and in teaching portion sizes on controlled caloric intakes. Besides the visual stimulation, putting the model in the person's hands makes a more active experience using another of the senses—touch. Plastic, life-sized food models may be purchased from sources, such as Nasco Nutrition Teaching Aids in Fort Atkinson, Wisconsin.

When discussing portion control of beverages or foods, show the diversity of sizes available. You may need a variety of sizes and shapes as well as disposable cups when portion size is important. If you are going to suggest 4- and 8-ounce servings, you should encourage using a measuring cup at home to train the eye to serve correct portion sizes. Practicing weighing portions is helpful, and dividing a box of cereal into the described portions is eye opening.

Advantages

- Realistic and colorful.
- Portable.
- Show and demonstrate portion sizes.

Limitations

- Cannot be seen in large groups.
- Items may be lost.

Photographs and Drawings

The professional may take photographs or have them done professionally. Photos can be enlarged to any size. They may be used on bulletin boards and computer screens. If you are photographing people, such as employees and clients, a signed form releasing the use of the photos without limitation is advisable.

Advantages

- Relatively inexpensive.
- Reflect real situations.
- Attract interest.

Limitation

- Distracting to pass around in groups.

Charts and Posters

Information may be presented in charts or on posters that are self-made or purchased. The U.S. Department of Agriculture's graphic design of dietary recommendations in the MyPyramid is an example **(Figure 15-2)**. Numerical data can be presented in bar charts, pie-shaped charts, or line graphs.

A table, easel, or tripod should securely hold the display. It is not necessary to read word for word from a visual. At most, you may tell why the visual is significant or paraphrase the content. If possible, remove it from audience view after discussing it.

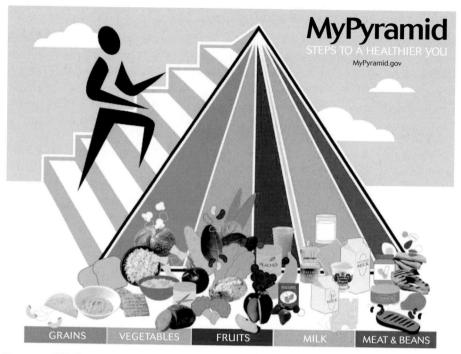

FIGURE **15-2**   MyPyramid. (Source: U.S. Department of Agriculture.)

Posters are also a medium for sharing research findings and other information at professional meetings. Often the posters are divided into specific segments that are prepared on separate sheets. They may be attached onto mounting boards at the meeting site or be freestanding tabletop posters.[13] Guidelines for poster sessions from the American Dietetic Association are outlined in **Figure 15-3**.

Advantages

- Inexpensive.
- Portable for short distances.

Limitations

- Cannot be seen except in very small groups (15 to 20 people).
- Homemade charts may be overcrowded with content.
- Become worn with repeated use.

Bulletin or Display Boards

Bulletin boards or display boards can spark interest in a topic. They should be totally self-explanatory. The concept should be simple, and the display should visually attract attention. The average adult spends 45 seconds looking at a display.[14] Focus on one theme with

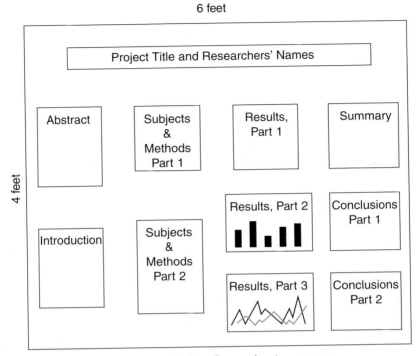

*Layout of a typical poster display. Remember to express
information with graphs, charts, or tables whenever possible.
Place important information at eye level or higher on the poster.*

FIGURE **15-3**   Guidelines for Poster Sessions.

three or fewer messages including the "take-home" message. Limit the number of words
and use a type size of 18 to 24 point. Use catchy headings, graphics, and photographs.[14]

Advantages

- Inexpensive.
- Require minimal preparation.

Limitations

- Cannot be used with large groups.
- Not generally portable.

Chalkboard or Whiteboard

Everyone has seen the chalkboard or whiteboard used and misused. When the writing is
legible and large enough to be seen, it is a good supplement to a presentation. Limit talking to the board rather the audience while writing. If this is a problem for the presenter,
a display of overhead transparencies or slides is preferable. Chalkboards, whiteboards, and
flip charts all foster participation.

Advantages

- Inexpensive.
- Easy to use.
- Allows audience opinions to be written down.
- Spontaneous.

Limitations

- Requires good timing so that one does not talk to the board.
- Not good in large groups.
- Poor spelling and handwriting are liabilities.

Flip Charts

If a chalkboard or whiteboard is unavailable, a flip chart with a display easel may substitute. Flip charts have a number of large sheets of paper fastened together. You can write or draw with crayon or black or colored felt pens, being sure to select ones that do not bleed through the paper. Writing should be large and bold to be seen—at least 1 inch high or more for every 20 to 30 feet of audience space. Inexperienced presenters may want to ask someone to do the writing for them.

Each sheet is turned at the top after completion. Finished sheets can also be torn off and attached to a wall. When you need a record of points made by the audience, a flip chart is preferable to a chalkboard because the sheets can be carried from the meeting. Alternately, one can prepare the sheets in advance and reveal them sequentially while standing facing the audience. This allows for the creative use of color, clip art, glitter, fabric, and other materials. It is advisable to leave a blank page when the audience focus should be on the presenter.

Advantage

- Informal and inexpensive.

Limitations

- Awkward to carry very far.
- Cannot be seen in larger groups.
- Require legible handwriting.
- Require practice to write quickly while speaking.
- May be too informal for some purposes.

Overhead Transparencies

Although rapidly becoming extinct, transparencies are a great visual complement to a presentation. The speaker stands, not sits, beside the projector facing the audience, being careful not to block the view of the screen.

Some speakers like to have a title or other visual on the projector as the audience assembles. To assist the audience, number the points on the transparency in the order in which you are discussing them and in order of importance. If all items are of equal importance, bullets (•) are more generic. When not in use, the machine should be turned off or a generic slide shown.

Keep in mind that the average overhead projector surface is 10 × 10 inches, transparencies are 10 × 12, and most paper is 8.5 × 11, so the actual message areas is about 7.5 × 9.0 to 9.5 inches.[3,7] A border needs to be left around all the edges.

A more professional look may be obtained by typing the information. A readable font is essential, and large type size must be used. About 30 points or ¼ inch is good, but you need to check the room size to be sure.[7] See Box 15-1 for samples of font styles and type sizes. Graphs or charts from scientific and professional journals, enlarged cartoons, and other data may be presented easily in this form. Be sure to include the source of the material. Photographs do not reproduce well except with a digital camera that will place pictures into a computer graphics file to be printed on a transparency.

Advantages

- Easy to use and inexpensive.
- Allows you to maintain eye contact with the audience, which helps to control attention.
- Use normal room lighting.
- Can be written on while talking.

Limitations

- In a large, deep room, may not be seen in the back.
- Easy to overcrowd information.
- Bulb may burn out (carry an extra).
- Availability is limited
- Seems old-fashioned

Print Handouts

Health care professionals tend to give patients and clients a great deal of information verbally. By the time they get home, most have probably forgotten at least half of the information. Trainers may do the same with new employees. Materials in print may be personalized using word processing and desktop publishing software.

Putting key points in writing so that clients, patients, employees, and other audiences can refer to them later solves this problem. In teaching about modified diets, for example, oral counseling is frequently supplemented with written materials, including the foods to eat often and those to limit, recipes suggestions, and web sites to visit. Printed materials are effective in reinforcing individual counseling sessions and group classes. When planning employee training, the presenter may consider giving an outline of the content with space for note taking or a list of the main points to be remembered. Listeners will be writing instead of listening unless you distribute copies of the information on the slides.

In teaching about normal nutrition, for example, the MyPyramid and the Dietary Guidelines for Americans may be distributed. Government agencies and private organizations produce printed materials for a wide range of audiences, or you can make your own. If you are using materials produced by others, determine the right to reproduce the materials. If the material is copyright-free, just acknowledge the owner. If the material is copyrighted, obtain permission to reproduce the material. There may be a charge for this based on the number of items being used and the purpose of the use. Some materials may need to be purchased for distribution.

One-page instructional sheets written in short, simple words in active voice assist clients, even when more detailed materials are also being given. These one-page sheets can be posted on the refrigerator or hung at the office to remind clients of what to do and when to do it. Small give-away items such as pens, magnets, puzzles, and games may also be useful to remind the person of your message.

For written materials, assess the readability or grade level, since some adults have low literacy skills. According to the U.S. Department of Education, 1 in 10 Americans has "below basic" English skills.[15] About 15% of adults are not high school graduates.[16] Some are recent immigrants with limited ability in English. Printed materials in other languages may be needed. Educational materials must be understandable to the people for whom they are intended. Therefore, nutrition educators need to select or develop printed materials that are easily comprehended.

Since the 1920s readability tests have been used. They measure word and sentence length and difficulty. Several readability formulas are available, both as software programs and in print, to help assess the audience's readability, grade level, or both.[17] The SMOG, FOG, Flesch, Raygor, and Fry tests are examples. The SMOG criteria are listed in **Table 15-1**. Because of the scientific and technical nature of health communications, vocabulary and wording of patient education materials may be incomprehensible to many adults. Readability formulas should be used to assess the approximate educational level a person must have to understand the material. Readability formulas, however, are only part of the process; developers should also "pilot-test," or try out materials on sample clients, or use more formal focus groups to find out if they will be understood by the target audience.[17]

Advantages

- Audience can refer to the information later at home or at work.
- Good when information has to be remembered.
- Helps the person to focus attention and follow points.

Limitations

- People may never look at the handout again.
- Time spent in preparing materials.
- Literacy level of users varies.

Slides and Computer-Based Presentations

Although slides are now rarely produced through traditional photography, most are computer-generated using such programs as Microsoft's PowerPoint or Corel. Most word-processing software packages have a presentation program that assist in producing slides. Typed-in words and pictures, graphs, and animations are cut and pasted into the presentation. Graphics, animations, and pictures use a considerable amount of space on a disk, so use them to make a point, not just because they are available. In some cases, slides are available for purchase or from publishers promoting the use of their materials.

With traditional slides in a remote-control projector, the presenter can advance the presentation while talking. Professionals begin and end with a black slide or a title/logo

T A B L E **15-1** | SMOG Readability Formula

1. Count off 10 consecutive sentences near the beginning, in the middle, and near the end of the text. If the text has fewer than 30 sentences, use as many as are provided.
2. Count the number of words containing 3 or more syllables (polysyllabic) including repetitions of the same words.
   a. Hyphenated words are considered as one word.
   b. Numbers that are written out should be counted. If written in numerical form, they should be pronounced to determine if they are polysyllabic.
   c. Proper nouns, if polysyllabic, should be counted.
   d. Abbreviations should be read as though unabbreviated to determine if they are polysyllabic. However, abbreviations should be avoided unless commonly known.
3. Look up the approximate grade level on the SMOG Conversion Table below:

Total Polysyllabic Word Count	Approx. Grade Level (+1.5 Grades)
0–2	4
3–6	5
7–12	6
13–20	7
21–30	8
31–42	9
43–55	10
56–72	11
73–90	12
91–110	13
111–132	14
133–156	15
157–182	16
183–210	17
211–240	18

From "SMOG grading: A new readability formula" by G. McLaughlin, 1969, Journal of Reading, 12(8), pp. 639-646. Adapted with permission.

slide to avoid the white glare of the screen without an image. If a very short part of the presentation does not include a slide, a black slide can be inserted there instead of turning the projector or computer off and on.

Most slide presentations are now computer-based. The computer, generally a laptop, is connected to a projection device. An LCD projector (liquid crystal display) or an LMD, which uses mirrors, displays the images on a screen. Projectors vary in resolution, brightness, ability to zoom, weight, portability, and cost.

Advantages

- Small and easy to carry.
- Can change the sequence as appropriate.
- Good for both large and small groups.

Limitations

- Equipment may malfunction.
- Need to dim room lighting; the better the projection, the less dimming needed.
- Cost to purchase or rent the projector.

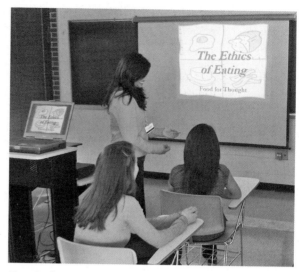

The title of one's presentation may be displayed as the audience gathers.

Audio Recordings

Cassette tapes, CD-ROMs, DVDs, and iPODS can be prerecorded to illustrate key educational points. Long recordings may be more appropriate for individual listening than for a group presentation, but short audios can be very effective in a large group. Testimonials, several sentences from a key leader, or a commercial or radio segment can be used as a springboard for many messages. When recording audio use an informal, conversational tone of voice with slow, clear enunciation. Listen to the recording before using it to assess whether the sound quality is acceptable. Background noise on the recording can be very distracting.

Advantages

- Easy to use.
- Portable.
- Allow repetition and reinforcement.
- Good for low-literacy groups.

Limitations

- Need a good-quality microphone for recording.
- Do not allow for questions and answers.

Video Recordings or Screencasts

The combinations of sights and sounds from videos are pleasing to most people. Purchased or rented videos should be previewed to check for appropriateness. Many groups, such as the American Dietetic Association, American Heart Association, American Diabetes Association, National Dairy Council, Educational Foundation of the

National Restaurant Association, drug companies, government agencies, and private media companies offer visual materials. An LCD projector with video signal capacities and monitor are generally necessary for audience viewing. Because audiences tend to view passively, they should be told what to look for before viewing, and preplanned activities or discussion questions should follow. A video or CD may be viewed alone at the learner's own pace or viewed repeatedly to enhance learning. The presenter may put a video on pause to stop for discussion. Short video clips can highlight key points and help segment the talk.

Capturing demonstrations and then placing on a CD or a streaming video on a web site can reinforce techniques and procedures in a step-by-step process. Whether you are illustrating how to easily remove the skin from chicken or how to interact with a client, the use of video can be a good learning tool for both learning and reinforcing learning.

Many employee programs for orientation and training use video formats, sometimes with printed workbooks or learner's guides. If the employee views a video alone, discussions with the instructor should follow to explain the relationship of the video to the job. Videos can be placed on a CD-ROM or a video server and connected to a web-based site, where demonstrations of learning can occur. The learner watches the video and periodically or at the end is asked questions about the content to assess learning. Many employee education and orientation programs are moving to web-based training as a portion of their training because it is convenient and available to all employees rather than those available on a particular day; also, competencies can be documented. Customized unit-based training is also easier to facilitate via technology-based training. The employee or client can be directed to complete only the modules pertinent to the current role, providing on-demand or "just-in-time" training. Videos should augment the learning. Teacher-facilitated discussion after the video should reinforce the concepts and promote active discussion. Short videos to take home after the presentation or counseling reinforce learning. This is especially useful for procedures such as preparing baby formula or conducting self-care.

While not replacing other education, a new form of complementary education is "on-the-job video gaming." It is a small but growing market with much potential in teaching technical skills.[18]

"Screencasts," a term developed by Jon Udell of *Infoworld* magazine,[19] are basically online movies. They are produced, edited, narrated, and posted online. Similar techniques apply. Create short 3- to 8-minute presentations, keep them simple, and use key messages with graphics and demonstrations. Talk, don't read, when you create. Other more specific suggestions include using a USB microphone and Flash format, which is available on most computers. Finally, be professional but do not worry about being perfect.[19] If taping clients or employees, obtain a written release of use without limitations.

Advantages

- Realistic, enjoyable, and dramatic.
- Include both sight and sound stimulation.
- When a story is told, people retain information better.

- For learning, can be viewed repeatedly and "just in time."
- Can have an emotional impact and help to change attitudes.

Limitations

- May not fit the purpose and objectives.
- May be expensive to buy or produce.
- Require equipment at production site.
- Complex issues may be misinterpreted unless discussed.

Mixed Media

The dietetics professional should consider using more than one of the previously discussed visuals in a presentation, such as a combination of handouts along with slides. Alternatively, you may use actual foods, handouts, and the chalkboard. Music to illustrate a point and a brief video may help. Many combinations are possible. Think of the message, and select the visual media that best fits the session. The focus is on the learners' needs.[20] A study by Hoelscher and colleagues found effective nutrition interventions using a variety of techniques. The key was adequate dissemination through the target population.[21]

PURCHASING PREPARED MEDIA MATERIALS

The question often arises about whether to prepare your own media materials or use existing materials. The most basic answer is to use the least expensive media to accomplish the goals with the best quality possible.[20] The anticipated longevity of the material before it is outdated and the number of times you will use the material should influence the decision. The cost of purchased versus self-made media needs to be considered in terms of time, quality, and expertise. With so many presentations posted on the web, searching the web for presentations is valuable. If the materials fit the needs of the group, try to obtain permission to use the materials, referencing the original source. Many organizations and the government encourage individuals to use their materials without permission, but with proper acknowledgment.

The availability of technical expertise in design and production are essential, especially for audio and video production. The availability of prepared pamphlets or videos to meet the objectives is also important. In addition, the cost to reproduce the material is a consideration.

Regardless of who produces the media, the materials should be assessed for readability, first impressions, content, and format. Is the content accurate? Does it address the needs of the audience? Is the material legible and readable? Have you pilot-tested the material on the target audience? **Box 15-3** lists some points to consider when evaluating materials.[22,23] It is important to evaluate media as you use them. Eventually, you want to know what proves most effective in the shortest time frame in learning and retention, thus providing efficiency.

BOX **15-3**

Evaluating Nutrition Education Materials.[23]

General Evaluation Practices

Distribute nutrition education materials to clients

Use a variety of printed nutrition education materials

Thoroughly preview nutrition education materials

Use a formal checklist to evaluate nutrition education materials

Develop new nutrition education materials

Pilot-test modified or new nutrition education materials

Use nutrition education materials provided by a reputable source

Request feedback relative to nutrition education materials from clients

Conduct a client assessment before providing dietary guidance

Consider the client's age

Consider the client's gender

Assess the client's education level

Consider the client's ethnicity and cultural background

Consider the client's lifestyle

Consider the client's socioeconomic status

Assess the client's reading ability

Readability Criteria

Readability level

Length of sentences

Length of paragraphs

Number of syllables per word

Use of examples

Use of jargon, cliches, or idioms

Word appropriateness

Legibility

Style and typeface

Size of print

Highlighting of specific information

Active or passive words

First, second, or third person

Typographical errors

Content Criteria

Addresses the needs of the client

Age appropriateness

Applicability of information

Consistency of information

Objectivity of information

Gender appropriateness

Implications of information

Motivational messages

Accuracy of information

Summarizes information

Credibility of information

Number of content errors

Date of publication

Flow of concepts

Ethnicity or cultural appropriateness

Scientific basis of information

Practicality of information

Focuses on behavioral change

Continuity of information

Format Criteria

Color scheme

Photographs

Layouts

Use of white space

Use of highlighting techniques

Quality of copy

Captures attention

Interactive

Complexity of details

Illustrations

Illustrations that support messages

Attractiveness

Quality of paper

Use of charts, graphs, and tables

Margin justification

GIVING PRESENTATIONS

After preparing both the presentation and the visuals, several practices are critical to success. The presenter needs to practice the presentation and the media. Have a friend or colleague provide feedback. If no one is available, practicing in front of a mirror is a possibility, although not as effective. Videotaping the presentation is a great method of seeing how to enhance the presentation. Preferably, practice in the actual setting of the presentation. As a presenter, try to arrive 30 minutes in advance to make sure that handouts are available and get instructions on how to run the equipment, lower the lights in the room, and the like.

EVALUATING RESULTS

Educational evaluation is treated in detail in Chapter 12. It is important to obtain feedback about your presentation. Some educational programs use written evaluation forms. **Figure 15-4** provides a sample evaluation form to assess the quality of a group teaching session. If a written form is not used, inquire verbally about audience reactions afterward. Any suggestions may be used as a basis for revising and improving the materials. Although it is probably not possible for novices, experienced presenters can watch the audience for nonverbal reactions during the presentation.

There is no doubt that media enhance learning and retention from presentations and educational sessions as well as having the potential to enhance the speaker's professional image. If you are not using at least five to eight visuals, you may be considerably less effective.

Computers and the Internet are having a profound impact on education and teaching in the 21st century. People read fewer books and newspapers and may dislike the concentrated effort that reading requires. News events are instantaneously available on the Internet or on television. People want information right away, in small segments, and in easy-to-use formats. The availability of educational materials on the Internet will continue to accelerate.

Projecting to the future, computer-based education will become the norm for learning techniques and testing. High-quality videos of cooking demonstrations, exercises, and procedures such as inserting a feeding tube will assist in group and individual educational sessions. As more animations and video clips become available, the computer, e-mail, and cell phones will become more integral parts of most counseling sessions. Downloading information will augment handouts so that clients or employees can review techniques, such as insulin administration, "just in time" for use in their home or office. The impact of instrumental media will grow in the next decade.

GROUP TEACHING EVALUATION FORM

Name _____   Signature _____

Date _____   Rotation Site: _____

Evaluated by: _____

Topic _____   Audience: Pt/Staff/RDs/Other

CRITERIA	RATING	COMMENTS
	5 4 3 2 1	

1. Observes social amenities: introduces self; ensures that audience is comfortable
2. Explains purpose of "class" to group
3. Speaks clearly and loudly
4. Uses grammar/language properly
5. Hold interest of group
6. Adjusts content of talk to educational level of group
7. Incorporates group participation as part of lesson
8. Follows a logical order in imparting information
9. Emphasizes key points
10. Summarizes at end of presentation
11. Allows time for questions
12. Encourages questions
13. Answers questions
14. Presents lessons approprate to time allotment
15. Is familiary with space and equipment
16. Prepares visuals/other aids to enhance presentation
17. Uses visial aids large enough to see clearly
18. Uses visual aids effectively
19. Plans and uses some method to evaluate learning
20. Provides resources/handout information for those who want further information
21. Content: thoroughness of lesson
22. Accuracy of lesson
23. Overall effectiveness of lesson

KEY
    5 = Consistently demonstrates skill
    4 = Demonstrates majority of skill
    3 = Adequately progressing with skill development
    2 = Needs emphasis
    1 = Unable to demonstrate skill

TOTAL AUDIENCE COMMENTS

AUDIENCE INITIALS

Used with permission of UMDNJ-SHRP Department of Primary Care.

FIGURE **15-4** Group Teaching Evaluation Form.

CASE STUDY 1

At 9:00 AM, Julie gathered her flip chart and magic markers and headed for her office door. She was conducting an employee training session that began at 9:00 AM. As she entered the training room, she said to the 20 participants, "Oh well, I'm here. Let's begin by watching a short video."

As Julie inserted the video into the videocassette recorder (VCR), she realized that the carriage was broken and she would not be able to show it. Frustrated and embarrassed, Julie said, "Nothing in this company works right. I guess I'll have to ask them to bring me another VCR."

After calling Media Services to obtain another VCR, Julie turned to the group and said, "I was in a hurry this morning, and I forgot my handouts for the session. It will just take me a few minutes to go back to my office to get them."

1. What should Julie have done to create a more positive image of herself and to improve this training session?

CASE STUDY 2

Doris Burns, RD, works for a large corporation in the corporate wellness center. Recently, the center nurse mentioned that several employees have high blood pressure. She asks Doris to join her in planning a health education program for them. In considering various approaches, they decide to have a booth for a week in the employee cafeteria, where they can display information and answer questions over the lunch break (11:00 AM–1:00 PM).

1. Write an objective for nutrition education in hypertension.
2. Based on the objective, what types of nutrition education media materials should Doris have available at the booth?

REVIEW AND DISCUSSION QUESTIONS

1. What benefits does the use of visual media provide in presentations?
2. What should be considered in planning visuals?
3. Why should the readability of printed materials be assessed?
4. Why is it important to evaluate visual media as one uses them?
5. When training employees, why is it preferable to train them using the real object, such as a meat slicer, dish machine, cash register, or other equipment?
6. What are some advantages of using computer-assisted formats for training and education?
7. What is the "rule of six?"
8. Why should a presenter arrive at the presentation 30 minutes before it starts?
9. List 15 criteria for evaluating a presentation.
10. When would you use synchronous versus asynchronous learning? What is the value of each method?

SUGGESTED ACTIVITIES

1. Think about your earliest experiences in school. Can you remember any visual materials used by a teacher? Describe as much as you can remember and your age at the time.
2. Prepare a chart or poster depicting one idea. Write a description of your objectives and intended audience. Write a critique of your visual explaining how you used art and design principles to enhance quality.
3. If a video camera is available, prepare a video or screencast of a new employee procedure or a technique the employee needs to learn about, such as kitchen sanitation, food handling, hand washing, and the like; or tape preparation of a recipe for a modified diet or a session on normal nutrition.
4. Create a computerized slide presentation, inserting at least one graphic.
5. Assign one student or a group of students to learn to use various types of equipment (overhead projector, slide projector, VCR, LCD projector, etc.) Each should write a task analysis (see Chapter 12) for the equipment and then train others in its use.
6. Select a commercially prepared CD. Evaluate it in terms of its intended audience, objectives, effectiveness, art and design principles, and cost.
7. View an educational program on television. Evaluate it using an evaluation form from the instructor.
8. Find two food labels. Describe how one could use the labels in teaching.
9. Select two educational pamphlets. Critique the content using a readability formula, if available. Critique the visuals as well. Determine whether the pamphlets can be reproduced and find out what the cost will be.

WEB SITES

USE OF MEDIA AND VISUALS

http://www.ala.org   Information on copyright (search on word "copyright")

http://www.copyright.gov   Information about copyright

http://www.microsoft.com/office/powerpoint/default.asp   or   http://www.actden.com/pp
   Information about PowerPoint; tips for making presentations and free clip art

http://www.pcwb.com   Information about media equipment

http://www.powerfulpresentations.net   Information about visuals for presentations

http://www.streamingmedia.com/tutorials   Tutorial on media streaming

http://uuhsc.utah.edu/pated/authors/readability.html   Information about measuring readability

SOURCES OF FREE EDUCATIONAL MATERIALS

http://www.ars.usda.gov/main/main.htm

http://www.fda.gov

http://www.nci.nih.gov

http://www.nhlbi.nih.gov/health/pubs/index.htm

http://www.nichd.nih.gov/publications/pubs.cfm

http://www2.niddk.nih.gov

http://ods.od.nih.gov/Health_Information/Vitamin_and_Mineral_Supplement_Fact_sheets.aspx
http://www.supermarketsavvy.com
http://www.usda.gov/wps/portal/usdahome

REFERENCES

1. Rankin SH, Stallings KD. Patient Education: Principles & Practice. Philadelphia: Lippincott Williams & Wilkins, 2001.
2. The seven sins of visual presentations. Presentation helper. Available at: http://www.presentationhelper.co.uk. Accessed July 10, 2007.
3. Heinich R, Molenda M, Russell JD, et al. Instructional Media and Technologies for Learning, 5th ed. Englewood Cliffs, NJ: Prentice-Hall, 1996.
4. Bjerkness S. The next step: making sense of education. DCE Newsflash. Diabetes Care Educ Newsletter 2002;23:15.
5. King C. Use Visual Aids to Enhance . . . Not Destroy . . . Your Presentations. Available at: http://creativekeys.net/PowerfulPresentations/articles1011.html. Accessed July 10, 2007.
6. King WL. Training by design. Train Dev 1994;48: 52–56.
7. Bashir S. Guidelines for Presentations. SBTC. Available at: http://www.sbtc.biz/notes/Guidelines-for-Presentations-EN.pdf . Accessed July 10, 2007.
8. Hernandez J. A recipe for food safety training. Food Manage 2002;36:84, 87.
9. Sandmann, L. Diabetes Education Kiosk for Latinos Summative Evaluation. Available at: http://www.coe.uga.edu/class/resources/Diabets_Education_Kiosk_for_Latinos_FinalEval.pdf. Accessed July 10, 2007.
10. Casazza K, Ciccazzo M. The method of delivery of nutrition and physical activity information may play a role in eliciting behavior changes in adolescents. Eating Behav 2007;8:73–82.
11. Izquierdo RE, Knudson PE, Meyer S, et al. A comparison of diabetes education administered through telemedicine versus in person. Diabetes Care 2003;26:1002–1007.
12. Fuller C, Keller L, Olson J, et al. Helping preschoolers become healthy eaters. J Pediatr Health Care 2005;19:178–182.
13. Coulston AM, Stivers M. A poster worth a thousand words: how to design effective poster session displays. J Am Diet Assoc 1993;93:865–866.
14. Ralph L. Displays that work. Econnect Communication, 2002. Available at: http://www.econnect.com.au/pdf/quicktips/presentation/pdf. Accessed July 10, 2007.
15. Blooomberg. Low US literacy rate costs billions. The Financial Express, December 17, 2005. Available at: http://www.tc.edu/news/article/htm. Accessed July 10, 2007.
16. U.S. Census Bureau News. Available at: http://census.gov. Accessed July 10, 2007.
17. Everything you ever wanted to know about readability tests but were afraid to ask. Available at: http://www.gopdg.com/plainlanguage/readability.html. Accessed July 10, 2007.
18. On-the-job video gaming. Business Week, March 27, 2006.
19. Weber B. Screencasting for beginners. Available at: http://www.presenteruniversity.com/visuals_screencasting.php. Accessed July 10, 2007.
20. Turmel WW. Technology in the classroom: Velcro for the mind. In: Piskurich GM, Beckschi P, Hall B, eds. The ASTD Handbook of Training Design and Delivery. New York: McGraw-Hill, 2000.
21. Hoelscher DM, Evans A, Parcel GS, et al. Designing effective nutrition interventions for adolescents. J Am Diet Assoc 2002;102(Suppl 3):S52–S63.
22. Tagtow AM, Amos RJ. Extent to which dietitians evaluate nutrition education materials. J Nutr Educ 2000;32:161.
23. Pennington J, Hubbard V. Nutrition education materials from the National Institutes of Health: development, review and availability. J Nutr Educ 2002; 34:53.

Counseling Guidelines—Initial Session

Step	Topic	Questions to Ask	Questions to Avoid
1	Candidly review problems of dietary change.		
	1. Review overall rationale and objectives for recommended diet.		"Do you have any opinion about this diet?"
	2. Acknowledge difficult nature of dietary change.	"What are your thoughts and feelings about changing your food intake?"	
	3. Listen to patient's concerns about the recommended diet.		
2	Build some commitment to solve problems.		
	1. Indicate your willingness to work with patient.		
	2. Clarify to patient that he or she must assume primary responsibility for making dietary changes.		
	3. Propose program of frequent meetings for the next 3 months, close observation of diet, phone contact.		
	4. Emphasize slow but steady approach to change.		
	5. Obtain patient's verbal commitment to meet any of your proposals.	"What aspects of this program are you willing to try now?"	"Do you want to try anything now?"
3	Plan some specific changes in diet during the coming month.		
	1. Emphasize good points of 3-day record.[a]		
	2. Look at record to identify needed dietary changes.		
	3. Probe patient for more ideas.		

4. Pinpoint one aspect of diet pattern to change.
5. Acknowledge patient's desire for radical and fast changes in diet, but reemphasize that the most successful approach is slow and steady.
6. Help patient set realistic dietary change goals (e.g., one meatless evening meal per week, substitution of a salad bowl for usual main entree at one lunch per week).

"What do you see that could be changed or improved?"

"Do you see anything to change?"

"What are realistic goals for you?"

"Is this a realistic goal?"

4 Plan how to make a change successful.
1. Identify obstacles that are likely to interfere with achieving goal. Consider problems in the following areas:
  a. Physical environment (e.g., what foods are available in house, snacking in front of TV in evening, absence of reminders on refrigerator or dining table).
  b. Social environment (e.g., influential people, such as spouse, children, business associates, whose approval and support or criticism can affect achievement of dietary change goal).

"What obstacles are likely to interfere with your plans?"

"Are any problems going to interfere with plans?"

"What can you change in your home, office, or car that will help you achieve your goals?"

"Do you need any reminders?"

"Who can help, what can they do, and what can I do to help during the next few weeks?"

"Do you need any help?"

(Continued)

363

c. Cognitive or private environment (e.g., what patient says to himself or herself when confronted with personal thoughts such as the following: What others will say about planned behavior; thoughts of failure or disappointment when he or she is not perfect in planned behavior).	"What encouraging things can you say to yourself when confronted with these inevitable thoughts?" "Will you give yourself encouragement?"
5 Plan how to keep track of progress. Devise an unobtrusive and convenient way for patient to keep a record of desired or target behavior (e.g., count egg cartons, measure side of vegetable oil container, attach pencil and paper to refrigerator, table, wallet).	"How are you going to keep track of (target behavior)?" "Can you keep track of (target behavior)?"
6 Plan counseling continuity and support.	"When is it convenient for us to discuss your progress?" "When can we schedule our next appointment?" "What would you like to discuss next time?" "Would it be possible for someone to come with you at our next visit?" "Do you want me to contact you sometime?"
7. Make certain that spouse, if present, is involved in answering questions, providing ideas, and discussing potential problems and solutions.	

aBefore initial counseling session, patient should be given materials and instructions for completing a 3-day food diary.
Adapted from and reprinted with permission from Wilbur CS. Nutrition Counseling Skills. Audiocassette series 5. Chicago: American Dietetic Association, 1980.

Nutrition Diagnostic Terminology

INTAKE — NI

Defined as "actual problems related to intake of energy, nutrients, fluids, bioactive substances through oral diet or nutrition support"

Energy Balance (1)

Defined as "actual or estimated changes in energy (kcal)"

- ☐ Unused — NI-1.1
- ☐ Increased energy expenditure — NI-1.2
- ☐ Unused — NI-1.3
- ☐ Inadequate energy intake — NI-1.4
- ☐ Excessive energy intake — NI-1.5

Oral or Nutrition Support Intake (2)

Defined as "actual or estimated food and beverage intake from oral diet or nutrition support compared with patient goal"

- ☐ Inadequate oral food/beverage intake — NI-2.1
- ☐ Excessive oral food/beverage intake — NI-2.2
- ☐ Inadequate intake from enteral/parenteral nutrition — NI-2.3
- ☐ Excessive intake from enteral/parenteral nutrition — NI-2.4
- ☐ Inappropriate infusion of enteral/parenteral nutrition (use with caution) — NI-2.5

Fluid Intake (3)

Defined as "actual or estimated fluid intake compared with patient goal"

- ☐ Inadequate fluid intake — NI-3.1
- ☐ Excessive fluid intake — NI-3.2

Bioactive Substances (4)

Defined as "actual or observed intake of bioactive substances, including single or multiple functional food components, ingredients, dietary supplements, alcohol"

- ☐ Inadequate bioactive substance intake — NI-4.1
- ☐ Excessive bioactive substance intake — NI-4.2
- ☐ Excessive alcohol intake — NI-4.3

Nutrient (5)

Defined as "actual or estimated intake of specific nutrient groups or single nutrients as compared with desired levels"

- ☐ Increased nutrient needs (specify) — NI-5.1
- ☐ Evident protein-energy malnutrition — NI-5.2
- ☐ Inadequate protein-energy intake — NI-5.3
- ☐ Decreased nutrient needs (specify) — NI-5.4
- ☐ Imbalance of nutrients — NI-5.5

Fat and Cholesterol (5.6)

- ☐ Inadequate fat intake — NI-5.6.1
- ☐ Excessive fat intake — NI-5.6.2
- ☐ Inappropriate intake of food fats (specify) — NI-5.6.3

Protein (5.7)

- ☐ Inadequate protein intake — NI-5.7.1
- ☐ Excessive protein intake — NI-5.7.2
- ☐ Inappropriate intake of amino acids (specify) — NI-5.7.3

Carbohydrate and Fiber (5.8)

- ☐ Inadequate carbohydrate intake — NI-5.8.1
- ☐ Excessive carbohydrate intake — NI-5.8.2
- ☐ Inappropriate intake of types of carbohydrate (specify) — NI-5.8.3
- ☐ Inconsistent carbohydrate intake — NI-5.8.4
- ☐ Inadequate fiber intake — NI-5.8.5
- ☐ Excessive fiber intake — NI-5.8.6

Vitamin (5.9)

- ☐ Inadequate vitamin intake (specify) — NI-5.9.1

☐ Excessive vitamin intake (specify) — NI-5.9.2

☐ A ☐ Riboflavin
☐ C ☐ Niacin
☐ D ☐ Folate
☐ E ☐ B6
☐ K ☐ B12
☐ Thiamin ☐ Other

Mineral (5.10)

☐ Inadequate mineral intake (specify) — NI-5.10.1
☐ Excessive mineral intake (specify) — NI-5.10.2

☐ Calcium ☐ Phosphorus
☐ Iron ☐ Potassium
☐ Magnesium ☐ Zinc
☐ Other (specify) _____

CLINICAL — NC

Defined as "nutritional findings/problems identified as related to medical or physical conditions"

Functional (1)

Defined as "change in physical or mechanical functioning that interferes with or prevents desired nutritional consequences"

☐ Swallowing difficulty — NC-1.1
☐ Biting/Chewing (masticatory) difficulty — NC-1.2
☐ Breastfeeding difficulty — NC-1.3
☐ Altered GI function — NC-1.4

Biochemical (2)

Defined as "change in capacity to metabolize nutrients as a result of medications, or surgery, or as indicated by altered lab values"

☐ Impaired nutrient utilization — NC-2.1
☐ Altered nutrition-related laboratory values — NC-2.2
☐ Food-medication interaction — NC-2.3

Weight (3)

Defined as "chronic weight or changed weight status when compared with usual or desired body weight"

☐ Underweight — NC-3.1
☐ Involuntary weight loss — NC-3.2
☐ Overweight/obesity — NC-3.3
☐ Involuntary weight gain — NC-3.4

BEHAVIORAL ENVIRONMENTAL — NB

Defined as "nutritional findings/problems identified that relate to knowledge, attitudes/beliefs, physical environment, access to food, or food safety"

Knowledge and Beliefs (1)

Defined as "actual knowledge and beliefs as related, observed or documented"

☐ Food- and nutrition-related knowledge deficit — NB-1.1
☐ Harmful beliefs/attitudes about food- or nutrition-related topics (use with caution) — NB-1.2
☐ Not ready for diet/lifestyle change — NB-1.3
☐ Self-monitoring deficit — NB-1.4
☐ Disordered eating pattern — NB-1.5
☐ Limited adherence to nutrition-related recommendations — NB-1.6
☐ Undesirable food choices — NB-1.7

Physical Activity and Function (2)

Defined as "actual physical activity, self-care, and quality-of-life problems as reported, observed, or documented"

☐ Physical inactivity — NB-2.1
☐ Excessive exercise — NB-2.2
☐ Inability or lack of desire to manage self-care — NB-2.3
☐ Impaired ability to prepare foods/meals — NB-2.4
☐ Poor nutrition quality of life — NB-2.5
☐ Self-feeding difficulty — NB-2.6

Food Safety and Access (3)

Defined as "actual problems with food access or food safety"

☐ Intake of unsafe food — NB-3.1
☐ Limited access to food — NB-3.2

Date Identified	Date Resolved

(Continued)

#1 Problem _____

Etiology _____

Signs/Symptoms _____

#2 Problem _____

Etiology _____

Signs/Symptoms _____

#3 Problem _____

Etiology _____

Signs/Symptoms _____

Used with permission from the American Dietetic Association (Edition 2008).

Nutrition Intervention Terminology

Problem _____	
Etiology _____	
Signs/Symptoms _____	

Nutrition Prescription
The patient's/client's individualized recommended dietary intake of energy and/or selected foods or nutrients based on current reference standards and dietary guidelines and the patient's/client's health condition and nutrition diagnosis. *(specify)*
_____
_____

Intervention #1 _____
　Goal (s) _____

Intervention #2 _____
　Goal (s) _____

Intervention #3 _____
　Goal (s) _____

FOOD AND/OR NUTRIENT DELIVERY　　ND

Meal and Snacks (1)
Regular eating event (meal); food served between regular meals (snack).

- ☐ General/healthful diet　ND-1.1
- ☐ Modify distribution, type, or amount of food and nutrients within meals or at specified time　ND-1.2
- ☐ Specific foods/beverages or groups　ND-1.3
- ☐ Other *(specify)* _____　ND-1.4

Enteral and Parenteral Nutrition (2)
Nutrition provided through the GI tract via tube, catheter, or stoma (enteral) or intravenously (centrally or peripherally) (parenteral).

- ☐ Initiate EN or PN nutrition　ND-2.1
- ☐ Modify rate, concentration, composition or schedule　ND-2.2
- ☐ Discontinue EN or PN nutrition　ND-2.3
- ☐ Insert enteral feeding tube　ND-2.4
- ☐ Site care　ND-2.5
- ☐ Other *(specify)* _____　ND-2.6

Supplements (3)

Medical Food Supplements　ND-3.1
Commercial or prepared foods or beverages that supplement energy, protein, carbohydrate, fiber, fat intake.

Type
- ☐ Commercial beverage　ND-3.1.1
- ☐ Commercial food　ND-3.1.2
- ☐ Modified beverage　ND-3.1.3
- ☐ Modified food　ND-3.1.4
- ☐ Purpose *(specify)* _____　ND-3.1.5

Vitamin and Mineral Supplements (3.2)
Supplemental vitamins or minerals.

- ☐ Multivitamin/mineral　ND-3.2.1
- ☐ Multi-trace elements　ND-3.2.2

- ☐ Vitamin　ND-3.2.3
  - ☐ A
  - ☐ C
  - ☐ D
  - ☐ E
  - ☐ K
  - ☐ Thiamin
  - ☐ Other *(specify)* _____
  - ☐ Riboflavin
  - ☐ Niacin
  - ☐ Folate
  - ☐ B6
  - ☐ B12

- ☐ Mineral　ND-3.2.4
  - ☐ Calcium
  - ☐ Iron
  - ☐ Magnesium
  - ☐ Other *(specify)* _____
  - ☐ Phosphorus
  - ☐ Potassium
  - ☐ Zinc

Bioactive Substance Supplement (3.3)
Supplemental bioactive substances.

- ☐ Initiate　ND-3.3.1
- ☐ Dose change　ND-3.3.2
- ☐ Form change　ND-3.3.3

❏ Route change	ND-3.3.4
❏ Administration schedule	ND-3.3.5
❏ Discontinue	ND-3.3.6

(specify) _____

Feeding Assistance (4)
Accommodation or assistance in eating.

❏ Adaptive equipment	ND-4.1
❏ Feeding position	ND-4.2
❏ Meal set-up	ND-4.3
❏ Mouth care	ND-4.4
❏ Other *(specify)* _____	ND-4.5

Feeding Environment (5)
Adjustment of the factors where food is served that impact food consumption.

❏ Lighting	ND-5.1
❏ Odors	ND-5.2
❏ Distractions	ND-5.3
❏ Table height	ND-5.4
❏ Table service/set up	ND-5.5
❏ Room temperature	ND-5.6
❏ Other *(specify)* _____	ND-5.7

Nutrition-Related Medication Management (6)
Modification of a drug or herbal to optimize patient/client nutritional or health status.

❏ Initiate	ND-6.1
❏ Dose change	ND-6.2
❏ Form change	ND-6.3
❏ Route change	ND-6.4
❏ Administration schedule	ND-6.5
❏ Discontinue	ND-6.6

(specify) _____

NUTRITION EDUCATION   **E**

Initial/Brief Nutrition Education (1)
Build or reinforce basic or essential nutrition-related knowledge.

❏ Purpose of the nutrition education	E-1.1
❏ Priority modifications	E-1.2
❏ Survival information	E-1.3
❏ Other *(specify)* _____	E-1.4

Comprehensive Nutrition Education (2)
Instruction or training leading to in-depth nutrition-related knowledge or skills.

❏ Purpose of the nutrition education	E-2.1
❏ Recommended modifications	E-2.2
❏ Advanced or related topics	E-2.3
❏ Result interpretation	E-2.4
❏ Skill development	E-2.5
❏ Other *(specify)* _____	E-2.6

NUTRITION COUNSELING   **C**

Theoretical Basis/Approach (1)
The theories or models used to design and implement an intervention.

❏ Cognitive-Behavioral Theory	C-1.2
❏ Health Belief Model	C-1.3
❏ Social Learning Theory	C-1.4
❏ Transtheoretical Model/ Stages of Change	C-1.5
❏ Other *(specify)* _____	C-1.6

Strategies (2)
Selectively applied evidence-based methods or plans of action designed to achieve a particular goal.

❏ Motivational interviewing	C-2.1
❏ Goal setting	C-2.2
❏ Self-monitoring	C-2.3

❏ Problem solving	C-2.4
❏ Social support	C-2.5
❏ Stress management	C-2.6
❏ Stimulus control	C-2.7
❏ Cognitive restructuring	C-2.8
❏ Relapse prevention	C-2.9
❏ Rewards/contingency management	C-2.10
❏ Other *(specify)* _____	

COORDINATION OF NUTRITION CARE   **RC**

Coordination of Other Care During Nutrition Care (1)
Facilitating services with other professionals, institutions, or agencies during nutrition care.

❏ Team meeting	RC-1.1
❏ Referral to RD with different expertise	RC-1.2
❏ Collaboration/referral to other providers	RC-1.3
❏ Referral to community agencies/ programs *(specify)* _____	RC-1.4

Discharge and Transfer of Nutrition Care to New Setting or Provider (2)
Discharge planning and transfer of nutrition care from one level or location of care to another.

❏ Collaboration/referral to other providers	RC-2.1
❏ Referral to community agencies/ programs *(specify)* _____	RC-2.2

Used with permission from the American Dietetic Association (Edition 2008).

Nutrition Monitoring and Evaluation Terminology

During nutrition monitoring and evaluation, practitioners list the signs and symptoms from the PES statement that are the targets of the nutrition intervention. Then, practitioners list the nutrition interventions and goals/expected outcome along with the indicators and criteria to provide evidence for the nutrition monitoring and evaluation. There may be more than one indicator per goal and one indicator may be used for multiple goals.

Nutrition Intervention(s) and Goal/expected outcome(s)	Indicator(s)	Criteria	Signs/Symptoms from PES statement(s)
Intervention			
#1 Goal			
#2 Goal			
Intervention			
#3 Goal			
#4 Goal			
Intervention			
#5 Goal			
#6 Goal			

NUTRITION-RELATED   **BE**
BEHAVIORAL- ENVIRONMENTAL OUTCOMES

Knowledge/Beliefs (1)

Improved understanding of nutrition concepts and change in beliefs and attitudes that increase the probability that the patient/client will successfully implement nutrition prescription/goal.

Beliefs and attitudes (1.1)

- Readiness to change   BE-1.1.1
- Perceived consequence of change   BE-1.1.2
- Perceived costs versus benefi of change   BE-1.1.3
- Perceived risk   BE-1.1.4
- Outcome expectancy   BE-1.1.5

- Conflict with personal/family value system   BE-1.1.6
- Self-efficacy *(breastfeeding, eating, weight loss)*   BE-1.1.7

Food and nutrition knowledge (1.2)

- Level of knowledge *(e.g., none, limited, minimal, substantial, and extensive)*   BE-1.2.1

(Continued)

☐ Areas of knowledge   BE-1.2.2
(food/nutrient requirements, physiological functions, disease/condition, nutrition recommendations, food products, consequences of food behavior, food label understanding, self-management parameters)

Behavior (2)
Patient/client activities and actions necessary to achieve nutrition-related goals.

Ability to plan meals/snacks (2.1)
☐ Meal/snack planning ability   BE-2.1.1

Ability to select healthful food/meals (2.2)
☐ Food/meal selection   BE-2.2.1

Ability to prepare food/meals (2.3)
☐ Food/meal preparation ability   BE-2.3.1

Adherence (2.4)
☐ Self-reported adherence   BE-2.4.1

Goal setting (2.5)
☐ Goal setting ability   BE-2.5.1

Portion control (2.6)
☐ Portion size eaten   BE-2.6.1

Self-care management (2.7)
☐ Self-care management ability   BE-2.7.1

Self-monitoring (2.8)
☐ Self-monitoring ability   BE-2.8.1

Social support (2.9)
☐ Ability to build and utilize social support   BE-2.9.1

Stimulus control (2.10)
☐ Ability to manage behavior in response to stimuli   BE-2.10.1

Access (3)
Availability of a sufficient quantity of safe, healthful food.

Access to food (3.1)
☐ Access to a sufficient quantity of healthful food   BE-3.1.1
☐ Access to safe food   BE-3.1.2

Physical Activity and Function (4)
improved physical activity and ability to engage in specific tasks (e.g., breast feeding).

Breastfeeding success (4.1)
☐ Initiation of breastfeeding   BE-4.1.1
☐ Duration of breastfeeding   BE-4.1.2
☐ Exclusive breastfeeding   BE-4.1.3
☐ Breastfeeding problems   BE-4.1.4

Nutrition-related ADLs and IADLs (4.2)
☐ Acceptance of assistance with eating   BE-4.2.1
☐ Ability to use adaptive eating devices   BE-4.2.2
☐ Time taken to eat and consume meals   BE-4.2.3
☐ Ability to shop for food   BE-4.2.4
☐ Nutrition-related ADL   BE-4.2.5
☐ Nutrition-related IADL   BE-4.2.6

Physical Activity and function (4.3)
☐ Consistency/frequency   BE-4.3.1
☐ Duration   BE-4.3.2
☐ Intensity   BE-4.3.3
☐ Strength   BE-4.3.4

FOOD AND NUTRIENT INTAKE OUTCOMES   FI

Energy intake (1)
Total energy intake from all sources, e.g., food, beverages, supplements, and via enteral and parenteral routes.

Energy intake (1.1)
☐ Total energy intake   FI-1.1.1

Food and Beverage (2)
Foods and food groups and fluids from all sources, e.g., food, beverages, supplements.

Fluid/Beverage intake (2.1)
☐ Oral Fluids Amounts   FI-2.1.1
(water, coffee/tea, juice, milk, soda)
☐ Food derived fluids   FI-2.1.2
☐ IV Fluids   FI-2.1.3
☐ Liquid meal replacement   FI-2.1.4

Food intake (2.2)
☐ Food variety   FI-2.2.1
☐ Number of food group servings   FI-2.2.2
(grains, fruits, vegetables, milk/dairy, meat/protein substitutes)

☐ Healthy Eating Index (HEI)	FI-2.2.3
☐ Children's Diet Quality Index	FI-2.2.4
☐ Revised Children's Diet Quality Index	FI-2.2.5

Enteral and Parenteral (3)
Specialized nutrition support intake from all sources, e.g., enteral and parenteral routes.

Enteral/parenteral nutrition intake (3.1)
☐ Access	FI-3.1.1
☐ Formula/solution	FI-3.1.2
☐ Discontinuation	FI-3.1.3
☐ Initiation	FI-3.1.4
☐ Rate/Schedule	FI-3.1.5

Bioactive Substances (4)
Alcohol, plant stanol and sterol esters, soy protein, psyllium and β-glucan, and caffeine intake from all sources, e.g., food, beverages, supplements, and via enteral and parenteral routes.

Alcohol intake (4.1)
☐ Drink size/volume	FI-4.1.1
☐ Frequency	FI-4.1.2

Bioactive substance intake (4.2)
☐ Plant sterol and stanol esters	FI-4.2.1
☐ Soy protein	FI-4.2.2
☐ Psyllium and β-glucan	FI-4.2.3

Caffeine intake (4.3)
☐ Total caffeine	FI-4.3.1

Macronutrients (5)
Carbohydrate, fiber, protein, and fat and cholesterol intake from all sources, e.g., food, beverages, supplements, and via enteral and parenteral routes.

Fat and cholesterol intake (5.1)
☐ Total fat	FI-5.1.1
☐ Saturated fat	FI-5.1.2
☐ Trans fatty acids	FI-5.1.3
☐ Polyunsaturated fat	FI-5.1.4
☐ Monounsaturated fat	FI-5.1.5
☐ Omega-3 fatty acids	FI-5.1.6
(marine/plant derived, alpha-linolenic acid)	
☐ Dietary cholesterol	FI-5.1.7

Protein intake (5.2)
☐ Total protein	FI-5.2.1
☐ High biological value protein	FI-5.2.2
☐ Casein	FI-5.2.3
☐ Whey	FI-5.2.4
☐ Soy protein	FI-5.2.5
☐ Amino acids	FI-5.2.6
☐ Essential amino acids	FI-5.2.7

Carbohydrate intake (5.3)
☐ Total carbohydrate	FI-5.3.1
☐ Sugar	FI-5.3.2
☐ Starch	FI-5.3.3
☐ Glycemic index	FI-5.3.4
☐ Glycemic load	FI-5.3.5

Fiber intake (5.4)
☐ Total Fiber	FI-5.4.1
☐ Soluble Fiber	FI-5.4.2
☐ Insoluble Fiber	FI-5.4.3
(fructo-oligosaccharides)	

Micronutrients (6)
Vitamins and mineral intake from all sources, e.g., food, beverages, supplements, and via enteral and parenteral routes.

Vitamin intake (6.1)
☐ A	☐ Riboflavin
☐ C	☐ Niacin
☐ D	☐ Folate
☐ E	☐ B6
☐ K	☐ B12
☐ Thiamin	
☐ Other (specify) _____	

Mineral/element intake (6.2)
☐ Calcium	☐ Potassium
☐ Iron	☐ Sodium
☐ Magnesium	☐ Zinc
☐ Phosphorus	
☐ Other (specify) _____	

NUTRITION-RELATED SIGN/ SYMPTOM OUTCOMES   S

Anthropometric (1)
Measures such as weight, body mass index (BMI) percentile/age, waist circumference, and length.

(Continued)

Body composition/Growth (1.1)
- ☐ Body mass index (kg/m²) — S-1.1.1
- ☐ IBW or UBW percentage — S-1.1.2
- ☐ Growth pattern — S-1.1.3

(head circumference, length/height, weight for length/stature, BMI percentile/age, also see Weight change)

- ☐ Weight/weight change — S-1.1.4

(e.g. % change, weight gain/day)

- ☐ Lean body mass, fat free mass — S-1.1.5
- ☐ Mid-arm muscle circumference — S-1.1.6
- ☐ Body fat percentage — S-1.1.7
- ☐ Triceps skin fold — S-1.1.8
- ☐ Waist circumference — S-1.1.9
- ☐ Waist-hip ratio — S-1.1.10
- ☐ Bone age — S-1.1.11
- ☐ Bone mineral density — S-1.1.12

Biochemical and Medical Tests (2)

Lab values or medical tests such as glucose, lipids, electrolytes, and fecal fat test.

Acid-base balance (2.1)
- ☐ pH, serum — S-2.1.1
- ☐ Bicarbonate — S-2.1.2
- ☐ Partial pressure of carbon dioxide in arterial blood — S-2.1.3

Electrolyte and renal profile (2.2)
- ☐ BUN — S-2.2.1
- ☐ Creatinine — S-2.2.2
- ☐ BUN : creatinine ratio — S-2.2.3
- ☐ Glomerular filtration rate — S-2.2.4
- ☐ Sodium — S-2.2.5
- ☐ Chloride — S-2.2.6
- ☐ Potassium — S-2.2.7
- ☐ Magnesium — S-2.2.8
- ☐ Calcium — S-2.2.9
- ☐ Calcium, ionized — S-2.2.10
- ☐ Phosphorus — S-2.2.11
- ☐ Serum osmolality — S-2.2.12
- ☐ Parathyroid hormone — S-2.2.13

Essential fatty acid profile (2.3)
- ☐ Triene: Tetraene ratio — S-2.3.1

Gastrointestinal profile (2.4)
- ☐ Amylase — S-2.4.1
- ☐ Alkaline phophatase — S-2.4.2
- ☐ Alanine aminotransferase — S-2.4.3
- ☐ Aspartate aminotransferase — S-2.4.4
- ☐ Gamma glutamyl transferase — S-2.4.5
- ☐ Bilirubin, total — S-2.4.6
- ☐ Ammonia, serum — S-2.4.7
- ☐ Prothrombin time — S-2.4.8
- ☐ Partial thromboplastin time — S-2.4.9
- ☐ INR *(ratio)* — S-2.4.10
- ☐ Fecal fat — S-2.4.11

Glucose profile (2.5)
- ☐ Glucose, fasting — S-2.5.1
- ☐ Glucose, casual — S-2.5.2
- ☐ HgbA1c — S-2.5.3
- ☐ Pre-prandial capillary plasma glucose — S-2.5.4
- ☐ Peak postprandial capillary plasma glucose — S-2.5.5

Lipid profile (2.6)
- ☐ Cholesterol, serum — S-2.6.1
- ☐ Cholesterol, HDL — S-2.6.2
- ☐ Cholesterol, LDL — S-2.6.3
- ☐ Triglycerides — S-2.6.4

Mineral profile (2.7)
- ☐ Copper, serum — S-2.7.1
- ☐ Iodine, urinary excretion — S-2.7.2
- ☐ Thyroid stimulating hormone — S-2.7.3
- ☐ Zinc, plasma — S-2.7.4

Nutritional anemia profile (2.8)
- ☐ Hemoglobin — S-2.8.1
- ☐ Hematocrit — S-2.8.2
- ☐ Mean corpuscular volume — S-2.8.3
- ☐ RBC folate — S-2.8.4
- ☐ Red cell distribution width — S-2.8.5
- ☐ Serum B12 — S-2.8.6
- ☐ Serum methylmalonic acid — S-2.8.7
- ☐ Serum folate — S-2.8.8
- ☐ Serum homocysteine — S-2.8.9
- ☐ Serum ferritin — S-2.8.10
- ☐ Serum iron — S-2.8.11
- ☐ Total iron-binding capacity — S-2.8.12
- ☐ Transferrin saturation — S-2.8.13

Serum protein profile (2.9)
- ☐ Albumin — S-2.9.1
- ☐ Prealbumin — S-2.9.2
- ☐ Transferrin — S-2.9.3
- ☐ Phenylalanine, plasma — S-2.9.4
- ☐ Tyrosine, plasma — S-2.9.5

Respiratory quotient (2.10)
- ☐ RQ — S-2.10.1

Urine profile (2.11)
- ☐ Urine color — S-2.11.1
- ☐ Urine osmolality — S-2.11.2
- ☐ Urine specific gravity — S-2.11.3
- ☐ Urine tests — S-2.11.4
  (e.g., ketones, sugar, protein)
- ☐ Urine volume — S-2.11.5

Vitamin profile (2.12)
- ☐ Vitamin A, — S-2.12.1
  (serum or plasma retinol)
- ☐ Vitamin C, — S-2.12.2
  (plasma or serum)
- ☐ Vitamin D — S-2.12.3
  (25-Hydroxy)
- ☐ Vitamin E — S-2.12.4
  (plasma alpha-tocopherol)

- ☐ Thiamin — S-2.12.5
  (activity coefficient for erythrocyte transketolase activity)
- ☐ Riboflavin — S-2.12.6
  (activity coefficient for erythrocyte glutathione reductase activity)
- ☐ Niacin — S-2.12.7
  (urinary N'methyl-nicotinamide concentration)
- ☐ Vitamin B6 — S-2.12.8
  (plasma or serum pyridoxal 5'phosphate concentration)

Physical Examination (3)
Physical exam parameters such as such as edema, nausea, vomiting, bowel function, skin integrity, and blood pressure.

Nutrition physical exam findings (3.1)
- ☐ Cardiovascular-pulmonary — S-3.1.1
  (pulmonary edema)
- ☐ Extremities, musculo-skeletal — S-3.1.2
  (e.g., nails, subcutaneous fat, muscle)
- ☐ Gastrointestinal — S-3.1.3
  (e.g., nausea, vomiting, bowel function)
- ☐ Head and neck — S-3.1.4
  (e.g., tongue, mouth, and hair changes)

- ☐ Neurological — S-3.1.5
  (e.g. confusion, fine/gross motor)
- ☐ Skin — S-3.1.6
  (e.g., appearance, turgor, integrity)
- ☐ Vital signs — S-3.1.7
  (blood pressure, respiratory rate)

NUTRITION-RELATED PATIENT/CLIENT-CENTERED OUTCOMES — PC

Nutrition Quality of Life (1)
Patient/client's perception of his/her nutrition intervention and its impact on life.

Nutrition quality of life (1.1)
- ☐ Food impact — PC-1.1.1
- ☐ Physical state — PC-1.1.2
- ☐ Psychological factors — PC-1.1.3
- ☐ Self-image — PC-1.1.4
- ☐ Self-efficacy — PC-1.1.5
- ☐ Social/interpersonal factors — PC-1.1.6
- ☐ Nutrition quality of life score — PC-1.1.7

Satisfaction (2)
To be added.

Used with permission from the American Dietetic Association (Edition 2008).